WHAT YOUR DOCTOR
MAY *NOT* TELL YOU ABOUT™
MENOPAUSE

"Buttressed by impressive data, the book presents an easy-to-follow program that enables women to stay energized, sexually vibrant, and unafflicted with 'female problems' before, during, and far beyond menopause."

—*SONOMA COUNTY INDEPENDENT*

"It covers not only menopause, but PMS, infertility, and osteoporosis. One of the best books describing the true facts about the female body and its functions."

—*BROWARD NEWS*

"With a penetrating eye for truth and a courageous disregard for self-interest, John Lee makes clear sense out of the confusing area of women's hormone therapy. In the process he demonstrates the best remedy for our health care crisis: a physician whose first priority is the patient's welfare."

—PHILIP INCAO, M.D.,
FAMILY PRACTICE PHYSICIAN

Also by John R. Lee, M.D. and Virginia Hopkins

What Your Doctor May Not *Tell You About Premenopause*
What Your Doctor May Not *Tell You About Breast Cancer*

WHAT YOUR DOCTOR MAY *NOT* TELL YOU ABOUT™
MENOPAUSE

REVISED AND UPDATED

The Breakthrough
Book on *Natural* Hormone Balance

JOHN R. LEE, M.D.
with VIRGINIA HOPKINS

**WARNER
WELLNESS**

NEW YORK   BOSTON

Publisher's Note:

The information in this book can be a valuable addition to your doctor's advice, but it is not intended to replace the services of trained health professionals. You are advised to consult with your health care professional with regard to matters relating to your health, and in particular regarding symptoms that may require diagnosis or immediate attention.

Revised and Updated
Copyright © 1996 by John R. Lee and Virginia Hopkins
Revised edition copyright © 2004 by John R. Lee and Virginia Hopkins
All rights reserved. Except as permitted under the U.S. Copyright Act of 1976, no part of this publication may be reproduced, distributed, or transmitted in any form or by any means, or stored in a database or retrieval system, without the prior written permission of the publisher.

Originally published with the subtitle *The Breakthrough Book on* Natural *Progesterone*

Warner Wellness
Hachette Book Group USA
237 Park Avenue, New York, NY 10169
Visit our Web site at www.HachetteBookGroupUSA.com.

Warner Wellness is an imprint of Warner Books, Inc.

Printed in the United States of America

First Warner Books Edition: May 2004

10 9 8 7 6 5 4

Warner Wellness is a trademark of Time Warner Inc. or an affiliated company. Used under license by Hachette Book Group USA, which is not affiliated with Time Warner Inc.

Library of Congress Cataloging-in-Publication Data

Lee, John R., M.D.
      What your doctor may not tell you about menopause : the breakthrough book on natural hormone balance / John R. Lee, with Virginia Hopkins.—Rev. and updated.
      p. cm.
      Originally published with the subtitle "the breakthrough book on natural progesterone."
      Includes bibliographical references and index.
      ISBN 0-446-69142-9
      1. Menopause—Hormone therapy. 2. Progesterone—Therapeutic use. 3. Menopause—Complications—Alternative treatment. I. Hopkins, Virginia. II. Title.

RG186.L44 2004
618.1'75061—dc22   2003057698

Cover design by Diane Luger
Book design by Charles A. Sutherland

CONTENTS

FOREWORD

I first heard of natural progesterone 25 years ago. Twenty-three years out of medical school and in my 20th year of family practice in Mill Valley, California, I had been invited to present a report on hypoglycemia to the Orthomolecular Medical Society in San Francisco. After giving my paper, I returned to the audience to listen to the next presentation, a talk by Ray Peat, Ph.D., of Oregon. His subject was natural progesterone, its many roles in human health, and a criticism of the medical profession for having ignored this important hormone in the care of women's health. As I recall, Dr. Peat argued that giving unopposed estrogen (estrogen replacement without progesterone) to women after menopause (when periods stop) was, in short, the wrong thing to be doing. The force of his argument, the scientific knowledge he laid out, and the references he provided were a clear challenge to the prevailing practice of most of us in the room. We had all been taught that menopause (when the ovaries stopped making their hormones) led to a variety of female complaints that represented estrogen deficiency. We had believed it obvious to treat such patients with estrogen. Yet here was a Ph.D. in biochemistry telling us we were wrong.

Taking the opportunity to snare Dr. Peat immediately after his talk, I spent the next hour or so with him exploring the subject further and getting his list of references. In the months that followed, I read as many of the papers he had listed as I could find. The evidence was strong that Dr. Peat was right: Giving estrogen alone just did not make good sense. In the process of this research, I came upon more and more evidence that not only was progesterone an important hormone at all adult ages for both men and women but also that unopposed estrogen put women at risk of undesirable, potentially lethal side effects.

Just a year or so before, it had become evident that women using estrogen were at five to six times greater risk of endometrial cancer (cancer of the uterus) than women not using estrogen. In effect, women and their doctors had to make a cruel choice between using estrogen to prevent osteoporosis and increase their risk of uterine cancer or not using it and risk an earlier hip fracture. Further, many of my women patients on estrogen had experienced water retention, headaches, and tender, swollen breasts, in addition to becoming heavier no matter how they dieted.

The turning point came for me when I was confronted with patients I had known for years who now had progressive osteoporosis and could not take estrogen because of a history of breast cancer, uterine cancer, diabetes, vascular disorders, gallbladder disease, obesity, or a host of other problems for which estrogen was either totally or partially contraindicated. During these years our community had access to dual photon bone absorptiometry (DPA), a test that accurately measures bone mineral density. Osteoporosis could now be measured. I remembered that Dr. Peat had told of an over-the-counter cream (Cielo, it was called then) that contained good amounts of easily absorbed natural progesterone and was available at local health food stores. Since it had been used in cosmetics as a skin moisturizer for years and I found no references indicating any safety problems, I considered the progesterone cream safe to use.

So, in late 1979, I began recommending progesterone cream to my osteoporotic patients who could not use estrogen. Using annual serial DPA bone density tests, I followed the bone condition of these patients. To my considerable surprise, the bone mineral density tests showed that my patients using progesterone cream showed significant *increase* (average 15 percent) whereas my patients on estrogen alone showed no increase but either remained stable or actually *decreased*. In addition, the progesterone patients told me of one condition after another that had improved since they started using the cream. Their backaches had gone away, they slept better, they had more en-

ergy, they could lose weight more easily, their skin was less dry and less wrinkled, and their libido, which had more or less evaporated over the years, was now revived. And among those with a history of cancer, *none* had developed any recurrence or late metastases.

The increase in bone mineral density was particularly remarkable. In researching the medical literature, I could find no study reporting any similar results. Even the vaunted estrogen has never been found to increase bone mineral density; it only slows the bone loss of osteoporosis. And that meager benefit occurs only in the five- to six-year period around menopause time, after which osteoporosis bone loss continues at a rate of about 1.5 percent a year whether one takes estrogen or not. Fractures prevented, as advertised by the estrogen promoters, are actually only fractures delayed. It therefore seemed obvious to me to add natural progesterone cream to my patients already using estrogen. When I did, the same bone benefits appeared.

There was a problem, however. On adding progesterone, some of the patients complained of increased estrogen side effects such as water retention, fuller breasts, and weight gain. These all resolved when the estrogen dosage was reduced. This was my introduction into the mysteries of hormone balance. Each of these two important hormones increases the effect of the other. In nature's wisdom, the two hormones are meant to work together. Year after year, as I dealt with patient after patient, I learned more and more about the multiple ways in which these hormones affect the body. Things that once were mysterious became clear; things I thought I knew I discovered were more remarkable than I had dreamt. And, most wonderful of all, my treatment of hormonally related illnesses became based on understanding the underlying cause rather than on symptom-based prescriptions.

My library of books and papers on osteoporosis, breast cancer, menopause, uterine cancer, fibrocystic breasts, pregnancy, menarche, PMS, and hormones came to fill my shelves and accumulate in piles around my desk. In time, I wrote several papers on what I had observed in my patients. They found publication not in our U.S. mainstream journals (which demand placebo-controlled, double-blind studies), but in Australian, Canadian, English, and "alternative" journals. I talked to my colleagues and gave talks at our hospital staff meetings. The reception was warm but their looks of perplexity gave me to understand that I had hit what others have called "cognitive dissonance." While unable to dispute my work, my colleagues could not understand how the knowledge I presented was missing from their own education and the textbooks (and the pharmaceutical advertising) on which they relied. In their minds, the file marked "progesterone" was filled with advertising about synthetic progestins, which are not the same thing.

In 1993 I wrote a small book entitled *Natural Progesterone: The Multiple Roles of a Remarkable Hormone* in an attempt to explain to my colleagues everything I had learned about progesterone and women's hormone balance. Without any advertising, this little book has become a publishing success. In spite of its technical medical language, word has spread about this book and thousands of women, looking for the answers they haven't been getting anywhere else, have bought it. The informal networking among women on the subject of menopause and hormone balancing is a wonder to behold.

I teamed up with Virginia Hopkins to write this expanded and updated version of the book in lay language so that you would have easier access to information about the benefits of progesterone and hormone balance in a form that is straightforward, readable, and easy to use. We want you to know about the history and politics of the medical and drug establishment, to be extremely well informed about synthetic hormone replacement therapy, to understand the biochemistry and dynamics of your own hormones and how they get out of balance, and most of all, to learn how to prevent hormone imbalance and how to stay healthy. We have given you many guidelines for determining whether your hormones are out of balance as well as detailed information about how to use natural progesterone and other hormones. We want to empower you to question your doctors intelligently; if you read this book from cover to cover, you are likely to be better informed on the subject of progesterone than they are. We hope that as you discover for yourself the truth of what is written here, you will insist that your doctor read it too, and continue the quiet but powerful revolution in knowledge and practice that is taking place regarding hormone replacement therapy.

Since we first wrote this book in 1995, tremendous changes have occurred in conventional medicine's approach to hormones. When this book was first published, I was scorned and ridiculed by my colleagues for suggesting that hormones could be absorbed through the skin; now there are FDA-approved estrogen and birth control patches that deliver hormones through the skin. Just a few years ago, hormone replacement therapy (HRT) with a combination of estrogen and a progestin was widely advertised as helping menopausal women with everything from heart disease to Alzheimer's; now, thanks to the Women's Health Initiative study and the Million Woman study from the United Kingdom, we know that these synthetic hormone cocktails increase the risk of heart disease, stroke, breast cancer, and gallbladder disease.

In the past decade, first dozens and then hundreds of courageous physicians have begun to use progesterone and other natural hormones in their clinical practices, with great success. In fact, these are the busiest physicians I know, and I might add, the happiest, because their patients are healthy and happy. In this new edition of *What Your Doctor May* Not *Tell You About Menopause*, we have much more information to share with you about how hormones interact with each other and how they can be used to promote optimal health. We have many new studies to share and new questions to answer.

There is a great thirst for knowledge in this field. Many women have known for years that they are not being served properly by the treatments their doctors give them, and these concerns have been validated over and over again by research. Women know something is wrong when 650,000 (or more) hysterectomies per year are performed in the United States. They know they are not victims of some mistake of Mother Nature. They know that a hormone that is supposed to cure them should not also promote cancer. Women are far more knowledgeable, intelligent, and intuitive than their doctors give them credit for. A revolution in women's health care is under way, spurred by the efficacy of using natural hormones to help restore balance.

But the full story of hormone replacement and hormone balancing has yet to be told. I'm sure that more discoveries and insights are ahead. Medicine is an ever-emerging science. With this new edition, I hope to share with you what I've learned and to add to the knowledge base that presently exists. It is a culmination of 30-plus years of practice, more than 20 years specifically studying progesterone and other hormones, the reading of countless books and articles on the subject, and conversations with hundreds of doctors and thousands of women in my practice, as well as the thousands of people who have contacted me to share their experiences. It is my firm belief that our doctors need to be reeducated in the realities of their female patients' hormone matters, and now that it is acknowledged that conventional HRT may be harmful and ineffective, there's a better chance that they'll listen. There is no teaching force for doctors more formidable or effective than knowledgeable, intelligent, assertive women. The book is dedicated to them.

This book would not have been possible without the expert assistance of my coauthor, science writer Virginia Hopkins. Her tireless dedication to the project, her communication and writing skills, and her attributes of applied women's wisdom have been indispensable not only to my understanding but to the understanding all readers will achieve concerning this important subject.

—John R. Lee, M.D.

INTRODUCTION

The change. Every adult woman in North America and other industrialized countries knows what these words refer to: the "change of life" that occurs with menopause. Those who have entered into menopause know it by their own experience; others know the experience of their mothers, an older sister, or a friend. They have heard the stories of the hot flashes and night sweats, the mood swings, the vaginal dryness, and the sagging breasts and fatter hips. They vow (and pray) to somehow never let it happen that way to them. They fear the loss of sexual enjoyment that menopause may portend. They see older women shrunken and bent with osteoporosis, and cannot visit an older friend in a nursing home without some dread that this may be their destiny, too.

But they also know from other older women, who are vigorous and full of life, that this deterioration is not universal with all women. What, they wonder, makes the difference and what can be done to remain vital and healthy? Menopause, after all, is not a disease but only a transition between one's childbearing years and the large segment of life that follows when one no longer need be concerned with monthly menstrual bleeding and the possible responsibilities of pregnancy. Womanly intuition tells them that menopause is not a mistake of Mother Nature, a design error from which there is no escape. Women in many other cultures appear to make this transition without all the problems we see here. Are they merely more stoic or do they have no audience for their complaints? Do they in fact sail through the change without any particular problem? Is there a difference and, if so, what makes it so?

Many writers on the subject of menopause remind us that the

general lack of medical history detailing menopausal changes in ages past can be explained by the shorter average life span common in earlier times. They point out that many mammals remain fertile throughout their lives and perhaps Mother Nature intended women to simply die when they were no longer able to carry children. This argument implies that our longer average life span is an unnatural extension of life created by our food abundance and improved medical care. Such reasoning is fallacious and should be put to rest.

Average life span does *not* mean that the average person died at such and such an age. It merely means that the age of death for a sufficiently large number of people born during a certain time period was recorded and used to calculate a numerical average. If, for example, during this time period half of the children died before age 2 and all the others lived to be 80, the average life span would be about 40 years. Or if no children died and everyone lived until 40 and then died, their average life span would also be 40 years. As it turns out, our longer life span is due almost solely to the decrease in childhood deaths from infectious diseases.

There were plenty of older women in European and American cultures during previous centuries. The average life span of our first seven presidents was longer than that of our most recently dead seven presidents. Saint Patrick, of Irish fame, is credited with living from A.D. 385 to 461 and this (76 years) was not thought to be particularly unusual at the time. Socrates was given poison hemlock to bring about his death in 399 B.C. when he was 70 years old. His contemporary, Plato, lived from 427 to 347 B.C. (80 years) and was not thought to be remarkably old. Though these examples are male, there is no time in history when women did not typically outlive males. I think we can safely discard the average life span argument as a basis for the lack of historical reports of menopause as a crisis in women's lives.

Others might argue that women's illnesses were not of sufficient importance to be included in medical writings of ages past. This, too, does not wash. Even though the typical doctor-historian was male, he would not refrain from writing about his success in treating such an important female malady if it existed.

Another argument I have heard is that the women's rights movement has used their media access to overstate the case regarding menopause problems. I have heard men exploit this argument to claim that U.S. women are spoiled. This also is nonsense, as anyone who treats these women can tell you. Any woman who goes through pregnancy and the delivery of a baby without undue complaint has got to be regarded as a strong and stoical person. When such a person tells me she is extremely distraught by uncontrollable hot flashes, night sweats, mood swings, depression, and the fear of osteoporosis, I tend to believe her.

The fact we must face is that women today are indeed suffering from a real menopausal disorder of which we have only a rudimentary understanding and for which our present mainstream treatments are simply not satisfactory. Our treatment with supplemental estrogen may reduce hot flashes and treat vaginal dryness, but it does so at the risk of inducing a higher incidence of endometrial cancer and breast cancer; it also causes unwanted fat and water retention. Consider the financial implications. Turning menopausal symptoms into a disease of estrogen deficiency resulted in Premarin's being one of the top 10 prescription drugs sold in the United States. Until recently, let any American woman of menopausal age complain to her doctor of any symptom and the odds were she would receive a prescription for Premarin and a progestin. Any symptom that persists after estrogen supplementation is considered trivial or cause for a tranquilizer prescription or a referral to a psychiatrist.

This symptom/drug approach points the way to what is amiss in mainstream medicine today. It suffers from a fixation on the drug treatment of health problems. The typical medical treatment program for almost any given health problem follows a war metaphor: Find the villain and destroy it. If a villain cannot be found, look for the destruction left in its wake. That is, treat the disease by killing it or, failing that, treat the symptoms. This was not the metaphor of conventional medicine of past centuries. Treatment concepts were previously directed at restoring balance in terms of physical, nutritional, emotional, environmental, and even spiritual factors.

Disease is often a late manifestation of a process that has its origin long before symptoms developed. This is certainly true of coronary heart disease, osteoporosis, breast and other cancers, fibroids, hypertension, arthritis, and many, many others. Mainstream medicine focuses on the disease as it becomes symptomatic, not on the initial asymptomatic stages. If we are to make any advance in health care, it will come as a result of understanding initial causes, not in waiting to treat the later symptomatic phase. A recent study in monkeys showed that diabetes and cardiovascular disease occurred rarely in monkeys that had been fed to remain slim, but almost exclusively in those monkeys allowed to get fat, even if they later had been put on a diet to lose their fat. Is this not a clue to guide us in the rearing of our own children?

Parallels abound throughout our present health care problems. The majority of illnesses being treated today in the United States stems from preventable causes. A well-researched report in the *New England Journal of Medicine* states that *preventable illness makes up approximately 70 percent of the burden of disease and the associated costs*. By shifting our view from the mainstream disease oriented categories to underlying causes, it is found that preventable causes account for eight of the nine leading categories and for 980,000 deaths per year.

We stand at the confluence of profound changes. Our present medical system is symptom-fixated and driven by misplaced economic incentives, but it now faces stiff competition from alternative practitioners. Women's health problems clustered under the banner of hormone balance are epidemic and not well addressed by mainstream medicine. Women are emerging from under a cloud of historic medical neglect and are rightly demanding new and more effective approaches. It is my hope that this book will provide guidance in this needed effort.

Since writing my book *Natural Progesterone: The Multiple Roles of a Remarkable Hormone*, in 1993, and writing the first edition of this book, in 1995, I have had thousands of letters and phone calls from women describing the condescending, insensitive attitudes of their doctors in dealing (not very effectively) with their premenopause and menopause problems. A revolution is under way. Despite the lucrative incentives that sustain the present system, change will come because women demand it.

PART I

THE INNER WORKINGS OF HORMONE BALANCE

CHAPTER 1

THE CRUX OF THE MATTER: MENOPAUSAL POLITICS AND WOMEN'S HORMONE CYCLES

Not so long ago, *menopause* was a word you did not say out loud in public, and you had to go to a medical library to find a book on the subject. Go into a typical bookstore these days and you'll find literally dozens of titles on menopause. They range from praising the wonders of estrogen and hormone replacement therapy to personal stories of the ups and downs some women experience during the "change of life," and there are now many other books written on the subject of natural hormones. What was once a taboo subject has become a mainstay of talk shows and women's magazine articles.

Menopausal Politics

With 30 million menopausal women in North America and some 20 million baby boomer women in menopause or on the brink of it, it's no wonder this is a major topic of discussion. What *is* a wonder is how we have managed to make menopause, a perfectly natural part of a woman's life cycle, into a disease. It has only just dawned on us that menstruation, pregnancy, and childbirth are not diseases; now we need to realize that menopause is not a disease despite millions in advertising dollars spent by drug companies to convince us otherwise. The pharmaceutical companies have not failed to notice the huge population of premenopausal women in the pipeline, a financial gold mine in the making. Premarin, a form of hormone replacement therapy made from pregnant mare's urine by the Wyeth-Ayerst Company, was one of the top-selling prescription medicines in the United States until the 2002 Women's Health Initiative (WHI) study showed that PremPro (a combination of Premarin and a progestin) increased the risk of breast cancer, strokes, and gallbladder disease. Although Premarin/PremPro generated more than $2 billion in sales in 2001 and represented 22 percent of Wyeth's pharmaceutical sales, more recently, sales of Premarin/PremPro have declined about 25 percent.

In 1995, when I first wrote this book, I stated, "A large percentage of advertising and research dollars are spent trying to convince women that estrogen will cure everything from heart disease to Alzheimer's, but there is scant evidence for any of these claims and reams of evidence that synthetic estrogens are highly toxic and carcinogenic." Now the WHI has proven me correct on this, and many millions of women are searching for a safe alternative to PremPro. In my opinion, it's not so much the estrogens per se that are toxic and carcinogenic, it's estrogens used in excess, and with progestins instead of natural progesterone. But you will learn a lot more about this as you read further.

The good news is that women have become guarded and skeptical about having new drugs pushed on them. After being told that DES, a hormone that was supposed to guard against miscarriages, was safe, hundreds of thousands of women discovered the hard way that it caused cancer in their children. Women were told that Valium was a safe and effective remedy for depression and anxiety, only to find out that it was addictive. Then their physicians tried to convince them that once they had reached menopause they should automatically go on hormone replacement therapy featuring synthetic estrogens and progestins, only to find it could increase their risk of deadly diseases rather than save them from the aging process. It is telling that only 10 to 15 percent of menopausal women chose to use conventional HRT despite intense pressure from doctors and the media. The real tragedy is that many thousands of women may have died or been permanently harmed because they used HRT, when the natural forms of these hormones, used wisely and in moderation, could have been, and still could be of very real benefit. In the chapters that follow, we will look more closely at how estrogen and progesterone work in a woman's body and the politics of pushing drugs to women.

What Is Menopause?

Strictly speaking, menopause is the cessation of menses, the end of menstrual cycles. The unpleasant "symptoms" of menopause that some women suffer, such as hot flashes, vaginal dryness, and mood swings, are peculiar to industrialized cultures and, as far as I can tell, they are virtually unknown in agrarian cultures. In native cultures menopause tends to be a cause for quiet celebration, a time when a woman has completed her childbearing years and is moving into a deeper level of self-discovery and spiritual awareness. She is becoming a wise old woman. In these cultures menopausal women are looked up to and revered. They are sought out for advice and their opinions are heavily weighed in the decision-making process of the community. How strange that sounds to us! We know menopause as a death knell, the end of a woman's sexuality, a descent into a dried-up and painful old age of arthritis and osteoporosis. How did this experience of menopause come to be? I believe it's a combination of poor diet, unhealthy lifestyle, environmental pollutants, cultural attitudes, the incorrect use of synthetic hormones, and advertising. But first, let's look at what happens in a woman's body as menopause approaches.

The Rise and Fall of Hormones During the Menstrual Cycle

In a normal menstrual cycle, every 26 to 28 days, the ovaries, which hold a woman's eggs, receive a hormonal signal from the brain that it's time to get some eggs ready to be fertilized. Anywhere from a few to a few hundred eggs begin to mature inside sacs called *follicles*. After 10 to 12 days one egg has moved to the outer surface of the ovary and the follicle bursts, releasing the egg into the fallopian tube for its journey to the uterus.

As the egg is ripening in the ovary, the uterus is ripening in preparation for the possibility of growing a fetus. The uterine lining thickens and becomes engorged with blood that will nourish the growing embryo. If no fertilized egg implants itself in the uterus, it sheds its lining. This shedding is the blood of menstruation. Then the cycle begins again, with the signal from the brain telling the ovary to ripen an egg (see Figure 1).

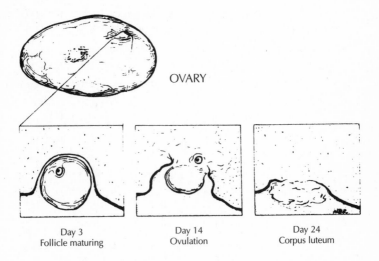

OVARY

| Day 3 | Day 14 | Day 24 |
| Follicle maturing | Ovulation | Corpus luteum |

Figure 1: Ovulation of a follicle

Estrogen (from *estrus*, meaning "heat" or "fertility") is the dominant hormone for the first week or so after menstruation, stimulating the buildup of tissue and blood in the uterus as the ovarian follicles simultaneously begin their development of the egg. Around the time of ovulation, estrogen causes changes in the vaginal mucus, making it more tolerant of male penetration during sexual activity and more hospitable to sperm. At this phase in the menstrual cycle, the vaginal mucus tends to somewhat resemble uncooked egg whites. Watching for this change in mucus combined with a rise in body temperature is one of the best nonlaboratory methods for identifying the time of ovulation.

About twelve days after the beginning of the previous menstruation, the rising estrogen level peaks and then tapers off just as the follicle matures and just before ovulation. After ovulation the now-empty follicle becomes the *corpus luteum* (so named because of its appearance as a small yellow body on the surface of the ovary). The corpus luteum is the site of progesterone production, which dominates the second half of the menstrual month, reaching a peak of about 20 milligrams (mg) per day.

Progesterone production during this phase of the cycle, along with estrogen, leads to a refinement and "ripening" of tissue and blood in the uterus. Progesterone also contributes to the changes in the vaginal mucus seen at the time of ovulation. The rise of progesterone at the time of ovulation causes a rise of body temperature of about one degree Fahrenheit, a finding often used to indicate ovulation.

If pregnancy does not occur within 10 to 12 days after ovulation, estrogen and progesterone levels fall abruptly, triggering menstruation, and the cycle begins anew. If pregnancy occurs, progesterone production increases and the shedding of the lining of the uterus is prevented, thus preserving the developing embryo. As pregnancy progresses, progesterone production is taken over by the placenta and its secretion increases gradually to levels of 300 to 400 milligrams per day during the third trimester.

Premenopause

A woman's hormone balance can begin to shift at anywhere from her mid-30s to her late 40s, depending on a variety of factors such as heredity, environment, how early or late she began menstruating, whether she had children and if so at what age and how many, and her lifestyle. Was she exhausted trying to juggle career and family? Was she eating junk food, caffeine, sugar, and alcohol or whole grains, fresh vegetables, and fruits? Has she taken vitamins? Has she lived in the city or country? Was she exposed to toxins in the workplace? Hormone balance is intimately connected to stress levels, nutrition, and the environmental toxins encountered daily. We will discuss all of these factors more thoroughly in the chapters to come.

The ability of the follicles to mature an egg and release it may begin "sputtering," so to speak, a decade before actual menopause, creating menstrual cycles in which a woman does not ovulate, called *anovulatory* cycles. If she isn't ovulating, she isn't producing progesterone from the ovaries and she may begin experiencing menopausal symptoms such as weight gain, water retention, and mood swings. Menstrual cycles can continue even without the progesterone, however, so most women aren't aware that the lack of progesterone is causing their symptoms. I call this phase *premenopause*. I will be discussing premenopause symptoms in more detail in Chapter 11, and have also written an entire book on the subject called *What Your Doctor May* Not *Tell You About Premenopause*. The phase right around the time of menopause, when hormones and brain signals to the ovaries are fluctuating, is called *peri*menopause.

It used to be true that the majority of women began menopause in their mid-40s to early 50s. In the last generation, however, things appear to have changed. Women now may have anovulatory periods starting in their early 30s and yet do not experience cessation of periods (menopause) until their 50s. During this time, the ovaries continue to produce estrogen sufficient for regular or irregular shedding, creating what I term "estrogen dominance," which will be discussed in detail throughout the book.

Some women may go for years with irregular cycles and slowly wind down, or may just suddenly stop menstruating one month and never menstruate again. They may be overwhelmed with unpleasant symptoms or hardly notice what has happened other than not having to worry about birth control or tampons every month. How menopause is experienced is as individual and unique as each human being.

During the many months of anovulatory periods, estrogen

production may become erratic, with surges of inappropriately high levels alternating with irregular low levels. Periods of vaginal bleeding may become erratic, some much heavier than others. When estrogen surges, women undergoing these changes may notice breast swelling and tenderness, mood swings, sleep disturbance, water retention, and a tendency to put on weight. These may be the symptoms of estrogen dominance caused mainly by lack of ovulation and thereby lack of progesterone while their estrogen levels are still in the "normal" range. Their doctors may check their estradiol levels and their follicle stimulating hormone (FSH) and luteinizing hormone (LH) levels, but rarely does it dawn on them that their patients' progesterone levels are too low. In taking the usual blood tests, the doctor may find the estrogen normal that day or even a bit on the low side and FSH levels a bit too high. On another day the estrogen might be elevated and FSH levels normal. If the former is found, the doctor may even prescribe some estrogen on the theory that the patient is nearing true menopause. The woman usually finds that this does not help her and often makes things worse.

More often, the doctor ascribes her complaints to emotional causes or simply some defect of Mother Nature that women must endure. In later chapters, I will discuss this phenomenon in more detail. For the present, we will merely say that a rising percentage of women are experiencing premenopausal woes that are related to their hormones. The details concerning environmental toxins, nutritional factors, stress, adrenal hormones, exercise, and weight will be found in the chapters ahead.

CHAPTER 2

THE DANCE OF
THE STEROIDS

The word *steroids* may conjure up visions of muscle-bound bodybuilders and unpleasant side effects, but steroid is really a generic name for dozens of body regulators (hormones) made from chole*sterol*. Cholesterol, the basic building block for the steroid hormones, gives them all a similar structure. An analogy would be a basic clothing ensemble. You begin with a beige jacket and matching slacks. Add a blouse, a necklace, and some pumps and you have a business outfit for a corporate office. Make it black and add a scoop-neck silk blouse, cut the jacket at the waist, and you're ready for a night on the town. Or make the jacket and slacks navy blue, add a button-down shirt, some epaulets and gold braid, and you have a military uniform. The basic suit stays the same, but the additions, subtractions, and other alterations make the difference in the role you play. In the same sense, all the steroid molecules resemble cholesterol in their basic structure. Switch a few atoms around and the role of the hormone can change dramatically.

Without sufficient cholesterol, we can't make sufficient steroid hormones. (If you would like to see how biochemists picture the cholesterol molecule, turn to the appendix on page 425.) Some of the other more familiar steroids are estrogen, progesterone, testosterone, the corticosteroids, and dehydroepiandrosterone (DHEA). The steroid drugs that bodybuilders use are called anabolic steroids. *Anabolic* means that they have a "building" function rather than a "taking apart" function. Testosterone, for example, helps build up muscle mass, as do some other androgens (male hormones). Although the workings of the steroids are subtle and complex, a slight imbalance can have major effects. Learning a bit about steroid hormones can give you an enormous advantage in making informed decisions about hormone replacement therapy. What I am about to tell you here, most doctors forgot a long time ago, but the information is fundamental to truly understanding hormone balance.

The first step in the body's manufacture of steroid hormones from cholesterol happens in tiny energy packets called *mitochondria* found within every cell of the body except red blood cells. From cholesterol, the mitochondria make a hormone called *pregnenolone*, which can then be transformed into progesterone or 17-OH-pregnenolone. Then, from these two steroids, progesterone and 17-OH-pregnenolone, all the other steroid hormones can be made by relatively minor molecular modifications, depending on body need. In this sort of production, one steroid is transformed into another. Many of the steps along the steroid pathway are active hormones in their own right even though they also serve by being transformed into yet other hormones (see Figure 2).

Although the steroid hormones are remarkably similar in shape, each of them has markedly different effects, and these differences arise from very slight variations in their molecular structure. Let's look at some of the major players in this constantly shifting milieu of steroid hormones.

The Cast of Major Players

Pregnenolone   Synthesized from cholesterol by mitochondria of all the cells of the body (except red blood cells), this molecule is the precursor to all steroid hormones.

Progesterone   A precursor to most of the steroid hormones, it is responsible for a myriad of important jobs from maintaining pregnancy to regulating menstrual cycles. Made primarily in the ovaries, it is described in detail in later chapters.

17α-OH-progesterone   A variant of progesterone, it leads to

cortisol production in the adrenal cortex and to androstenedione from which all other sex hormones are made.

DHEA (dehydroepiandrosterone)   A precursor to the androgens, testosterone, and the estrogens, DHEA is important to
protein building and repair. Most likely it has other important jobs as well that are still being discovered. It is made primarily in the adrenal glands. DHEA levels decline
dramatically as we age, making it a primary biomarker of
aging.

Androstenedione and Androstenediol   Androgenic (masculinizing) hormones, they are precursors to testosterone and the
estrogens. Produced in the ovaries and the adrenals from either progesterone or DHEA, they are the source of estrogen
production after menopause or loss of one's ovaries.

17-OH-pregnenolone   A modification of pregnenolone created in the adrenal cortex, testes, and ovarian follicles, it is
used in the adrenal cortex and testes to create DHEA. In the
ovaries it is an alternate step for 17µ-OH-progesterone production.

Testosterone   A male sex hormone that stimulates the growth
of male characteristics and the production of sperm, it also is
a precursor to the estrogens. It is made primarily in the testes
but also in much smaller amounts by the ovaries.

Estrone, Estradiol, and Estriol   Female sex hormones known
as estrogen, they are primarily responsible for the growth of
female characteristics in puberty and regulating the menstrual cycle. They are made primarily in the ovaries but also
from androstenedione in fat cells, muscle cells, and skin even
after menopause.

Corticosterone, Cortisol   They help regulate numerous bodily
functions including glucose and energy balance; they also
moderate inflammation and immune responses throughout
the body. They are made in the adrenal glands.

Aldosterone   Made in the adrenal glands, it controls sodium
and potassium levels in the blood and is important in regulating electrolytes and blood pressure.

Their position in the biosynthesis pathway is indicated in Figure 2.

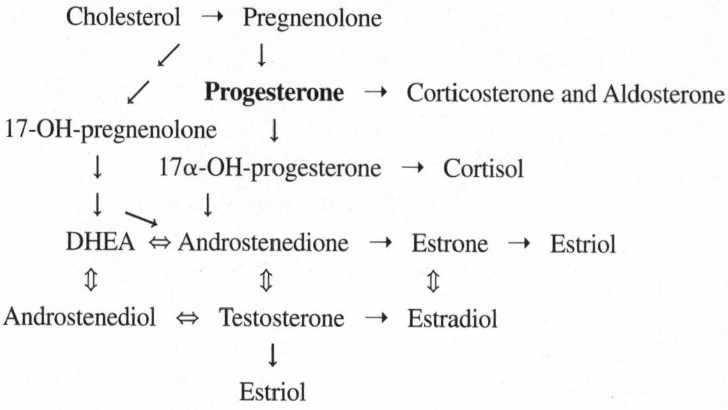

Cholesterol → Pregnenolone
          ↙   ↓
       ↙   **Progesterone** → Corticosterone and Aldosterone
17-OH-pregnenolone   ↓
   ↓   17α-OH-progesterone → Cortisol
   ↓ ↘   ↓
DHEA ⇔ Androstenedione → Estrone → Estriol
  ⇕   ⇕   ⇕
Androstenediol ⇔ Testosterone → Estradiol
                ↓
              Estriol

Figure 2: Basic steroid hormone pathways in the ovary, testis, and adrenal gland. Each arrow in the pathway diagram represents the work of a specific enzyme. The arrow symbol was chosen because it indicates the direction of the action. Only in a few instances is an action reversible, as indicated by the double arrows.

Choreographing the Dance

The steroid hormones shown in Figure 2 are made primarily in the ovaries of women, the testes of men, and the adrenal glands of both sexes. As far as we know, all of the steroid hormones are made from cholesterol. This is one of the reasons it is so important *not* to go on a no-fat or no-cholesterol diet. Although our body can manufacture about 75 percent of our cholesterol from other foods we eat, the remaining 25 percent comes directly from cholesterol-containing foods. Eliminate cholesterol entirely and hormone imbalance may result. Low cholesterol in the elderly has been linked to depression and suicide. As in most things, moderation and balance are the answer. The transformation from one hormone to another requires enzymes, which in turn require vitamin and mineral *cofactors*. A substance that is the source of another substance is called the *precursor*. (If you would like more detailed biochemical information about the enzymes in the steroid pathways, please see the appendix on page 425.)

The Journey Along the Steroid Hormone Pathway

As I describe the pathways in words, follow my description on the diagram in Figure 2.

The journey begins on the upper left corner with pregnenolone having been derived from cholesterol. The flow of hormones then progresses from pregnenolone along one of two major pathways: one to the left and down through the adrenal DHEA pathway, or straight down through progesterone in both the ovarian and adrenal glands. Both pathways lead to what we call *metabolic end points*. Aldosterone, cortisol, and the estrogens are the final stops, or metabolic end points, on the steroid hormone pathways.

With the exception of the end point hormones, all of the steroid hormone molecules are capable of being converted into some other molecule. Testosterone, for instance, can be a precursor of the estrogen called estradiol, and androstenedione can be a precursor of either testosterone or estrone, another estrogen. Estrone and estradiol can be interchanged into each other via a redox (reduction/oxidation) system in the liver. Progesterone is a precursor in several pathways, one leading to androstenedione and on to the estrogens and to testosterone, another to cortisol, and another to corticosterone and aldosterone. Similarly, DHEA is a precursor in the pathway leading to testosterone and androstenedione, the latter leading on to the estrogens but *not* to other corticosteroids.

The ebb and flow of steroid hormones along their pathways is a result of enzyme action monitored and controlled by biofeedback mechanisms evolved over eons of time in the limbic brain (hypothalamus). It is important to realize that enzyme (and hormone) function is dependent on precise molecular configuration. Enzymes are large molecules continuously created from blueprints in our chromosomes, which generally require specific vitamin and mineral cofactors to maximize their job of transforming one hormone into another. (That is why a healthy diet and vitamin/mineral supplements can be so effective in helping your body work right.) Each enzyme performs but one function, such as the splitting of a single chemical bond in a specific molecule. To perform that one function, an enzyme must precisely "fit" the structure of the molecule, like a complicated key-and-lock system. Molecular conformation, or the exact and specific structure of the molecules, is the key to the smooth running of these enzyme pathways.

Molecular conformation is the factor that distinguishes natural hormones most strongly from the synthetic versions sold by drug companies. Synthetic hormones have altered shapes not known in nature, created by the addition of atoms at unusual positions. Thus, synthetic steroids, such as those found in the typical hormone replacement therapy (HRT) prescription, are not subject to the usual enzymatic pathways. We don't naturally have enzymes designed to handle any of the synthetic steroids; their effects cannot be "tuned down" or "turned off" as needed, nor can they be efficiently excreted through the usual enzymatic mechanisms. Despite their advertisements, synthetic hormones are not equivalent to natural hormones. Harmony and balance, the hallmark of a healthy body, are lost when biologically active synthetic compounds are thrown into the dance of the steroids. The mischief they can create in the normal ebb and flow of vital steroid hormones is most likely responsible for a great deal of hormonal imbalance and resulting illness.

The Dance of the Steroids

Understanding steroids requires a vision into the unseen. Humans have the power to create reality beyond their normal experience. We do it all the time with music, books, stories, fantasies, dreams, and, yes, especially in science. Science is really the art of "seeing" forces and elements invisible to the normal senses. No physicist has ever seen an atom, yet she conjures an image to understand its behavior. We know that atoms join together to create molecules. Although the atomic bonding necessary to create molecules involves a sharing of electrons not well understood, we can still glean information from nature's hidden forces. We can learn to understand, to use, and even to create molecules. In the "movements" that follow, I will describe my vision of the world of the biological molecules we call steroid hormones, based on my understanding of biochemistry. I call this vision "the dance of the steroids." Think of it as action accompanied by music. Do not try to understand this vision with your logical, linear mind; allow your intuitive mind to grasp it for you.

Four Movements:
The Flow of Steroids in Our Bodies

Movement 1. *Andante con molto*

There is a land near but far away where busy workers by the millions are doing the work of the body in beautiful, flowing, complex harmony. These are the steroids, turning out products to match our needs, stabilizing, energizing, and nurturing our cells and tissues; ensuring repair and replication of vital body parts; protecting us against damage; and, for a great portion of our adult life, fostering the genesis and development of a new life to carry on the species after our own body ceases to exist. The landscape is alive with hustle and bustle but the prevailing mode is one of synchrony and balance, busy but harmonious. Life is throbbing in a ceaseless flow of energy. We sense the magnitude of activity, the surgings and ebbings of rhythms unseen, and the ungraspable complexity of it all. But at the same time we are aware of order, coordination, and purpose. Despite the complexity and energy apparent, there is an air of majesty and design.

Movement 2. Adagio

A collection of still photographs reveals workers at their benches, bakers busy in their shops, potters at their kilns, carpenters at their labor, homemakers in their nests, firemen at their stations, police standing vigilant, nurses doing their tending, and a host of activities beyond our understanding. At first glance, the workers all look identical. Closer examination reveals slight differences among the various classes of workers. They all seem to be made of the same parts but with minor variations in how the parts are put together. We see that without exception the minor differences among the workers strictly correlate with the work each is doing. Though all are steroids, each is designed with a specific job in mind. What at first appeared to us as chaos is only a fault in our understanding. Precision and synchrony are paramount.

Movement 3. Allegro con brio

Live video captures the hustle and bustle of myriad activities, the arrival of raw materials and the departure of finished products, and the ceaseless inflow of new workers and the outflow of workers apparently called elsewhere. Just off camera, we are told, are the cholesterol molecules having their parts rearranged to enter the scene as worker units. To our amazement, some workers will, in the blink of an eye, be suddenly transformed from baker to chef, from nurse to fireman, from carpenter to potter, without a hint of discontinuity or a missed beat in their activities. Their parts will have been suddenly rearranged and their functions switched simultaneously with their newly acquired form. This magical transformation is accomplished by shimmering protein globules (enzymes) passing among them, briefly embracing each selected worker molecule and, in a flash of electromagnetic energy, leaving them with slightly altered elements and new functions, impressing upon the whole scene a synchrony of design and purpose.

Movement 4. *Largo maestoso*

Some of the molecules, having reached an end point in their transformational process, are kept in balanced concentration by being gently swept along in an invisible current to distant parts (the liver) where, their work being done, they are wedded (conjugated) to bile acids and carried silently off our viewing screen. Scientists would say that they are inactivated by hydroxylation (in the case of estrogens) or hydrogenated and conjugated with glucuronic acid (in the case of progesterone) for excretion in bile. On the periphery of our video scene is a continuous magical influx of new worker units sufficient to meet the rise and fall of their essential functions. In this manner, excesses and/or deficiencies are well prevented and a sense of order pervades.

Now that your intuitive mind has had some fun, you can go back to your logical, linear mind. For those interested in the whole tableau of the biosynthetic pathways complete with their molecular structure, the known enzymes (and their vitamin and mineral cofactors) that perform the transformation, and the gland tissue(s) in which each step takes place, turn to the appendix on page 425. You will be able to follow the transformations by simply following the arrows. It is time now to get on with a look at the history of hormone replacement.

CHAPTER 3

THE HISTORY OF HORMONE REPLACEMENT THERAPY AND THE ESTROGEN MYTH

Estrogen replacement therapy (ERT) was first conceived in the late 1950s, the era of "better living through chemistry." These were the heady, innocent postwar years when enthusiasm for controlling the natural environment with chemicals was matched only by the eagerness of the chemical companies to find a profitable use for their products. Concurrently, pharmaceutical companies were discovering the financial gains to be made by a similar philosophy: For every human ailment there is a drug that will cure it. Plastics, pesticides, and antibiotics were going to save the human race.

Both the chemical and pharmaceutical companies were learning the value of cleverly disguised public relations campaigns in which articles extolling the virtues of a product were "planted" in magazines and newspapers. The media went along with this approach (and still do), reaping huge benefits in advertising dollars from these same companies. The public naïvely believed (and still do) that if they read it in a major publication, it must be true. Few industries have reaped more benefits from this public naïveté than pharmaceutical companies. The practice continues unabated to this day; the major women's magazines and the nightly TV news shows are a virtual pipeline of information for drug companies eager to push their products under the guise of editorial neutrality.

The burgeoning awareness in American industry that the

media could be easily manipulated to push their products took place in a cultural milieu that placed an emphasis on the nuclear family, with the father out earning a living and the mother at home with a baby on her hip and a batch of cookies in the oven. The ultra-feminine Marilyn Monroe was the cultural ideal of beauty. Women were thought to be at their best pleasing their husbands sexually and raising healthy, happy children. It's no coincidence that ERT was born just as the first big wave of American women raised to be happy homemakers was approaching middle age and menopause. Their children were leaving home, their hair was turning gray, and their breasts were sagging. Symbolically, their usefulness had come to an end: If they were no longer raising children, and no longer sexually attractive to their husbands, of what use were they? Psychological problems such as depression became common among women of this age. Millions of women became hooked on "mother's little helpers," Valium and other tranquilizers.

Menopause Becomes a Disease

Meanwhile, Ayerst, the first maker of a conjugated estrogen called Premarin, found the goose that laid the golden public relations egg in a Brooklyn, New York, gynecologist named Dr. Robert A. Wilson. With a list of sterling credentials as long as his arm, a dash of charisma, a zeal for keeping women young and feminine, and plenty of money from the pharmaceutical industry, Wilson hit the streets with the good news about estrogen. He used adjectives bordering on lurid to describe menopause deprecatingly as a time when women became dried-up, cranky, sexless old hags. His magic pill was going to save them from that "tragedy," keeping them "feminine forever." To make matters worse, it seems that almost everyone researching or writing about menopause from that point on quoted Wilson and unquestioningly accepted his information as fact, when in fact most of it was fiction.

If one were to pick a year during which ERT entered public consciousness, it might be 1964. The January 13, 1964, issue of

Newsweek carried a one-page story entitled "No More Menopause?" reporting on the work of Dr. Wilson, who was reported to have been studying menopause since the 1920s. He had reached the conclusion that "change of life" stemmed from a lack of the female hormones estrogen and progesterone.

Meanwhile, an enterprising and unhappily menopausal writer in London named Ann Walsh happened to read the *Newsweek* article with great interest. She was immediately struck by the great similarity between Wilson's description of what happens when one's ovaries stop functioning and her own disturbing set of symptoms. Walsh returned to the United States for a whirlwind tour of interviews with as many medical authorities involved in hormone research as she could track down. Their consistently cautionary tone about estrogen did not dampen her enthusiasm in the least. By late 1965 she produced a book titled *Now! The Pills to Keep Women Young! ERT The First Complete Account of the Miracle Hormone Treatment That May Revolutionize the Lives of Millions of Women!* Shortly thereafter, Dr. Wilson produced his own book, entitled *Feminine Forever*, copies of which were quickly disseminated to doctors' offices by Ayerst detail men (sales reps for pharmaceutical firms) throughout the United States, including my own office in Mill Valley, California. Even though Wilson's own research had led him to the conclusion that it was progesterone and estrogen that were missing in menopausal women, his book promoted only estrogen for hormone replacement therapy.

In the years of 1964 and 1965, the lay press suddenly blossomed with ERT articles. Following the January 1964 *Newsweek* article, there appeared the following:

Pageant (August 1964) "No More Menopause"
Ladies' Home Journal (January 1965) "The Truth About Female Hormones"
Good Housekeeping (April 1965) "Menopause: Is It Necessary?"
Time (April 16, 1965) "The Springs of Youth"
Cosmopolitan (July 1965) "Oh, What a Lovely Pill"
Vogue (August 15, 1965) "How to Live Young at Any Age— Straight Talk About Hormones from a Famous Doctor"

McCall's (October 1965) "E.R.T.: Pills to Keep You Young"
   (by Ann Walsh herself)

The economic impact of the ERT revolution was not lost on the financially minded: Even the *Wall Street Journal* carried a couple of lead articles on the subject. What woman wouldn't want to maintain her youth and femininity forever?

The Truth Behind the Hoopla

In truth, estrogen had been very poorly researched. Its approval as a prescription drug was based on a dubious study with a relatively small number of women in Puerto Rico who took birth control pills. The pill used at first was only a progestin, which was later found to be contaminated with estrogen-like substances. When estrogen was taken out of the birth control pills, they didn't work as well, so a synthetic estrogen was intentionally added. Twenty percent of the women in the study complained of side effects, but they were dismissed as neurotic. The three women who died while taking these pills were not autopsied to find out the cause of death. There has been ample evidence since then that these pills caused blood clots and strokes, but that evidence was dismissed and suppressed for the supposedly higher good of controlling the population explosion. Meanwhile, the pharmaceutical companies scrambled to find a combination of synthetic hormones that had fewer side effects. As Paula B. Doress-Worters said in a foreword to Sandra Coney's excellent book, *The Menopause Industry: How the Medical Establishment Exploits Women*:

> Hormone therapy has been called a product in search of a market. Most research on menopause is designed to demonstrate the desirability of medicalized interventions. Although the use of hormones to help women cope with common signs of menopause, such as hot flashes, has been known since 1937, hormone treatment was popularized for a mass market in the 1960s. It was promoted not sim-

ply as a palliative for the discomforts of menopause but also as a panacea for "psychological problems" supposedly related to the change of life. Such claims were unproven but were treated as common knowledge. These assertions promoted a stereotyped view of postmenopausal older women as asexual, neurotic, and unattractive. As a result, exogenous estrogen was approved for prescription use without adequate testing and soon became one of the five top-selling prescription drugs.

From 1965 to the mid-1970s, the ERT bandwagon sailed along with more and more women opting for the little pills that would keep them young. By 1975, however, a dark cloud emerged: Women on ERT were developing uterine (endometrial) cancer at a rate four to eight times greater than in untreated women. Multiple researchers confirmed the link between estrogen supplementation and uterine (endometrial) cancer. When the bad news hit the newspapers, sales of estrogen supplements dropped precipitously. Not only were women deciding not to start ERT and those on ERT deciding to quit, but physicians were understandably reluctant to prescribe it, despite its apparent virtues.

But the estrogen bandwagon was only temporarily stalled. After a spate of papers arguing the question of whether estrogen "caused" endometrial cancer or merely "promoted" it (a distinction lost on most female patients and their doctors), medical authorities pulled themselves together and switched from ERT to HRT (hormone replacement therapy).

The difference was the addition of the progestins (synthetic versions of progesterone). Fairly solid research existed or was soon accomplished to show that only "unopposed" estrogen was the culprit; estrogen combined with progestins actually prevented endometrial cancer. Endometrial cancer was unknown in women whose ovaries produced a proper balance of estrogen and progesterone. Research by Dr. R. Don Gambrell Jr. of the Medical College of Georgia and also by Dr. Lila E. Nachtigall at the Goldwater Memorial Hospital in New York City revealed that in women on a combined treatment program of estrogen with progestin, the incidence of uterine cancer was considerably less than in controls (women not receiving hormones).

The parallel fear of estrogen causing breast cancer was addressed in the same manner. Studies of women on HRT were reported to show less breast cancer than in women not on HRT. Whether this question was truly resolved or not (it wasn't), the ERT bandwagon was soon back on track as the HRT bandwagon.

The promoters of HRT also decided that estrogen and progestins could cure other ills and were soon declaring that HRT would also lower a woman's risk of heart disease and would prevent osteoporosis. These assertions were followed by massive marketing campaigns to "popularize" osteoporosis and educate women about it. I have had literally hundreds of women tell me that their doctors have "threatened" them ominously with predictions of heart disease and osteoporosis if they didn't take estrogen—regardless of whether they had any risk whatsoever for these diseases! The first assertion, that HRT protects women from heart disease, is not true, as you will discover throughout this book, nor does it reverse osteoporosis, but these myths persisted until very recently. Most people don't have the medical background to check and question the original research from which these assertions are made.

Somewhere early in the development of the HRT industry, progesterone was not only forgotten, it was mislabeled and mistaken as its distant cousins, the synthetic progestins. Even well-researched books on menopause tend to make this error: They never question whether the use of natural hormones might have some benefit, and they never question what happened to natural progesterone.

In rereading the early papers on estrogen replacement therapy I can sense the zeal and honest conviction of the authors. However, in retrospect, I can also see the narrowness of their views. They failed to ask some important questions, such as: Do women in other cultures experience the same menopausal symptoms and, if not, why not? Are there other causal factors operating here? What about side effects such as weight gain, water retention, migraine headaches, breast swelling, and fibrocystic breasts? Why do symptoms start before menopause, when estrogen levels are still high? Whatever happened to progesterone? What about HRT side effects of progestins? Within a specific culture, are symptom differences among women related to exercise, diet, or work environment? Their enthusiasm for estrogen seemed to blind them to this wider view.

It has been assumed that most women suffer from menopause symptoms. However, in checking the research, I can find no solid evidence to back up this assumption; most of it is anecdotal. My own hunch, based on 30 years of family practice and conversations with tens of thousands of women around the country, is that a small percentage of women suffer from severe enough hot flashes and vaginal dryness to warrant treatment with natural hormones. Then there is a large population of women in their mid-30s and on up suffering from the symptoms of estrogen dominance brought on by a sedentary lifestyle, a poor diet, birth control pills, HRT, and exposure to environmental estrogens. Many of these women can find relief simply through exercise and a good diet. Others can solve their problems with a few herbs, vitamins, and mineral supplements. Most of the rest find relief by using a natural progesterone cream. My observation is that estrogen is needed by only a very small percentage of women, and then often for only a short time.

Sandra Coney, author of *The Menopause Industry*, carefully researched the claims made about how ill menopausal women really are. She has also found *no* good evidence that the majority of menopausal women are unhealthy, suffer debilitating symptoms, or lose their sex drive. The majority of women showing up in doctors' offices with problems have had their uterus and/or ovaries removed, a very specific kind of menopause. Menopause as a disease has been largely fabricated by physicians and the pharmaceutical industry. Moreover, there is also no evidence to support the claims that estrogen alone retards aging, keeping women "young and feminine" forever. On the contrary, for most women it has unpleasant side effects ranging from annoying to life-threatening because it is prescribed in unnatural forms and in excess.

Perpetuating the Estrogen Myth

Given the above, one might ask: How does this estrogen-deficiency mind-set maintain its hold on the medical profession and the public? Is there some sort of censorship that controls what is published in our journals? The answer is yes and no. There is no formal censorship, but there is an economic incentive that has subtly persuaded the policies of advertisement-dominated journals to continue the estrogen myth. Consider the following by Jerilynn C. Prior, M.D., an endocrinology professor at the University of British Columbia, Vancouver, British Columbia, excerpted from an article she wrote entitled "One Voice on Menopause." Her words speak for themselves:

He spoke carefully, choosing his words, "Maybe you had better not write it, then. I'd hate to see you put effort into it and then be unable to have it published."

I had been invited to be an author for a short, practical chapter on osteoporosis for a monograph for family doctors about menopause treatment. I was telephoning the editor, a young academic gynecologist, to ask for guidelines about my chapter. As we talked, it became clear what I was expected to write: *All menopausal women need estrogen treatment to prevent osteoporosis.*

"Thank you anyway," he said. "Good-bye."

As I hung up the phone I felt a great mixture of feelings. At first I was relieved. I can certainly manage without an additional deadline! Then I was filled with a bitter chagrin—I was dismissed and neatly eliminated from the scene. I was not allowed to say what I thought was true and what I felt would be helpful for doctors and their patients. The worldview of this gynecologist left no place for honest scientific debate. When all those feelings had settled, I was angry. How dare he impose his view of the world on me and, for that matter, on women! With no hesitation, he had defined a natural phase of life, inevitable for half the world's population, as a disease.

I am the first to admit that I am not a menopause expert. I am only a perimenopausal woman with 15 years of practice in reproductive endocrinology who has conducted (and been able to publish a few) prospective studies of reproduction. My own experiences, the histories of my patients, and the science that is pertinent, prospective, and randomized leave me deeply skeptical that menopause is a medical liability and, most of all, that estrogen deficiency is the major problem. I am astonished, for example, at how little "science" prepared me for my own perimenopausal experiences. The current view that estrogen levels gradually decrease in cycles that become longer and then scant before the last flow is based on a study of eight selected women who had blood drawn daily across one cycle that was some unspecified duration into the four years of the usual menopause transition. In contrast to this, in the last two years I have had hot flashes and night sweats and I haven't missed one menstrual period. I continue to have cycles that are normal or short in interval, tend to be heavy in flow, and, with two exceptions, have been absolutely normal in ovulatory characteristics (normal luteal phase length of ten or more days).

What if I had told this editor that I believe I am currently experiencing estrogen excess? Otherwise, I find it hard to explain my short follicular phases, early and increased cervical mucus production, short cycles, breast enlargement, and nipple tenderness. Is my experience a figment of my imagination? What I have learned from my own experience, has, however, been reported. . . .

Neugarten, for example, found that the symptoms of perimenopausal women resembled those of adolescents more than those of postmenopausal women (with the exception that adolescents had fewer hot flushes). When breast tenderness, weight gain, bloating, and mood changes occur in adolescence, however, they are ascribed to high estrogen exposure. Yet, when these same symptoms are experienced during the transition to menopause, they are caused by "estrogen deficiency"!

I flashed back to my telephone conversation. He was not pleased when I said I thought menopause was a normal phase of every woman's life. No, it would be too confusing to write that. "The literature clearly indicates that menopause causes heart disease and osteoporosis. Also, it causes vasomotor symptoms, mood changes, decreased sex drive, and other problems," he said. I said I would write that each woman herself must make the final decision about whether or not to take hormone treatment. He responded glibly, "Of course, but doctors must tell each woman that she is estrogen deficient so she will make the right choice."

"How would you feel if you knew you were condemned to become diseased when you reached your late forties or early fifties?" I said.

He didn't answer. Instead he retorted, "If I were a woman, I would take estrogen."

"But some women don't feel well on estrogen," I protested.

"Estrogen treatment, I mean hormone treatment," he corrected himself, knowing my belief that progesterone is also an important female hormone, "is benign. Most women tolerate hormone treatment very well."

When I didn't answer, he went on, "I have colleagues coming from all over asking me to put their 40-year-old wives on estrogen so they won't get heart attacks."

"Why aren't the 40-year-old wives *themselves* coming?" I asked gently, now feeling helpless.

He didn't answer my question.

Perhaps, I thought to myself, those 40-year-old wives of physicians didn't feel diseased. Maybe they were more willing to take their chances for a heart attack than they were to risk endometrial cancer. "I think a lot of women are more afraid of endometrial cancer, which they believe they can avoid without treatment, than of osteoporosis, which they feel they probably won't get if they maintain a healthy lifestyle," I said.

"The risk for endometrial cancer is very small," he retorted quickly, "when progestins are given along with estrogen." Then he added, "And most women who get endometrial cancer will have totally curable lesions anyway." As if "a little" endometrial cancer were just a nuisance. . . .

I also remember mentioning to him that I didn't think there was sufficient evidence for the notion that estrogen treatment prevented heart attacks. In all the many trials, the women who were given and took estrogen treatment were healthier and had fewer known heart disease risks like obesity and sedentary lifestyles than the nonrandomized, nonblinded "control" women who didn't or wouldn't take estrogen. Before he could reply, I continued, "You know that the only double blind randomized controlled studies of conjugated estrogen treatment, studies that were performed in men, showed no prevention of heart attacks and sufficient various complications (pulmonary emboli and thromboses) that the trial was prematurely stopped. Furthermore, there was an unexplained but significantly increased cancer risk, for cancers of all types, in the estrogen-treated men."

"Yes, I know," he said flippantly. "That's why I'm not on estrogen."

It was no use. He was unshakable. His message was truth: *Menopause is an estrogen deficiency disease and must be treated with estrogen.* I have both a clear idea of what I am experiencing as a perimenopausal woman and a scientific understanding of reproductive endocrinology. Yet my experiences are dismissed since they don't fit the current notion. He is not the only one who is certain of the menopause truth. So are other influential physicians: "We suggest estrogen treatment for all women with any stigmata of hormone deprivation."

Yet what do we *really* know? . . . Can we predict a given woman's hormonal changes or experience based on her reproductive life, family history, weight, and exercise? No, we cannot. Instead we ascribe everything that happens in the years before the last period to "estrogen deficiency" and assume that women who don't fit the pattern are imagining things. In reality, we know more about the natural history of AIDS than we do about the menstrual transition!

As I put the phone down, I mused. At least this time I had had a fighting chance to get across a different view of menopause. I knew the booklet editor and he knew of my work. I was even asked to write the chapter. Yet, despite all of these factors in my favor, I was not heard. Although I am chronologically his senior and academically his peer, I had been given no say.

If my voice can be so easily and effectively silenced, are other women likely to be heard?

There you have it: A highly regarded female reproductive scientist, who by virtue of her personal experience, her own scientific studies, and professional knowledge of the relevant literature is dismissed from her task of writing a chapter on a subject she knows very well, the reason being that her conclusions do not fit the prevailing estrogen dogma. The same would be true of other experts whose conclusions differ from the "acceptable" line.

The HRT Chickens Come Home to Roost

By the mid-1990s, there was ample scientific evidence that HRT was not living up to its promise and even that it was probably doing more harm than good, but the many excellent studies showing this were ignored in favor of continuing hype from the drug companies about all the diseases that HRT could prevent. The majority of physicians were solid in their belief that every menopausal woman should be on HRT, even though only 25 percent of patients continued on it, because of the side effects. Many women, rather than being taken off the HRT when they complained of weight gain, bloating, breast tenderness, anxiety, depression and insomnia, were instead given sleeping pills and antidepressants, which made them feel even worse.

Then, in the summer of 2002, two major studies published

in the *Journal of the American Medical Association* (JAMA) finally changed the fixed mind-set of conventional medicine toward HRT. About that time I received an e-mail from a woman who had read one of my books and as a result had gone to her doctor and asked to be taken off of PremPro and put on natural hormones. His response was, "Now why in the world would you want to do that?" When she tried to explain he interrupted her, ended the visit, and left her with another prescription for PremPro. I have received literally thousands of letters with similar stories over the past decade.

The first blow to HRT came from the huge Women's Health Initiative (WHI) study, one part of which looked at the effects of the most common form of HRT, PremPro. This arm of the study was ended after five years (three years early) because of a clearly greater risk of invasive breast cancer, heart disease, and strokes among women using PremPro [Premarin (equine estrogens) plus Provera (a synthetic progestin)].

The study analyzed the health of 16,000 women aged 50 to 79 years. After five years, those using PremPro had a 29 percent higher risk of breast cancer, a 26 percent higher risk of heart disease, and a 41 percent higher risk of stroke.

To personalize these numbers a bit more, let's project them out into the general population: of the 6 million women who are reportedly using PremPro (this is a very conservative estimate and doesn't count the millions of women on other combinations of HRT), this would translate to approximately 4,200 women who would get breast cancer, 4,800 women who would get heart disease, and 10,800 women who would have a stroke in a five-year period because they were taking this form of HRT. If we extend these numbers out over a decade, nearly 40,000 women would be harmed (many of them killed) by taking these drugs. That's an epidemic, and it doesn't include all the women who suffer from weight gain, fatigue, depression, irritability, headaches, insomnia, bloating, low thyroid, low libido, gallbladder disease, and blood clots as result of taking the medication.

One of the most disturbing aspects of this scenario is that it was created due to the carelessness of conventional medical practice, which dictated—in my opinion, without good supporting evidence of safety and efficacy—that most women over 50 complaining about symptoms even remotely related to menopause be put on HRT. In most cases their hormones weren't measured to find out which ones they needed or how much, and they were subjected to a one-dose-fits-all mind-set that created overdoses of estrogen for millions of them. Furthermore, the efficacy of progesterone in hormone replacement has been largely ignored in favor of the patentable (and therefore more profitable) synthetic counterparts known as progestins.

Shortly after the WHI study was halted, another study was released, this one from the Breast Cancer Detection Demonstration Project, part of a nationwide breast cancer screening program, and it showed that estrogen-only hormone replacement (ERT) increases the overall risk of ovarian cancer by more than threefold. Given what we've known for at least 20 years about unopposed estrogen's cancer-promoting properties on a woman's reproductive system, the concept of giving only estrogen to women without a uterus should never have taken hold in medical practice in the first place.

In spite of overwhelming evidence that conventional HRT may do more harm than good, the drug companies have not given up the fight to convince American women to take it. One of the most common ways that undesirable results of medical research are hidden or skewed is by the clever manipulation of statistics. Conveying information is not as straightforward as most people imagine. It is a highly manipulative art form that can, on the one hand, convey full and even profound understanding but, on the other hand, can obscure or misrepresent the truth without actually being a lie. Clever people make a good living at doing the latter as, perhaps, in the world of advertising or selling real estate, or in politics, for example, where it is considered a valuable asset. In the hard sciences, such as physics and chemistry, misrepresentation and obscuration are less common since, if uncovered, the damage to one's reputation is quite severe. In the health sciences, the picture is somewhere in-between.

A few months after the results of the PremPro arm of the

WHI were released, I watched a very popular talk show one afternoon that was ostensibly about breast cancer. One of the guests, a woman doctor well known for avidly promoting HRT in the media, continued to insist that HRT was very safe, highly beneficial, and that the WHI results were essentially nothing to worry about. Her only nod to the study was to suggest that maybe women should use HRT for only a few years around the time of menopause, and not think of it as a lifetime prescription. She justified her lack of concern by interpreting the statistics from the WHI in a way that was technically correct, but terribly misleading. She did this by claiming that the 26 percent increase (a 42-woman difference) in breast cancer during the study was actually not all that important since the 42 extra cancer cases out of 8,000 women on the HRT is a small number, and represents only 0.5 percent of the 8,000 women in the study.

To the unwary, this sounds like an insignificant percent. However, at the time, there were over 6 million women using the PremPro compound in the United States. Six million is 750 times greater than 8,000. If the ratio holds nationwide, the 42 extra cases in the WHI study indicate a possible increase of 31,500 cases of breast cancer clearly correlated with PremPro. This is one reason why the study was stopped early! No "treatment" that could possibly cause an extra 31,500 cases of breast cancer should be used. And this does not count the significantly increased incidence of stroke and gallbladder disease.

To add insult to injury (literally) the real-world numbers are certainly much higher than this, because the women selected for the WHI study were carefully screened and eliminated if they had any history of heart disease, diabetes, stroke, or breast cancer, which is not representative of how the majority of women have been prescribed HRT in doctors' offices.

Nor do these numbers account for the fact that 40 percent of the women who originally enrolled in the study dropped out, mostly due to side effects. And what happened to the 40 percent of women who dropped out of the study early? According to an article by *New York Times* science writer Gina Kolata, the National Institutes of Health (NIH) reported that "Those women who stopped taking the hormones after enrolling in the study had more breast cancer than those who never took the hormone. . . . Dr. Richard Rodes, the director of the National Institute on Aging, said, 'People who are presuming that there is no increased risk unless you have been taking hormones for four or five years are overinterpreting the study.' " In other words, we really don't know that HRT is safer if you take it for only a year or two. Buyer beware.

The time has come to clear the air and face reality. That is in part the purpose of this book. Mainstream medicine has been firmly entrenched in its belief that menopause connotes the onset of an estrogen deficiency disease that requires estrogen treatment. This, as you will discover, is not only scientifically inaccurate but is a parochial, patriarchal, and narrow-minded view that acts to retard a deeper and more constructive understanding of the problem. In the chapters to come, you will discover a better answer.

CHAPTER 4

WHAT IS ESTROGEN?

Estrogen is a household word, thanks to the universal medical practice over the past 30 or so years of prescribing hormone replacement therapy to menopausal women. In spite of this, the amount of just plain wrong information out there about estrogen among women and their doctors is staggering. This chapter shares the facts about estrogen as I have come to know them.

A key to hormone balance is the knowledge that when estrogen becomes the dominant hormone and progesterone is deficient, the estrogen becomes toxic to the body; thus does progesterone have a balancing or mitigating effect on estrogen. There are few Western women truly deficient in estrogen; most become deficient in progesterone. I have been accused of bashing estrogen, but I have only been responding to the blindness of the medical profession toward the need for real progesterone in hormone replacement therapy. There is nothing inherently wrong with estrogen. Sufficient estrogen is essential to good health and is dangerous only when it is present in excess or without being balanced by progesterone and in some cases, other hormones as well. There are many women who clearly need a little bit of estrogen supplementation menopausally—they're usually petite and slim, and a true deficiency can be easily confirmed with a salivary hormone level test.

In a normally functioning premenopausal woman, the majority of estrogens are made in the ovaries from progesterone and/or from androgens (male hormones). After menopause, most estrogens are made in body fat from male hormones that are still being made by the ovaries and the adrenals. This is why menopausal women with more body fat have higher estrogen levels, and those who are slim are often estrogen deficient.

Estrogens and progesterone have seemingly opposing functions but are simultaneously antagonistic to each other and very interrelated, somewhat like yin and yang. Progesterone tends to balance out many of the negative side effects of estrogen and at the same time can't function properly in the body without the help of estrogen.

But before we go any further into the estrogen story, there is a semantic problem to clear up. When estrogen was first discovered, researchers assumed it was *the* estrus-producing hormone. As time went on, more types of estrogen were discovered and each one was given a specific chemical name. Thus the word *estrogen* became the name of the *class* of hormones, each having some estrogenic action and each having its own name, such as estrone, estradiol, or estriol, for example. Estrogen is not the name of one hormone, but the name of a group of similar hormones. Let's use apples as an analogy. There is no one apple named apple. There are apples named Winesap, Delicious, and Jonathan, each describing a specific type of apple. So it is with estrogens. In the same sense, there is no estrogen named estrogen. It is common in medical and popular literature about hormones for the author to erroneously refer to estrogen as a hormone that performs this or that function. This is an error that leads to many misconceptions about the estrogens, given the fact that each type of estrogen has a different function in the body. Just as it is possible to make some generalizations about apples, we can make some generalizations about estrogens, but we should avoid thinking they're all the same.

In the case of progesterone, however, we are talking about only one specific hormone. Thus progesterone is both the name of the class and the single member of the class. As the body uses progesterone, it produces derivatives and metabolites, such as 17α-OH-progesterone, that have certain unique functions or actions that are not, strictly speaking, due to progesterone.

One metabolite (produced in the liver's metabolization of progesterone) is allopregnanolone, which, if present in sufficient amounts, has an anesthetic effect on brain cells. Each of these various derivative and metabolites are given a name, and none are identical with progesterone. The same is true of testosterone and all the various androgens.

Although the word *estrogen* generally refers to the class of hormones produced by the body with similar estrus-like actions, there are also estrogens found outside the body.

*Phyto*estrogens refer to plant compounds with estrogen-like activity. They are usually considerably weaker than one's own estrogens and compete for the same estrogen receptors throughout the body. Thus they have often been used successfully to decrease symptoms of estrogen excess.

*Xeno*estrogens (meaning foreign estrogens) refer to other environmental compounds (usually petrochemical) that generally have very potent estrogen-like activity and thus can be considered very toxic. Though briefly described next, they will be discussed more thoroughly in later chapters.

The fourth type of estrogens we will be discussing are the *synthetic estrogens* made by the pharmaceutical companies. These have had their molecular structure altered so they can be patented. Like the xenoestrogens, they tend to be more potent than the body's own estrogens, and more toxic.

An example of synthetic estrogen is diethylstilbestrol (DES). This drug resembles a phytoestrogen called P-anol, found in fennel and anise plants. The DES variation resembles two molecules of P-anol linked end to end and is fully as potent as the body's own estradiol. DES can be inexpensively synthesized and is highly active when taken orally. In the past it was used for regulation of the menstrual cycle, in oral contraceptives, and to prevent premature labor. However, while the P-anol found in plants is harmless when the body is exposed to small quantities, DES has been implicated in certain types of cancer (vaginal and cervical cancer in daughters and testicular cancer in sons of mothers who were given DES during pregnancy). It has been superseded by other, presumably less dangerous synthetic estrogen compounds. Because estrogen causes fat buildup, DES was also used extensively in beef cattle to fatten them up more quickly for slaughter.

A common feature of estrogenic substances is what is known in chemistry circles as the *phenolated A-ring* of the molecule. (See the appendix on page 425.) We can think of this A-ring as a molecular key that opens the door to some cells. This A-ring, as it is found in estrogens, is not present in the other steroid hormone molecules, including progesterone, testosterone, or corticosterone. Most likely, it is this phenolated A-ring that distinguishes the estrogenic substances and gives them their specific actions in the body. This same A-ring is common among the xenoestrogens found in petrochemical derivatives (plastics, herbicides, pesticides, industrial by-products such as dioxins) that are pervasively polluting our environment. Some of these are extremely potent estrogenic substances even at nanogram doses. (A nanogram is a billionth of a gram—an inconceivably small amount to most of us.) There is mounting evidence that exposure to xenoestrogens may be a significant causal factor in breast cancer, the decline in male sperm production, testicular cancer, and prostate cancer.

How and Where Estrogens Are Made and Used in the Body

A Few Interesting Factoids About Estrogens

Estrone, estradiol, and estriol are the three most important estrogens made in the female human body. Estrone is referred to as E_1, estradiol as E_2, and estriol as E_3. In the nonpregnancy state, estrone and estradiol are produced by the ovary in quantities of only 100 to 200 micrograms per day, and estriol is only a scant by-product of estrone metabolism. During pregnancy, however, the placenta is the major source of estrogens; estriol is produced in milligram quantities, while estrone and estradiol are produced in microgram amounts, with estradiol excreted in the smallest amount.

After menopause, estrone continues to be made by conversion of the adrenal steroid, androstenediol, primarily in body fat and muscle cells. The more fat, the more estrone is made. Indeed, some obese women produce more estrogen after menopause than thin premenopausal women. Yet obese women are not immune to the problem of hot flashes.

Estriol made by the placenta is made from a hormone called DHEA (dehydroepiandrosterone), supplied from either the mother or the adrenal cortex of the fetus. Because of fetal participation in estriol formation, estriol measurements can be a sensitive indicator of placenta and/or fetal well-being. The placenta also becomes the major source of progesterone, producing 300 to 400 milligrams per day during the third trimester. Estriol and progesterone therefore are the major sex steroids present during pregnancy.

Estriol is the estrogen most beneficial to the vagina, cervix, and vulva. In cases of postmenopausal vaginal dryness and atrophy, which predisposes a woman to vaginitis and cystitis, estriol supplementation seems to be the most effective (and safest) estrogen to use in treating these conditions.

Estrogen and Cell Division

Estrogens in general tend to promote cell division, particularly in hormone-sensitive tissue such as the breast and uterine lining, and this is the key to why they can cause cancer. Among the three estrogens, estradiol is most stimulating to the breast and estriol the least. Estradiol is 1,000 times more potent in its effects on breast tissue than estriol. Studies of two decades ago clearly found that overexposure to estradiol (and estrone to a lesser extent) increases one's risk of breast cancer, whereas estriol is protective.

Synthetic ethinyl estradiol, commonly used in estrogen supplements and contraceptives, is even more of a breast cancer risk because it is efficiently absorbed by mouth and slow to be metabolized and excreted. The longer a synthetic estrogen stays in the body, the more opportunity it has to do damage. Since this factor of slow metabolism and excretion is true of all synthetic estrogens, one would think that, in all cases of estrogen supplementation, the natural hormones would be superior.

The brand names of some of the ethinyl estrogen/progestin combinations used as birth control pills are:

Alesse	Neolova
Apri	Nordette
Brevicon	Norinyl
Demulen	Ortho Cyclen
Desogen	Ortho-Cept
Estrostep	Ortho-Novum
Jenest	Ovcon
Levlen	Ovral
Levlite	Tri-Levlen
Levora	Tri-Norinyl
Loestrin	Triphasil
Lo/Ovral	Trivora
Mircette	Zovia
Modicon	

How Estrogen Affects a Woman's Body

Estrogen is responsible for the changes that take place at puberty in girls, such as growth and development of the vagina, uterus, and fallopian tubes. It causes enlargement of the breasts and contributes to molding (fatty content) of female body contours and maturation of the skeleton. It is responsible for the growth of underarm and pubic hair and pigmentation of the nipples and areolae.

There are no doubt good evolutionary reasons for some of estrogen's seemingly negative actions on the body such as water retention and weight gain. If we think of estrogen in terms of procreation and survival of the fetus, it would seem advantageous to the baby for the expectant mother to be able, in times of famine, to store body fat. Thus the effects of estrogen include far more than its action in creating the female body form and its stimulation of the uterus and breasts. During times of severe famine when a woman would be nutritionally unable to carry a pregnancy to term, estrogen production decreases to prevent fertility. During times of consistent dietary abundance, however, estrogen's effects are potentially harmful. When women consume considerably more calories than needed, estrogen production increases proportionately to supernormal levels and may set the stage for estrogen dominance and exaggerated estrogen decline at menopause. In the United States and most industrially advanced countries, diets are rich in animal fats, sugar, refined starches, and processed foods, providing calories in excess of need and leading to estrogen levels in women twice as high as those in women of the more agrarian third-world countries.

Estrogen Dominance

It is clear that excess estrogen, when unopposed or not balanced by progesterone, is not something wholly to be desired. Stated differently, it is clear that many of estrogen's undesirable side effects are effectively prevented by the presence of progesterone. I would propose that a new syndrome be recognized: *estrogen dominance*. This syndrome, with symptoms familiar to most women in industrialized countries, commonly occurs in the following situations:

1. *Conventional hormone replacement therapy* (due to excessively high doses of estrogen and the use of progestins instead of progesterone)
2. *Premenopause* (early follicle dysfunction resulting in a lack of ovulation and thus lack of progesterone well before the onset of menopause)
3. *Exposure to xenoestrogens* (cause of early follicle dysfunction)
4. *Birth control pills* (with excessive estrogen component and suppression of one's own hormone production)
5. *Hysterectomy* (can induce subsequent ovary dysfunction or atrophy)
6. *Postmenopause* (especially in overweight women)

Thanks to the nearly universal misconception in Western medicine that estrogen deficiency brings about all menopausal symptoms, it is the custom to prescribe unopposed estrogen for women who do not have a uterus (i.e., have had a hysterectomy). Equally unfortunate is the fact that premenopausal estrogen dominance is simply ignored.

A peculiarity of Western industrialized societies is the prevalence of uterine fibroids, breast and/or uterine cancer, fibrocystic breasts, PMS, ovarian cancer, premenopausal bone loss, and a high incidence of osteoporosis in menopausal women. I believe that most of these are the symptoms of estrogen dominance.

The following is a list of symptoms that can be caused or made worse by estrogen dominance:

acceleration of the aging process
allergies
anxiety
autoimmune disorders such as lupus erythematosus and thyroiditis and possibly Sjögren's disease
breast tenderness
breast cancer
decreased sex drive
depression
fat gain, especially around the abdomen, hips, and thighs
fatigue
fibrocystic breasts
foggy thinking
gallbladder disease
hair loss
headaches
hypoglycemia
increased blood clotting (increasing risk of strokes)
infertility
insomnia
irritability
memory loss
migraines (especially premenstrually)

miscarriage
osteoporosis
premenopausal bone loss
PMS
seizures (related to menstruation)
strokes
thyroid dysfunction mimicking hypothyroidism
uterine cancer
uterine fibroids
water retention, bloating

The Myth of Estrogen in Hormone Replacement Therapy

Until the recent WHI results (see Chapter 3), most physicians attempted to push hormone replacement therapy (HRT) featuring synthetic estrogens and progestins onto *all* menopausal women. Their enthusiasm for these drugs, however, was not backed up by the facts. Let's examine why these claims for HRT persisted for so long, in hopes of avoiding similar mistakes in the future.

The chief argument for postmenopausal estrogen supplementation was (and still may be) the deeply ingrained assumption of estrogen deficiency after menopause. This has been touted in pharmaceutical estrogen ads, consumer advertising for HRT in the mainstream media, many medical texts, lay publications, and by mainstream medical practitioners. Women are constantly told that their mood swings, depressions, hot flashes, vaginal dryness, loss of sex drive, and accelerating osteoporosis are indisputable evidence of estrogen deficiency. Menopause is treated as the onset of an estrogen deficiency disease.

It is true that menopause is known to be associated with decreasing estrogen levels, but what is not known is whether these decreased levels of estrogen do in fact cause all the symptoms of menopause. Carolyn DeMarco, M.D. (who has been in practice over 20 years specializing in women's health issues, is the author of *Take Charge of Your Body* and is a respected contributor to other publications and health councils) states, "There is no direct proof that estrogen lack causes heart disease or other ailments associated with the menopause." Germaine Greer, well-known feminist and author of *The Change*, writes, "The proponents of HRT have never proved that there is an estrogen deficiency, nor have they explained the mechanism by which the therapy of choice effected its miracles. They have taken the improper course of defining a disease from its therapy."

Dr. Jerilynn Prior, researcher and professor of endocrinology at the University of British Columbia in Vancouver, B.C., Canada, points out that no study proving the relationship between estrogen deficiency and menopausal symptoms and related diseases has yet been done. "Instead," says Dr. Prior, "a notion has been put forward that since estrogen levels go down, this is the most important change and explains all the things that may or may not be related to menopause. So estrogen treatment at this stage of our understanding is premature. This is a kind of backwards science. It leads to ridiculous ideas—like calling a headache an aspirin deficiency disease."

Although it is common experience that estrogen supplementation relieves many women of certain postmenopausal symptoms, it is not at all clearly established that estrogen deficiency per se was the cause. For example, none of the estrogen proponents have bothered to check progesterone levels before and after menopause. As Dr. Prior has pointed out, during menopause, progesterone decreases to 1/120 of baseline levels whereas estrogen decreases only to 1/2 to 1/3 of premenopausal baseline levels.

Western women tend to have a 10- to 15-year period prior to menopause when they are estrogen dominant and suffering from estrogen dominance symptoms, and some doctors are giving them more estrogen. Something is terribly wrong here!

Helene Leonetti, M.D., did a double-blind study of progesterone cream that was published in the journal *Obstetrics and Gynecology* in 1999, which showed that menopausal symptoms such as hot flashes responded very nicely to progesterone cream in 83 percent of the women in the progesterone cream group, while only 19 percent of women using the placebo got relief. A

Norwegian study published in the journal *Maturitas* measured hormone levels (except progesterone!) in postmenopausal women suffering from hot flashes and found that low testosterone and DHEA levels were significantly associated with hot flashes, and that normal or high levels of these hormones protected against hot flashes.

Would it not be wise to consider the effects of other hormones, including progesterone, when evaluating postmenopausal symptoms and related conditions such as osteoporosis, heart disease, depression, and loss of sex drive?

Dr. Graham Colditz, associate professor at the Harvard Medical School, is an eminent and respected authority on the breast cancer risks of estrogens. In a talk he gave in San Francisco in February 1994 at a meeting of the American Association for the Advancement of Science, he included an interesting graph of pre- and postmenopausal plasma levels of estrone plus estradiol. His graph showed typical *pre*menopausal levels to be 2.35 and untreated *post*menopausal levels to be 2 (the scale dimensions

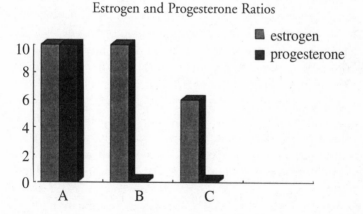

Estrogen and Progesterone Ratios

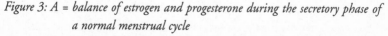

Figure 3: A = balance of estrogen and progesterone during the secretory phase of a normal menstrual cycle

B = relative production of estrogen and progesterone during an anovulatory premenopausal menstrual cycle

C = relative production of estrogen and progesterone after menopause

were not identified). This is a drop of only 15 percent—just enough to allow menstruation to stop. But 85 percent of a woman's estrogen is still present!

The graph in Figure 3 depicts the relative balance of estrogen and progesterone during a normal menstrual cycle, an anovulatory cycle, and after menopause.

In this graph, estrogen and progesterone are assumed to be in balance during the secretory phase of a normal menstrual cycle. In an anovulatory menstrual cycle, estrogen remains the same and progesterone production drops to very low levels. After menopause, estrogen production decreases 40 to 60 percent and progesterone remains at very low levels. Thus in anovulatory *and* menopausal conditions, estrogen dominance persists.

What Are "Normal" Estrogen Levels?

Another peculiarity of the Western mainstream medical practitioner concerning menopause disorders is the ignorance of the worldwide menopause picture. Among the less industrialized, more agrarian cultures, where women eat less and exercise more, menopause complaints are minor or unknown. The everyday languages of many of these cultures have no word for hot flashes. But as we have discovered in the past decade, the introduction of Western eating habits and industrialization, which results in less exercise and greater calorie intake, has contributed to the dramatic increase in the incidence of menopausal symptoms in Third World countries. In a recent study of menopausal symptoms from China, "professional" women tended to have plenty of menopause symptoms, while "farm" women had few.

Dr. Peter Ellison of Harvard University has measured women's ovarian hormones using saliva, making it relatively simple to study hormone levels in their natural settings. He has reported his findings of ovarian hormone levels in various populations of distinct genetic, ecological, and cultural backgrounds. He found that in Western populations premenopausal estrogen levels represent a high extreme of the spectrum and should be considered abnormal. Further, he suggests that these abnormal levels may relate to the current epidemic of breast and ovarian cancer.

Dr. Ellison believes there is a direct link between hormone levels and energy balance, meaning the balance between dietary energy intake and energy expended in work. A negative energy balance (a woman who does a lot of physical work and doesn't have enough to eat) will tend to lower hormone levels, presumably protecting her against the higher energy requirements of pregnancy. A positive energy balance (a woman who doesn't get much physical exercise and eats more than she needs) raises hormone levels. Ellison conjectures that the high hormone levels found in Western cultures are a reflection of overeating and underexercising common in these populations. Further, Ellison suggests the higher ovarian function common in Western populations results in a proportionately greater fall in hormone levels at menopause, and this may account for the greater incidence and severity of menopausal symptoms seen. In non-industrialized populations, the discrepancy between pre- and postmenopausal hormone levels is considerably less than in industrialized populations. Remember, postmenopausal estrogen levels do not drop to zero, they merely drop to the level that will not produce a blood-rich uterine lining to be shed (menstruation). If Dr. Ellison's hypothesis is correct, it may mean that prevention of menopausal symptoms could be accomplished by eating less and getting more exercise. It would be very useful to conduct a study of Western menopausal women in industrialized cultures to find out if there is a correlation between menopausal symptoms and various groups of women who differ substantially in terms of exercise and diet.

Our dietary problem includes not only the excess calories but also the nutritional quality of our foods. A diet rich in fatty meats, sugar, refined carbohydrates, hydrogenated oils, and processed foods is quite different from a plant-based diet high in fiber, nutrients, phytoestrogens, antioxidants, and complex carbohydrates. The now-popular high protein diets that emphasize high-quality proteins, fresh vegetables, reduced starchy carbohydrates (bread, corn, potatoes), and almost no sugar also differ vastly from the typical Western fare. Such diets directly affect hormone production. In an article titled "Oestrogen Overdose" by Gail Vines in *British Vogue*, Lyliane Rosetta, physiologist at the Université René Descartes in Paris, found that estrogen and progesterone levels fell in women who switched to a low-fat, high-fiber, plant-based diet with more legumes, even though they did not gain or lose weight and ate as many calories as women in the control group who had a traditional Western diet, high in fat and simple carbohydrates. It would be very interesting to test hormone levels in women on a high-protein, high-vegetable, low-carbohydrate, and low-sugar diet.

It is also interesting to note that as one researches the more authoritative texts on hormones, one finds a vastly different view of the supposed estrogen "deficiency" status of postmenopausal women from that promoted by the pharmaceutical companies. The following quote from *Novak's Textbook of Gynecology* (11th edition, Williams & Wilkins, 1987) is representative of the views of the experts who are not being paid to promote estrogen:

> Thus it would seem that although menopausal women do have an estrogen milieu that is lower than that necessary for reproduction, it is not negligible or absent but is perhaps satisfactory for maintenance of support tissues. The menopause could then be regarded as a physiologic phenomenon that is protective in nature, protective from the undesirable reproduction and the associated growth stimuli.

In plain language, this means that in most menopausal women, estrogen levels are below that necessary for pregnancy but sufficient for other normal body functions, as well as being a whole lot safer. The estrogen "deficiency" hypothesis as an explanation of postmenopausal symptoms or health problems is thus not supported by the facts of estrogen blood levels, by worldwide ecologic surveys, or by endocrinology experts.

Menopause per se should be regarded as a normal physiologic adjustment reflecting a benign change in a woman's biological life away from childbearing and onward to a period of new personal power and fulfillment. The Western perception of menopause as a threshold of undesirable symptoms and progressive illness due to estrogen deficiency is an error unsupported by fact. More accurately, we should view menopause problems as an abnormality brought about by industrialized cultures' deviation from a healthy lifestyle.

CHAPTER 5

HORMONE BALANCE, XENOBIOTICS, AND FUTURE GENERATIONS

Throughout this book I will be referring repeatedly to xenobiotics or xenoestrogens, foreign substances originating outside
the body that have hormone- and estrogen-like activity in the
body, and thus a profound impact on hormone balance. I will
use the term "xenobiotics" as a generic reference to substances
with a hormone-like effect on the body and "xenoestrogens" to
specifically describe those with an estrogenic effect on the body.
These pollutants are also known as endocrine disruptors (the
endocrine system includes the glands that make brain hormones, reproductive system hormones, adrenal hormones, insulin and thyroid hormone, for example).

In the early 1990s, when I wrote my first self-published book
for doctors about natural progesterone, the suggestion that pollutants and chemicals could affect human reproductive organs,
and could affect an embryo in ways that could cause reproductive damage that would show up later in life, was met with
much scorn and skepticism by my colleagues. Now, just a
decade later, this fact is no longer even arguable; there are thousands of studies showing the hormonal effects of petrochemical
pollutants. Congressional committees have been formed to fund
and direct research on the subject, and new findings are coming
out almost weekly.

Nearly all xenobiotics are petrochemically based, meaning
"derived from petroleum oil." We live in a pervasively petrochemical world. Our machines run on petroleum fuels, many of

our buildings are heated with petroleum oil, and thousands, maybe millions of products, including plastics, microchips, medicines, clothing, foods, soaps, pesticides, and even perfumes, are made from petrochemicals or contain them. While these substances have undeniably improved our quality of life, the price we pay is pervasive petrochemical pollution of the air, water, soil, and our bodies.

The legacy of this pollution in living creatures, including humans, includes an epidemic of reproductive abnormalities, including steadily increasing numbers of cancers of the reproductive tract, infertility, low sperm counts, and the feminization of males. Estrogen is the female hormone and we are awash in a petrochemical sea of xenoestrogens. The potential consequences of this overexposure are staggering, especially considering that one of the consequences is passing on reproductive abnormalities to offspring.

By-products of manufacturing processes that use chlorine and compounds formed when chlorine interacts with organic matter, called *organochlorines*, are such a serious threat to our health and the environment, both as potent carcinogens (dioxins and PCBs) and as xenobiotics, that President William Clinton, the World Health Organization (WHO), and the United States–Canadian Joint Commission (IJC) called for a phaseout of the use of chlorine and chlorinated compounds.

Turning on the Hormone Switch

Why do some petrochemicals behave as potent estrogens? Something in their molecular structure contains the basic "key" that fits in the hormone receptor "ignition" of the cell, switching on hormonal action. John McLachlan, Ph.D., who was chief of the National Institute of Environmental Health Sciences (NIEHS) and is now director of the Tulane/Xavier Center for Bioenvironmental Research, explains that it is difficult to track these chemicals by traditional toxicology methods. Their effect may not show up until the next generation, and furthermore, we cannot judge a petrochemical's hormonal potential by any specific attribute of their molecular structure. McLachlan has therefore suggested the development of a "functional toxicology," in which chemicals are defined more by their function than by their chemistry. He recommends an array of panels made up of cells containing receptors for the hormones in question. Chemicals could be tested for their ability to occupy, activate, or turn off cell receptors.

McLachlan's vision of the future is that this information be included along with chemical information such as melting point, molecular weight, and solubility. Personally I'd like to see these effects listed on every can of bug spray, every box and bottle of weed killer, on the sides of the trucks that spray chemicals on lawns, on every box of detergent or tub and tile cleaner that contains nonylphenols, and everywhere else in our environment that we're exposed to these chemicals. If food manufacturers have to list calories, fat grams, and sodium on their labels, shouldn't chemical manufacturers be obliged to let us know when their product may cause reproductive abnormalities in our offspring?

As you remember, synthetic drugs tend to be far more potent than their natural derivatives. The xenoestrogens have the same property. In their estrogenic activity, these estrogens are considerably more potent than the estrogen made by the ovaries. In their effect on fish, some of them have been found to be potent estrogenic substances even at nanogram doses. A nanogram is a billionth of a gram, which is roughly the same proportion as a grain of sand to an Olympic swimming pool. If we extrapolate this to the human body, the amount of a xenoestrogen necessary to have an estrogenic effect is inconceivably small. A popular argument by those who feel that xenoestrogens are harmless is that the amounts we're exposed to from any one source are generally very tiny. What these people fail to take into account is the multitude of ways in which we are exposed to these substances every day.

McLachlan explains the various effects of hormonal mimics in Figure 4.

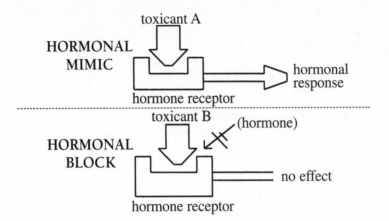

Figure 4: Some hormonal mimics (e.g., progestins and xenoestrogens) activate the receptor to stimulate the hormone effect while others will occupy the receptor and block the natural hormone from doing its work.

The Canary in the Coal Mine?

Xenobiotics come from many sources and have a multitude of biochemical effects on living creatures. Thanks to testing done by a wide array of scientists, we know beyond a doubt that xenobiotics are threatening the survival of many birds, reptiles, and mammals in North America. We would be wise to pay attention to what's happening with these animals. Miners used to take a canary in a cage down into the mine with them. If the sensitive canary suddenly keeled over and died, they hightailed it out of the mine, knowing the air was poisonous and that soon they too would be keeling over. The many animal species more sensitive than humans that are effectively being exterminated by overdoses of xenobiotics could be a large environmental version of the canary in the cage.

More recent research is showing that exposure to xenohormones suppresses the immune system, and in particular hampers T-lymphocyte function, and lowers the proportions and numbers of natural killer (NK) cells. These are two of your immune system's most important defenses. The latest studies are showing even more widespread damage to the immune system.

Infants of women who have been chronically exposed to xeno-hormones seem to be particularly susceptible to immune system damage through exposure in breast milk, and children are more susceptible than adults. Many of the xenobiotics activate the 1B1 enzyme, which converts estrogens to 4-catechols, the "bad" estrogens that can damage DNA and lead to breast cancer. Progesterone inhibits activity of 1B1, which would suggest that progesterone may protect against xenobiotic-activated estrogen metabolite formation.

The Impact on Future Generations

There is much evidence that xenobiotics harm future genera-tions. Studies done at the University of California, Davis, show that seagulls whose eggs are injected with estradiol hatch chicks that show the same birth defects as those exposed to DDT: chemically castrated males with feminized gonads and females with overdeveloped ovaries. Michael Fry, Ph.D., a professor at the University of California, Davis, Department of Avian Sci-ences, researches the toxic effects of airborne and waterborne organochlorine pesticides on the development and reproduction of birds. Some of the abnormalities he has found in birds ex-posed to xenobiotics include clubbed feet, crossed bills, huge thyroid glands, nests with more than the normal number of eggs (laid by more than one bird), a surplus of females, female-female pairing, feminization of male reproductive tracts, ovarian corti-cal tissue in testes, abnormal persistence of oviducts in males, and general failure to thrive. Experimental injection of organo-chlorines into gull eggs reproduced these abnormalities. Eggshell thinning in gulls occurs in eggs laid by adult birds that have been exposed to estrogenic chemicals while still embryos.

Scientists at the University of Florida in Gainesville found that both male and female alligators, born after a pesticide spill exposed their parents to a pesticide similar to DDT called dico-fol, have abnormally high levels of estrogen and low levels of testosterone. Additionally, the females have abnormal ovaries and follicles described as "burned out," and the males have abnormally small penises. Since the pesticide spill in Florida's Lake Apopka in 1980, the number of young alligators has been reduced by 90 percent. The implication is that the alligators there are no longer capable of reproducing.

In a May 1993 article in *Lancet*, researchers in Scotland and Denmark hypothesized that xenobiotics are responsible for a steadily declining sperm count in men. According to Niels Skakkebaek of the University of Copenhagen, sperm counts have dropped by more than 50 percent since 1940. Meanwhile, the rate of testicular cancer in the United States and Europe has more than tripled in the past 50 years and reproductive abnormalities such as undescended testicles have become increasingly common. The decline of sperm counts began at the same time that "better living through chemistry" became the national anthem of big business in America and Europe and we began being carelessly exposed to petrochemical pollutants.

By far the most susceptible cells to the effects of xenohormones are those in a developing embryo; when you are in the womb you are exquisitely sensitive to the effects of hormones. The parts of an embryo that are most susceptible (as far as we know now), are the reproductive organs. (There's a good chance that down the road we'll discover that the brain is equally sensitive to the effects of these substances.) Every day, millions of pregnant women unknowingly expose their unborn children to potentially damaging substances that may cause a lifetime of reproductive problems and abnormal reproductive development. It could be dioxins in that fish she just ate, or the pesticides just sprayed in the elevator or airplane she's riding in, the new carpet that's off-gassing fumes in her office, the nail polish remover she's using on her toenails, or the paint she's using to paint the new baby's bedroom.

It's likely that the class of pesticides known as organochlorines (of which DDT is the most notorious) are the most widely pervasive *and* potent form of estrogenic pollutants on the planet. According to the book *The Truth About Breast Cancer*, by Claire Hoy, "Greenpeace found that the one country that banned organochlorine pesticides—Israel—quickly went from breast cancer rates that were among the highest in the world to rates in keeping with those of other industrialized nations. It also found that U.S. counties with waste sites were 6.5 times more likely to have elevated breast cancer rates than those without waste sites, and that women with breast cancer tend to have higher levels of organochlorine pesticides and PCBs in their tissues than women without breast cancer." Organochlorines have since been shown repeatedly to cause mammary cancers in laboratory animals, but they remain a fundamental part of agriculture in the United States. In this way, perceived economic necessity takes the lives of women year after year.

Awareness can go a long way toward avoidance of xenohormones, but ultimately it will take political action at the grassroots level to change the big picture.

Safe Living in a Sea of Estrogens

Xenoestrogens, in addition to being highly estrogenic, are fat-soluble and nonbiodegradable, meaning that they easily pass through the skin and sit in fatty tissues, and that in the body and in the environment they don't break down over time. Because of the widespread use of petrochemical products they are difficult to avoid, but we can significantly reduce our exposure.

One source of oral intake of xenoestrogens is by way of animal fats, particularly red meat and dairy fats. In addition to the fact that these animals are often given estrogenic substances to fatten them up for market, they are also exposed when they eat grains that have been sprayed with pesticides. The xenoestrogens accumulate in their fat. Every 15 pounds of grain a steer eats produces 1 pound of beef, so there's a relatively high amount of these pesticides in the meat of these animals. Anyone who eats nonorganic meat and dairy products is eating these compounds and they are all potent estrogens. They can accumulate in our fatty tissues (breast, brain, and liver) and cause estrogen dominance, with all of its attendant symptoms. While I am not against eating meat, I do recommend that you eat hormone-free meat and dairy products, which are easily available these days.

Reproductive organ changes caused by xenobiotics have been reported by a long list of scientists in North America and Europe in everything from wrens and panthers to sturgeons and turtles. DDT, PCBs, or dioxins are often found in the tissues of these animals. But these are just three of the most potent xenobiotics that stay in the body for a lifetime. Other xenobiotics may not stay in the body but will have their effect passing through the body. The majority of other xenobiotics come to us through petrochemical pollution, including some from rather bizarre sources.

Sumpter and Charles Tyler of Brunel University in Uxbridge, England, exposed trout to effluent (treated sewage) at a variety of sites. After exposure, the fish tested positive for high amounts of a chemical called *vitellogenin*, indicating they had been exposed to an excess of estrogen. When the Tylers were unable to find an industrial source for these xenoestrogens, they finally theorized that it must be coming from the urine of women taking birth control pills containing the synthetic estrogen ethinylestradiol (EE). When they tested this hypothesis in the laboratory by exposing the fish to EE, they found that nanogram amounts of this estrogen could cause vitellogenin levels to spike in the trout. The implications of this discovery are immense, because synthetic estrogens are being dumped into waterways all over Europe and North America and have entered the food chain.

In the process of uncovering the source of the estrogen effect in these fish, the Tylers also discovered another ubiquitous source of xenoestrogens: nonylphenols, breakdown products of surfactants commonly used in detergents (including dishwashing liquids), cosmetics and other toiletries, as well as pesticides and herbicides. Although nonylphenols are not as potent as EEs, they are dumped in our waterways in much higher quantities. This is a good reason to buy "green" (i.e., environmentally safe) products when you go to the supermarket. Ironically, nonylphenols are found in the spermicides used for birth control in diaphragm jellies, on condoms, and in vaginal gels to facilitate dispersal. This directly exposes the vagina and cervix to xenoestrogens.

COMMON SOURCES OF XENOHORMONES

- Petrochemically derived pesticides, herbicides, and fungicides.
- Car exhaust.
- Solvents and adhesives such as those found in nail polish, paint remover, and glues.
- Emulsifiers and waxes found in soaps and cosmetics.
- Dry cleaning chemicals.
- Nearly all plastics.
- Phthalates, synthetic compounds that add flexibility to plastics, such as the plastic tubes and bags used in storing and delivering IV fluids to patients, and the rubbery toys children play with. Exposure to phthalates during embryo and perinatal life will also damage testes and ovaries just as the pesticides and solvents do.
- Industrial waste such as PCBs and dioxins.
- Meat from livestock fed estrogenic drugs to fatten them up.
- Waste from sewage treatment plants that contains nonylphenols, estrogenic breakdown products of detergents.
- Synthetic estrogens and progestins found in the urine of millions of women taking birth control pills and hormone replacement therapy that is flushed down the toilet and eventually works its way into the food chain.

Pesticides and Plastics

Even without the nonylphenols that are added to them, nearly all petrochemical pesticides, herbicides, and fungicides are potent xenobiotics. Billions of pounds of these substances are applied to our fruits and vegetables every year, and many of them don't go away; when you eat the fruit or vegetable you generally get a dose, albeit a small one, of pesticides along with it. A recent study of children's exposure to toxins found that children who eat organically grown fruits and vegetables have only one-sixth the concentrations of organophosphate pesticide by-products in their urine compared with children who eat produce sprayed by pesticides. This illustrates why I suggest that everyone eat organic fruits and vegetables as much as possible. The more we, as consumers, demand organic produce, the more likely it is to be grown that way. When farmers first switched back to organic methods a few decades ago, the produce tended to be small and not very nice looking compared with what we were used to. Now that organic farmers have had a couple of decades to practice, organic produce tends to be just as beautiful, even more tasty, and, because it is grown in rich, healthy soil, more nutritious than its contaminated counterpart.

We also use petrochemical pesticides in our homes in the form of bug spray, as well as on our lawns and gardens. There is absolutely no need to use these poisons around your home. There are a wealth of excellent books out on simple, easy, and cost effective methods of organic gardening and pest control. (See "Recommended Reading" on page 389.) Many communities in the United States have city- or county-sponsored classes on organic gardening and pest control.

Another nearly universal source of xenoestrogens is plastics. Some types of plastic shed xenoestrogens when they are heated. Because it would be nearly impossible to figure out which plastics shed xenoestrogens, the best approach is to assume they all do and behave accordingly. Don't routinely drink hot beverages from plastic cups and don't routinely microwave your food in plastic containers. If you don't buy coffee in plastic cups and frozen food in plastic containers, the manufacturers will eventually catch on and stop making them that way.

Solvents

A common source of potent xenohormones is the type of chemicals called *solvents*. All organic solvents are volatile liquids at room temperature and are lipophilic (fat-loving). They enter the body extremely easily through the skin, and they accumulate in lipid-rich tissues such as the brain, myelin (nerve sheath), and adipose (fat). In combination they may be additive, synergistic, or potentiated, meaning that their effects on the body could be vastly more potent and toxic in combination than separately.

Industries in which exposure to solvents is well known include automotive manufacturing and repair, paint and varnish manufacturing, the electronics industry, industrial cleaning, metal-part degreasing, and dry cleaning. In addition to the work environment, exposure via hobbies must be considered. The use of most glues and fiberglass also involve exposure to solvents.

One of the most insidious routes of solvent exposure and toxicity is through fingernail polish and fingernail polish remover. Young girls are especially susceptible to the toxic and xenohormonal effects of solvents, and yet they are the ones most likely to have a dozen different shades of fingernail polish in the bedroom.

Some of the immediate effects of exposure to solvents include CNS (central nervous system) depression, which would look like fatigue or depression; psychomotor or attention deficits, which would look like incoordination and inability to focus; brain swelling (headaches); central nervous system (CNS) capillary damage; and oxygen deprivation in the brain with possible permanent brain damage resulting in lowered cognitive abilities.

Long-term exposure to solvents can cause mood disturbances such as depression, irritability, fatigue, and anxiety, as well as inability to focus, incoordination, and short-term memory loss.

In addition, solvents can damage a developing fetus in very small amounts and should be studiously avoided in any amount by pregnant women. It should be required by law (and is in some states) that labels on nail polish contain warnings to pregnant women, and that beauty salons have warning signs in areas where nail polish is applied and removed.

SOME GENERAL CLASSES OF ORGANIC SOLVENTS

Check product labels for items in the following list (you might find them in cosmetics, nail polish and nail polish remover, glues, paints of all kinds, varnishes and other types of finishes, cleaning products, pesticides and herbicides, carpet, fiberboard and other processed woods, and even in clothing and mattresses).

aliphatic hydrocarbons (e.g., n-hexane)

halogenated hydrocarbons (e.g., carbon tetrachloride, trichlor-
ethylene)

alcohols (e.g., methanol, ethanol)

cyclic hydrocarbons (e.g., cyclohexane)

esters (e.g., ethyl acetate)

ethers (e.g., ethyl ether)

nitrohydrocarbons (ethyl nitrate)

ketones (e.g. acetone, methylethylketone)

glycols (e.g., ethylene glycol)

aromatic hydrocarbons (e.g., benzene)

aldehydes (e.g., acetaldehyde)

CLEANING UP YOUR HOUSE

- Throw away all pesticides, herbicides, and fungicides. Take a class in organic gardening and read up on natural pest control. *Do not* tent your house and fumigate it with pesticides, or "bomb" it, or have your lawn sprayed with chemicals.

- Check your cosmetics for toxic ingredients and try as much as possible to use "clean" cosmetics. It's unlikely that there is any truly nontoxic hairspray on the market. Throw away the nail polish and nail polish remover; it's toxic both when you breathe it and when you put it on your nails. We know of no safe nail polish at this time.

- Don't use fabric softeners; this puts petrochemicals directly onto your skin, which as you know by now is quite capable of absorbing all kinds of substances.

- Be aware that most scented products and perfumes are petrochemically based, and when you inhale them they go directly to your brain. Don't use petrochemically-based perfumes or air fresheners. Try some of the natural aromatic oils and combinations if you want to change how you, your house, or your car smell. In the same vein, use unscented laundry soaps and naturally scented shampoos and conditioners.

- Don't use tap or bottled water as a source of drinking

water; get a good quality filter for your whole house or for taps that are used for drinking and cooking water.

- Be aware that all plastics leach into the environment; some leach faster and some are more potent. The soft plastics such as are found in many baby toys and in some water bottles leach the most. *Do not* let your child chew on plastic toys.
- Do not microwave food in plastic containers and especially avoid microwaving food covered by plastic wrap.
- Eliminate or decrease consumption of foods most likely to be contaminated with these chemicals. If you eat red meat, poultry, eggs, meat and fish, it should be organic and/or hormone- and antibiotic-free.
- Avoid surfactants such as nonoxonyl (spermicides) found in many condoms and diaphragm gels.
- Consider that a new home or office can be a toxic soup of noxious gases coming from glues, fiberboard, new carpet, and new paint. If your new home makes you feel sick it is probably *not* all in your head; have the air tested. Chances are it's loaded with formaldehyde and solvent fumes. When you're pregnant or have an infant, it's not a good idea to move into a newly built home, remodel, or even paint. This can be challenging for a pregnant woman when the nesting instinct kicks in, but first consider the future health of your baby.

CLEANING UP YOUR OFFICE

- Be aware that new carpeting can give off noxious fumes.
- Be aware that any type of fiberboard can give off noxious fumes, especially when it's new. Most office furniture is made of fiberboard.
- Remember that copiers and printers that use toner and inks give off noxious fumes.
- If you work in an office building, be sure there is a firm policy in place that requires notification of building occupants when pesticides of any kind are being used. Take an

active interest in exactly what is being used, and why, and what the alternatives might be.

- Be aware that the air quality in office buildings can be a source of a wide range of toxins from fungi to xenohormones.

- Consider that computers, monitors, printers, and other electronic office equipment can give off very high levels of electromagnetic fields (EMFs). Though we haven't covered EMFs in detail in this book, we believe there is enough scientific evidence to justify avoiding them. The good news is that EMFs coming from electronic equipment tend to drop off within a few feet. Never sit for long periods of time right next to a computer hard drive or right behind a computer monitor. It's wise to invest in a handheld gauss meter and test both your office and your house for EMFs. (See Resources at the end of this book for how to find a gauss meter.)

Xenoestrogens and Future Generations

Excess estrogen exposure in humans in the first trimester of pregnancy can affect fetal sexual development. We first learned this painful lesson via the sons and daughters of women given DES (diethylstilbestrol) during pregnancy. DES is a synthetic estrogen that was given to women to prevent miscarriage, to treat breast cancer, and to reduce the symptoms of menopause. Between 1948 and 1971 it was taken by 2 to 6 million women in the United States and Europe. Some 50,000 pounds of DES were also dumped into livestock feed to fatten them up for market until it was banned in 1979 because it was showing up in supermarket beef in measurable amounts. (There are rumors that DES is still used illegally in livestock feed.) In the early 1970s, researchers looking for links to a high incidence of cervical cancers in young women traced it to their mothers, who were prescribed DES during pregnancy to prevent miscarriage. Further research has shown that the use of DES in pregnancy is also linked to testicular cancer in males, as well as infertility, birth defects, and other reproductive problems in both sexes.

Lurking as an unknown factor in the later development of one's sexual preference is the possibility of fetal influence by the xenobiotics found in our petrochemically polluted environment. Having now mentioned this factor in a number of talks I've given, I realize it may not be a politically correct position, but nevertheless I feel it is an important factor to consider. If xenobiotics can blur the distinctions between the sexes in seagulls and alligators at nanogram levels, how far-fetched is it to speculate that the same pollutants may be affecting humans in a similar fashion? Recently it has been found that daughters of mothers who had been given DES during pregnancy are not only more likely to develop vaginal and cervical cancer, but also to become bisexual or lesbians as adults.

I believe xenoestrogens are affecting our children in profound ways. Girls used to begin menstruation around age 16. Now they may start menstruating as early as 10 years old. We have come to think of this as normal. It's not. Some scientists claim this is a sign of better nutrition. My suspicion is that this early onset of puberty is caused by exposure to the xenoestrogens so prevalent in every part of our environment, from our meat supply to the air we breathe, combined with diets sadly lacking in the whole foods that contain the protective phytoestrogens. The long-term consequences of early menstruation are a longer lifetime exposure to estrogen, with an increased risk of hormone-driven cancers such as breast and uterine cancer.

It's time for us to wake up and pay heed to these warnings for the sake of future generations. You can play your part in protecting our grandchildren and great-grandchildren in the same ways you can protect yourself: by refusing to use pesticides, minimizing your use of plastics, purchasing hormone-free meat and organic produce, using "green" products for detergents and household cleaners, and, in general, using "natural" products in favor of petrochemical products. I realize using these types of products costs slightly more, but it seems a small price to pay to insure our future reproductive health.

If You Want to Know More

In the late 1990s Theo Colborn coauthored a groundbreaking book, *Our Stolen Future*, which details, in a rigorously scientific detective story, how synthetic chemicals have already done widespread damage to all types of wildlife and are in the process of damaging humans. Since that time, other excellent books on the topic of xenohormones and reproductive damage have been published, and if you're interested in delving further into this topic, we highly recommend reading them. They include:

• *Generations at Risk: Reproductive Health and the Environment*, by Ted Schettler, M.D., Gina Solomon M.D., et al. (MIT Press, 1999), which explains reproductive and developmental physiology, how toxins affect this physiology, and then gives guidelines for investigating possible exposure to toxins, and for creating change in your community and workplace.

• *Hormonal Chaos: The Scientific and Social Origins of the Environmental Endocrine Hypothesis*, by Sheldon Krimsky (Johns Hopkins University Press, 2000), focuses more on how the endocrine disruptor theory emerged and examines the ethics of a scientific, economic, and political community that has been trying to ignore these findings for decades, as well as the social and medical consequences of continuing to allow these substances to be dumped into the environment.

• *Pandora's Poison*, by Joe Thornton (MIT Press, 2000) focuses most on the issue of organochlorines (products made using chlorine gas, including pesticides, plastics, paper, PCBs, and dioxins) as the key substances most seriously affecting human physiology. Thornton specifically proposes how we can change chemical testing and environmental protection policies to—in effect—save ourselves.

• *Living Downstream*, by Sandra Steingraber (Vintage Books, 1997) combines meticulous science and lucid writing with the author's personal experience of fighting bladder cancer. The book will open your eyes to the ubiquity of petrochemical toxins accumulating in our environment.

Should we not be calling for a meaningful reduction in the use of petrochemical xenohormones that are now threatening not only our health but the normal development of human-kind? Xenohormones are ubiquitous in our diet and environment and already are recognized as the likely cause of the threatened die-off of a number of animal species in areas exposed to these toxic compounds. The fate of future generations of humanity may hinge on our ability to substantially decrease environmental contamination by the petrochemical xenohormones.

CHAPTER 6

WHAT IS NATURAL PROGESTERONE?

Progesterone is a primary hormone of fertility and pregnancy. Fertility has always fascinated humankind. Fertility and pregnancy symbols, rites, and icons abound in all cultures throughout human history. It is only since Old Testament times that fertility and pregnancy have *not* been a source of religion and worship in the Western world. Woman's ability to bleed every month without dying, as well as her ability to bring new life into the world, was regarded as sacred. These miraculous abilities no doubt inspired the goddess worship prevalent throughout the world for so much of early human history.

The regular occurrence of natural breeding times, annually in some animals and monthly in human females, provided the first real understanding of male and female roles in reproduction. These cycles of fertility were recognized several millennia before Christ. The early Greeks provided us with the medical word *oestrus* or *estrus*, which to them meant "frenzy," and to us now means a cyclic period of sexual activity. Other cultures used their words for heat to describe the fruitful breeding times of most mammals and human females. The causes of these cyclic occurrences of fertility and bleeding were unknown to the Greeks and regarded as sacred.

With the ascendancy of patriarchal cultures, females were assigned a different role in reproduction. Through the Middle Ages in Europe, women were considered merely the receptacle for the germinating seed of man, which would, by itself, create a new life. One has to wonder about the origin of this belief, since the female contribution to offspring is obvious in humans by simply observing the many children who strongly resemble their mothers. Not until the mid-1800s did scientists acknowledge that the female provided an equal share of the inherited characteristics of her offspring.

In 1866, Gregor Mendel, an obscure Austrian monk, published his paper on the hybridization of peas describing the equal importance of male and female factors to inherited characteristics of succeeding plant generations. Despite the impetus stemming from the independent but simultaneous publications in 1858 by Charles Darwin and A. R. Wallace, as well as Darwin's superb and very successful book *Origin of Species* (1859), all dealing with inherited factors of selection as the keystone of evolution, the prevailing view of male dominance in Western culture was still so great that Mendel's work was essentially ignored at the time. However, these genetic principles were rediscovered a generation later in 1900 by three scientists, Hugo de Vries, C. G. Correns, and Erich Tschermak-Seysenegg, each working independently in different countries.

The Discovery and Use of Progesterone

Not only did the science of genetics make a quantum leap during the early 1900s, but so also did the science of the biochemistry of reproduction. In 1900, the role of ovaries in hormonal control of the female reproductive system was established. In 1926 the hormone we now call *estrogen* was discovered in the urine of menstruating women, and scientists next observed that the concentration of the hormone varied with the phase of the menstrual cycle.

Many early researchers had correctly postulated that the ovary produced two hormonal substances. As early as 1897, researchers suggested that the small yellowish bodies (the *corpora lutea*) found on the ovary surface of pregnant females must serve a necessary function during pregnancy. In 1903 it was shown that destruction of the corpora lutea in pregnant rabbits caused abortion. With the discovery of the importance of the corpus luteum in hormone reproduction, the second hormone was soon identified. In 1929, the existence of the corpus luteum hormone was finally established, was proven to be necessary for a successful pregnancy, and thus was given the name progesterone (i.e., "pro-gestation").

As you'll recall, we now know that at birth ovaries contain hundreds of thousands of tiny sacs called *follicles*, each holding a potential egg (*ovum*). Each menstrual cycle results in the activation of 150 or so follicles to bring their egg to a mature state. When one of these follicles has moved to the outer surface of the ovary and released its egg (ovulation), it becomes the corpus luteum, the central manufacturing plant for progesterone.

For several years progesterone research was hampered by the small amount of progesterone that could be obtained from sows' ovaries. However, by the late 1930s, the placenta was found to synthesize progesterone in relatively large amounts, and this led to the harvesting of placentas after childbirth and quick-freezing them for extraction of progesterone in quantities sufficient for experimental work and clinical application. Then, in 1939, Russell E. Marker devised a method to convert sarsasapogenin, a sapogenin found in the sarsaparilla plant, into a progesterone-like compound. Soon thereafter he was able to convert disogenin from the wild yam (*Dioscorea villosa*) into progesterone with an excellent yield of 40 percent. With this method of production the price of progesterone fell from $80 per gram to $0.50 per gram.

Progesterone was found to be a fat-soluble compound that when given orally was relatively ineffective because most of it is quickly disposed of via the liver. When dissolved in vegetable oil and given by injection, progesterone is rapidly absorbed and thoroughly effective. Unfortunately, intramuscular injection proved to be locally irritating and painful, somewhat limiting its use. Physicians attuned to the intricacies of hormone balance, however, found progesterone to be remarkably effective in treating patients with what is now called PMS, ovarian cysts, and in preventing miscarriage. Progesterone is also well absorbed when given as a suppository in the rectum or vagina, and these methods of giving progesterone are still commonly used in Europe and Great Britain, although most women dislike their messiness. Katherina Dalton, M.D., of London has become world-famous for her highly successful treatments of PMS with transrectal progesterone.

In the early 1950s, active hormone-like substances were found in thousands of plant varieties. As previously mentioned, the sterol diosgenin is abundant in a variety of tropical wild yams with the Latin name *Dioscorea*, and can be converted in a laboratory into exactly the same molecule as human progesterone. (The wild yam is a different species from the yams we eat in North America. Our yams are not even true yams and have little to no plant steroid activity.) Furthermore, it was soon discovered that the diosgenin-derived progesterone could then be used inexpensively to create synthetic variations of progesterone (progestins) with potent progestational activity, as well as synthetic estrogens and testosterone, all with profitable commercial application. More recently, diosgenin is being extracted from soybeans, one of the largest agricultural crops in America.

Man-made hormones *not found in nature* are far more profitable for the pharmaceutical companies than natural hormones because, unlike natural substances, they can be patented. Thus pharmaceutical funding for progesterone research early on veered in the direction of creating new and patentable synthetic progesterone analogs made from the yam-derived natural progesterone. This led to the introduction of new classes of so-called progestational agents that lasted longer in the body and were more effective when taken orally. Such agents are referred to as progestins, progestogens, and gestagens, all meaning the same thing: "any synthetically derived compound with the ability to sustain the human secretory endometrium." The progestational agents do not provide the full spectrum of natural progesterone's biological activity, nor are they as safe. Despite their long list of safety concerns (see page 91), progestins have become popular because of their effectiveness in birth control and as protection against the estrogen-induced risk of endometrial cancer. It is a sad commentary on the pursuit of profit over women's well-being that the pharmaceutical companies take perfectly good natural hormones that our bodies know and can use, and alter them, creating synthetic compounds with similar hormonal effects but toxic side effects. Research on natural progesterone has in the past two decades been essentially nonexistent. Thus does industrial profit influence the path of science.

The pharmaceutical companies that sell these patented prescription products have been remarkably successful in confusing doctors about the meaning of "progesterone." The typical doctor thinks that the synthetic products are actually progesterone! Since the progestins carry the risk of a long list of undesirable and potentially dangerous side effects, doctors have become leery of prescribing what they think is the natural progesterone, which has virtually no known side effects in physiologic doses (the same amount made by the body). This error of confusing the specific hormone, progesterone, with the synthetic progestins is rampant throughout medical literature. Numerous authors and articles list the multiple health risks of the progestins as "progesterone" risks, and the unwary reader becomes progressively more confused and misinformed.

Ignorance about progesterone began years ago and was well under way when I graduated from medical school in 1955. For some time in my medical practice as a family physician, I was one of those doctors who prescribed estrogen. I had graduated from the University of Minnesota Medical School, completed a residency at Minneapolis General Hospital, spent a good portion of a year in practice with a wizard physician in a small town in Minnesota, completed two interesting years in the Pacific area as a medical officer in the U.S. Navy, and, in 1959, opened my own general practice of medicine in northern California. I felt confident and well trained. I was good at explaining the workings of birth control pills and had become an editor of a monthly medical journal. But I was still troubled by those women who came to me with premenstrual bloating, water retention, and emotional problems who told me that their previous doctor had treated them successfully with "progesterone shots." My treatments of diuretics, birth control hormones, or mild tranquilizers were usually unsuccessful, and our local pharmacies no longer carried injectable progesterone. The first modern era of natural progesterone had been short-lived and had come and gone before my time, swamped by the flood of synthetic hormones.

Recently, however, the advantages of natural progesterone have again become evident and its use in clinical situations is growing due to an increasing dissatisfaction among women taking the synthetic HRT regimens. Many physicians who once left the intricacies of hormone balance to gynecologists and endocrinologist consultants are (spurred by the demands of their patients) returning to their textbooks to relearn the lessons they have so long ignored. I receive hundreds of letters and e-mails every week from women, doctors, and other health professionals in North America and Europe who have used natural progesterone with great success in treating a wide variety of female health problems. There is a quiet revolution going on among those who have discovered natural progesterone and are happily and healthily using it.

Exactly What Is Progesterone?

In menstruating women, progesterone is one of the primary hormones made by the ovaries, the others being the estrogens and testosterone. As described previously, progesterone is made by the corpus luteum of the ovary, starting just before ovulation and increasing rapidly after ovulation. It is the major female reproductive hormone during the latter two weeks of the menstrual cycle. Progesterone is necessary for the survival of the fertilized ovum, the resulting embryo, and the fetus throughout gestation, when production of progesterone is taken over by the placenta.

Progesterone is made from the sterol pregnenolone, which is in turn made from cholesterol, which is made from acetate, a product of the breakdown of sugar and fat in the body. Within all cells of the body (except the red blood cells) are tiny power units called *mitochondria*, which convert cholesterol to pregnenolone, which in turn is converted to progesterone in the ovaries and adrenals. Progesterone is carried in the bloodstream where it is either used by the body or, as it passes through the liver, is excreted. In the ovaries, progesterone is the precursor of estrogen, testosterone, and of all the important adrenal cortical hormones.

From progesterone are derived not only the other sex hormones, including the estrogens, but also the corticosteroids, which are essential for stress response, sugar and electrolyte balance, and blood pressure, not to mention survival. With

Table 1. Comparing the Synergistic Effects of Estrogen and Progesterone

Estrogen Effects	Progesterone Effects
Creates proliferative endometrium	Maintains secretory endometrium
Breast cell stimulation (fibrocystic breasts[a])	Protects against breast fibrocysts
	Helps use fat for energy
Increased body fat and weight gain[a]	Natural diuretic
Salt and fluid retention	Natural antidepressant and calms anxiety
Depression, anxiety, and headaches[a]	
Cyclical migraines[a]	Prevents cyclical migraines
Poor sleep patterns[a]	Promotes normal sleep patterns
Interferes with thyroid hormone function[a]	Facilitates thyroid hormone function
Impairs blood sugar control[a]	Helps normalize blood sugar levels
Increased risk of blood clots[a]	Normalizes blood clotting
Little or no libido effect[a]	Helps restores normal libido
Loss of zinc and retention of copper[a]	Normalizes zinc and copper levels
Reduced oxygen levels in all cells[a]	Restores proper cell oxygen levels
Causes endometrial cancer[a]	Prevents endometrial cancer
Increased risk of breast cancer[a]	Helps prevent breast cancer
Increased risk of prostate cancer[a]	Decreased risk of prostate cancer
Slows bone loss	Stimulates new bone formation
Reduces vascular tone (dilates blood vessels)	Improves vascular tone
	Prevents autoimmune diseases
Triggers autoimmune diseases[a]	Increases sensitivity of estrogen receptors
Creates progesterone receptors	
Relieves hot flashes[c]	Necessary for survival of embryo
Prevents vaginal dryness and mucosal atrophy[c]	Precursor of corticosteroid biosynthesis
Increases risk of gallbladder disease[a]	Prevents coronary artery spasm and atherosclerotic plaque
Improves memory[c]	
Improves sleep disorders[c]	Sleepiness, depression[b]
Improves health of urinary tract[c]	Digestive problems[b]
Relieves night sweats[c]	

[a]Indicates that these effects may be caused by estrogen dominance, or an imbalance of estrogen caused by too little progesterone.
[b]Indicates that these effects may be caused by an excess of progesterone.
[c]Indicates that these effects may be caused by a deficiency of estrogen.
© Copyright 2001 Hormones Etc., Inc.

progesterone as a precursor to so many other hormones, it's easy to see why a progesterone deficiency can cause such a wide range of problems.

In short, the three major functions of progesterone are:

1. to promote the survival and development of the embryo and fetus.
2. to provide a broad range of intrinsic biologic effects.
3. to act as a precursor of other steroid hormones.

Progesterone is a central factor in the biosynthesis of other hormones, but its many functions in the body are far more extensive (see Figure 5). (For a complete biochemical drawing of the many roles of progesterone, see the appendix on page 425.)

Cholesterol   →   Pregnenolone
                        ↓
                   Progesterone

↙   ↓   ↘

Biosynthetic Pathways

androstenedione
testosterone
estrone, estradiol,
    estriol
all cortisol and
    corticosteroids
aldosterone

Reproductive Effects

secretory endometrium
survival of embryo
development of fetus
    throughout gestation
libido

Intrinsic Effects

mild diuretic
helps use fat for energy
natural antidepressant
helps thyroid hormone action
normalizes blood clotting
helps normalize blood sugar
    levels
normalizes zinc and copper
    levels
maintains proper cell oxygen
    levels
protects against breast cysts
protects against breast cancer
protects against endometrial
    cancer
moisturizes skin when used
    topically
counteracts estrogen side
    effects

Figure 5: The multiple roles of natural progesterone.

The Cycle of Progesterone Production

The levels of progesterone in a woman's body rise and fall dramatically with her monthly cycles. With the development of the corpus luteum and ovulation, the ovarian production of progesterone rapidly rises from 2 to 3 milligrams per day to an average of 22 milligrams per day, peak production being as high as 30 milligrams per day a week or so after ovulation. After 10 or 12 days, if fertilization does not occur, ovarian production of progesterone falls dramatically. It is this sudden decline in progesterone levels (as well as estrogen levels) that triggers menstruation (i.e., the shedding of the secretory endometrium—the lining of the uterus), leading to a renewal of the entire menstrual cycle.

Progesterone and Procreation

Progesterone is the hormone that makes possible the survival of the fertilized egg. It maintains the lining of the uterus, which the fertilized egg will attach to and from which the germinating egg and the resultant embryo will gain sustenance during its first stages of growth. As might be expected, the surge of progesterone at the time of ovulation is one source of sex drive, the urge to procreate, by which is meant the sexual drive to bring egg and sperm together. (Doesn't it make sense that Mother Nature would connect sex drive to the hormone that comes at ovulation?)

In pregnancy, progesterone is necessary to prevent the premature shedding of the uterine lining. Any drop in progesterone level or blockage of its receptor sites at this time will result in the loss of the embryo (miscarriage). This in fact is the action of the antiprogesterone compound and abortifacient RU-486.

As the placenta develops, it assumes and progressively increases the production of progesterone for the duration of the gestation period until the birth of the baby. During the third trimester, the placenta is producing progesterone at the rate of

300 to 400 milligrams per day, an astoundingly high level for hormone production, which is usually measured in *micrograms* per day. It is interesting to note that many women say that aside from the physical discomfort of carrying all that extra weight and the constriction of organs such as the bladder, they never felt better than in their third trimester of pregnancy, when progesterone production is very high!

At birth the level of progesterone production drops suddenly, contributing to postpartum depression in some women. Postpartum depression, should it occur, can often be effectively treated with natural progesterone.

Progesterone (unlike estrogen and testosterone) is devoid of secondary sex characteristics, meaning that its presence or absence does not affect male or female characteristics. Thus its effects in promoting the development of the fetus are independent of the baby's gender. The fetus is allowed to develop according to its own DNA code and is not affected by the hormones of the mother.

Progesterone increases energy production (probably by helping thyroid hormone work more efficiently), causing a slight rise in body temperature. This is called the *thermogenic* effect of progesterone and can be used to indicate ovulation for women who want to know when (and if) ovulation occurs.

The fall of progesterone levels at menopause is proportionately much greater than the fall of estrogen levels. Though estrogen falls only 40 to 60 percent from baseline on average, the decline in progesterone levels is 12 times greater, according to research done by Canadian endocrinologist Jerilynn Prior, M.D. Postmenopausal progesterone levels in some women are actually *lower* than those of males. This is an odd circumstance, considering the importance of progesterone as a precursor of all the steroid hormones. Furthermore, progesterone has many other important intrinsic functions that, one would think, need to be continued for good health. There is no reason to believe that postmenopausal women require less progesterone than men.

How Progesterone Affects the Body

Progesterone has many beneficial actions throughout the body. Table 1 on page 73 provides an indication of its diversity and importance. Since progesterone protects against the undesirable side effects of unopposed estrogen, whether occurring from within the body as a result of anovulatory cycles or as a consequence of estrogen supplementation or exposure to xeno-estrogens, these effects are included in the list. Estrogen dominance allows the influx of water and sodium into cells, causing water retention (bloating) and high blood pressure. Estrogen dominance also reduces the amount of oxygen present in the cells, opposes the action of thyroid, promotes histamine release (which causes allergy-type symptoms), promotes blood clotting (thus increasing the risk of stroke and embolism), thickens bile and promotes gallbladder disease, and causes copper retention and zinc loss. Estrogen unopposed by progesterone also decreases sex drive, increases the likelihood of fibrocystic breasts, uterine fibroids, uterine (endometrial) cancer, and breast cancer. All of these undesirable effects of estrogen are countered by progesterone. Restoring proper progesterone levels is what is known as restoring hormone *balance*.

Progesterone and Steroid Synthesis

Before discussing the third important function of progesterone, its role in making steroid hormones, it may be helpful to review how cholesterol and pregnenolone are made. Cholesterol is made by cells throughout the body, particularly in the liver, from acetate (a small two-carbon compound), a substance derived from the breakdown of sugars and fats. There is a common myth that eating cholesterol causes cholesterol levels to rise, but the truth is that eating too many refined carbohydrates such as sugar and white flour can cause cholesterol levels to rise. Some 75 percent of our total cholesterol is made from these foods rather than from cholesterol intake per se. A rise in cholesterol levels has more to do with how much sugar and refined starch we eat, whether we're getting enough fiber, vitamins, and minerals in our diets, how much we exercise, and what our stress levels are. Genetics also plays a large part in cholesterol levels.

The production of hormones is a dynamic, fluctuating system, constantly responding to changing body conditions and needs. Hormones are the control messengers for a vast, interrelated, ever-changing network of organ-system commands. As such, they must be continually synthesized for moment-to-moment situational needs and likewise must be metabolized and removed from the system when no longer needed in order for their presence to fall as their need diminishes. (The liver is constantly metabolizing and excreting hormones as they pass through in the bloodstream.) Progesterone, in addition to its own hormonal effects, is a main player in the creation of all these hormones. Various cells in key organs throughout the body use progesterone to create the other specific hormones as needed, specifically the adrenal corticosteroids, estrogen, and testosterone.

This precursor aspect of progesterone distinguishes it from many other hormones that are at a metabolic end point, meaning they are unable to be used further except to be broken down for excretion. The synthetic progestins so heavily promoted in hormone replacement therapy have undergone molecular alterations at unusual positions. As these strange, not-found-in-nature molecules travel down the hormone pathways, they occupy progesterone receptor sites, create actions different from natural progesterone, cannot be used as precursors of other hormones (as progesterone can), and are difficult for the body to metabolize and excrete. These molecular alterations carry a heavy burden of potential undesirable side effects. This, however, does not seem to deter the marketing of them. Physicians who are the targets of heavy pharmaceutical advertising (and unaware that natural progesterone is available) tend to accede to marketing pressure.

Natural progesterone is needed for the appropriate and balanced supply of all the steroid hormones. To overcome present marketing practices and restore natural progesterone to its proper place in the practice of medicine will apparently require reeducation of its diverse and important role in health by patients and doctors alike.

Progesterone and the Brain

Although progesterone is not a sex hormone per se in that its presence doesn't confer the attributes of maleness or femaleness, it is important to central nervous system (the brain and spinal cord) function as are other sex hormones. Progesterone is concentrated in brain cells to levels 20 times higher than that of blood serum levels. Such high concentrations in brain cells cannot be due to simple diffusion but require work on the part of brain cells. This alone strongly suggests that progesterone in brain cells serves some important purpose.

Progesterone has long been known to have a calming or mildly sedating effect. This effect is caused by a metabolite of progesterone called *allopregnanolone* that is active at GABA (gamma-aminobutyric acid) receptors. (GABA is an amino acid that acts as a neurotransmitter inhibitor and tends to have a calming effect.) Progesterone's sedation of the central nervous system is sufficiently potent in higher doses that it has been used as an anesthetic. When used in small doses, progesterone is commonly effective in restoring normal sleep patterns and promoting a sense of calm.

Professor Etienne-Emile Baulieu of France has done extensive research on the effects of progesterone in nerve cells. He has discovered that progesterone is synthesized from Schwann cells within the central and peripheral nervous system and as such is a neurosteroid. Furthermore, he found that progesterone and pregnenolone promote myelin repair. The myelin sheath protects nerve cells and is damaged in some neurological diseases such as multiple sclerosis.

Equally intriguing are studies done at Emory University on the effects of brain injury in rodents, which found that survival and recovery rates were higher in females than in males. However, when the male rodents were supplemented with progesterone, their survival and recovery from brain injuries paralleled that of female rodents. This benefit did not follow from estrogen supplementation. Emory neuroscientist Donald Stein found that when estrogen was high, the female rodents had "lots of symptoms" following brain injury, but rats with high progesterone and low estrogen displayed few or no symptoms from the same type of injury. In addition, Stein found that, in both male and female rats, injections of progesterone after the injury prevented swelling in the brain. Swelling is the major source of permanent damage after a brain injury, in both humans and rodents. The earlier the progesterone was given after the injury, the greater the protection. Stein believes it "may be possible to use progesterone to protect the brain following such injury." He also found that progesterone was protective in rodents after the equivalent of a stroke. This corresponds to epidemiologic (population) research showing that premenopausal women recover better from stroke than do men and menopausal women.

Stein is now leading a clinical trial (using people) of progesterone as a treatment for moderate to severe traumatic brain injury. Brain injury kills about 50,000 Americans every year and disables 80,000 more; it's obviously a serious and widespread problem, and there is currently little to no conventional medical treatment. The three-year study has been approved by the U.S. Food and Drug Administration and is funded by the National Institutes of Health (NIH). Stein believes that progesterone reduces the inflammation that frequently leads to dangerous brain swelling following head injury, and that it may also slow or block the formation of free radicals, which in a brain injury can cause substantial brain cell death. The progesterone used in the study will be given intravenously for three days. If the results of this pilot phase study are promising, the researchers anticipate that the study will be extended to additional level I trauma centers in other U.S. cities in future years.

If one of my loved ones had a brain injury, I would certainly see that they were given liberal doses of progesterone cream.

At this time, what we know about progesterone and the brain is that it is selectively concentrated in brain cells, has a calming effect, and has a beneficial effect on recovery from brain injury. And, as we shall see, progesterone has an important effect on libido or sex drive.

Progesterone and Sex Drive

The early proponents of estrogen replacement therapy (ERT) created a myth promising that estrogen would keep women "feminine" and sexually attractive "forever." Without the magic pill, they would turn into sexless hags and no longer be attractive to their husbands. It was a common misconception that older women were no longer interested in sex.

In my medical practice, many *pre*menopausal women told me that they were less interested in sex. Others, however, told me that as they approached menopause, they had become even more desirous of sex; it was their husbands whose sexual stamina was failing. The difference in the women, it seemed to me, related to whether or not they were experiencing estrogen dominance, that is, continued estrogen effects (monthly periods) without progesterone (anovulatory periods). The women losing interest in sex had water retention, fibrocystic breasts, depression, dry, wrinkling skin, and irregular, sometimes heavy periods. I gradually came to understand that these signs and symptoms were indicative of a progesterone deficiency caused by a failure to ovulate while estrogen continued to be produced, which is to say loss of sex drive correlates with progesterone deficiency, not estrogen deficiency. Women on estrogen replacement therapy coming to me for treatment of their osteoporosis also confided in me that they were unhappy with the fat accumulating at their hips and abdomen, their swollen breasts, and their loss of sex drive. Estrogen replacement had not restored their previous sex drive.

When these women used the progesterone cream supplementation I recommended, the story changed; they were delighted to report that their sex drive had returned. I received a Christmas card from one woman telling me that her bones were better, her skin was more youthful, and, by the way, her husband thanked me, too! I learned to ask my progesterone-using patients about their sex drives, and uniformly their eyes brightened and they told me their sex life was better after progesterone therapy than any time during the 10 to 15 years before menopause. Progesterone had restored normal sex drive.

My clinical experience with these patients was at odds with what I had learned in medical school. I had been taught that only estrogen and testosterone were vital to normal sex drive. Pharmacologic (abnormally large) doses of progesterone, when given to male rats and lizards, had been found to inhibit sexual behavior. But a 1994 study found that physiologic (much smaller) doses of progesterone had the opposite effect (i.e., it restored sex drive).

But what about females? In another recent study, female hamsters with their ovaries removed did not show sexual behavior unless areas of their brains vital for sex drive were stimulated by progesterone. When stimulated with estrogen alone, these brain areas did not stimulate normal sexual activity. When progesterone was added, sexual activity revived.

While I grant that hamsters are not humans, it is clear that, in most female mammals, the rise and fall of sex hormones coordinates sexual behavior so that mating is most likely to occur near the time of ovulation. This, after all, is the primary function of sex drive. This study thus shows that sex drive is a function of both estrogen and progesterone, and probably also of testosterone. The administration of estrogen in the absence of progesterone does not accomplish stimulation of sex drive. (I would like to see a study where progesterone alone was administered!) In humans, estrogen production falls only 40 to 60 percent at menopause, whereas progesterone falls to close to zero when ovulation no longer occurs. This explains the loss of sex drive in my premenopausal patients with estrogen sufficient for monthly periods (and in postmenopausal women on ERT) but lacking in progesterone and the resumption of normal sex drive when progesterone was added.

Among many researchers, testosterone is given credit for being the hormone attached to sex drive in both males and females. It is widely assumed that the increased sex drive in fertile women at ovulation correlates with a timely spurt of testosterone. In a test of this hypothesis, Drs. Ben C. Campbell and Peter T. Ellison of Harvard University measured daily salivary testosterone levels among regularly cycling women and did find a very small peak, as expected. In an interesting aside, to verify that the women were in fact ovulating, they also checked midcycle progesterone levels. To their surprise, 7 of the 18 women in the study (age range 24 to 42 years, average 29 years of age) did not ovulate, although they were menstruating. This is still further evidence that anovulatory cycles are common among relatively young, regularly cycling women in the United States.

It is important to be reminded again of the complex interplay and delicate balance of hormones in the human body and the difference between taking *physiologic* and *pharmacologic* doses of hormones. *Physiologic* (equivalent to normal body function) doses are meant to be replacement doses for a specific hormone deficiency. They are not meant to exceed normal bodily production and they promote no abnormal actions in the body. *Pharmacologic* (drug) doses, on the other hand, are considerably greater than normal production and lead not only to suppression of natural hormone production, but also to actions different from those found with normal hormone levels. In the case of progesterone, pharmacologic doses may actually inhibit sex drive whereas physiologic doses stimulate sex drive. In my practice I recommended a progesterone cream that supplied only about 15 to 30 milligrams per day, simulating normal progesterone production. Many physicians, for reasons I do not understand, opt for doses 10 to 20 times higher. When they report that they do not see the resurgence of sex drive as I have found with my patients, it is not a surprise to me.

Progesterone in Men

Progesterone is the precursor of testosterone and corticosteroids, meaning the body uses progesterone to make these other hormones. Progesterone in men is synthesized by their testes to produce testosterone and in their adrenals to produce corticosteroids. Progesterone levels in men are naturally much lower than in women during their fertile years. However, after menopause (or even 10 to 15 years before menopause), some women's progesterone levels fall below that of same-age men. Typically, healthy men continue to produce normal testosterone and corticosteroid levels into their 70s and 80s.

I recall reading in the *Medical Tribune* more than 15 years ago of a study involving progesterone supplementation in men. Progesterone given to college-age men resulted in no apparent change in general stamina, vigor, or sex drive. Testosterone levels fell, however, to levels low enough to inhibit sperm maturation. Since many testosterone receptors also accept progesterone (and with similar results), it is likely that a biofeedback mechanism in the brain reduces testosterone production when high levels of progesterone are present. Thus it appears that pharmacologic doses of progesterone in men act only as a contraceptive.

Among men with prostate cancer, it is common practice to castrate them either surgically or chemically to reduce their testosterone level as low as possible in the belief that this suppresses prostate cancer growth. The abrupt, almost total absence of testosterone creates a sort of male menopause, often complete with hot flashes. Disturbing as this is, it is perhaps more important that the lack of testosterone will bring on an acceleration of osteoporosis within just a year or so. Like progesterone, testosterone can stimulate new bone formation, increasing bone density, and a lack of it can cause osteoporosis.

Progesterone and testosterone are similar hormones in regard to new bone formation. They and the corticosteroids compete for the same osteoblast receptor sites on the bones, with testosterone and progesterone stimulating new bone formation, whereas corticosteroids inhibit it. If one wishes to prevent or treat the castration-induced osteoporosis, it is possible to safely supplement progesterone to replace testosterone in these men. While my experience in using progesterone under these circumstances is limited, and insufficient for statistical evaluation, the results to date have been encouraging. It is my hope that further research will emerge to better evaluate this potential benefit of progesterone.

CHAPTER 7

THE DRAMATIC
DIFFERENCE BETWEEN
PROGESTERONE AND
PROGESTINS

Many physicians still believe that the synthetic progestins such as Provera (medroxyprogesterone acetate) are the same as natural progesterone. This is a common and very unfortunate misunderstanding. Most doctors don't have the time to keep up on the latest drug research, so they rely on pharmaceutical company ads or representatives for their information. The pharmaceutical companies have no interest in selling natural progesterone because they can't patent it, so they have no interest in sponsoring research or passing on information about it. Thus we have a widespread misconception among American doctors that natural progesterone has the same side effects as the progestins—an error that is dramatically affecting the health and well-being of millions of American women. In fact, natural progesterone used in physiologic doses (no greater than what the body normally should be making) has virtually no side effects, while the synthetic progestins have many.

There have been some excellent studies done on natural progesterone, which are referenced on pages 402–403. A small but interesting study was done when Joel Hargrove et al. (1989) compared oral progesterone to Provera (medroxyprogesterone acetate). Both were combined with different forms of estrogen in menopausal women. The group on progesterone found symptomatic improvement of menopausal symptoms, improved cholesterol levels, the absence of menstruation without the typical progestin and estrogen-related problems of abnormal tissue growth in the uterus, and no side effects. All 10 of the women taking progesterone and estradiol wished to continue their hormone treatment, while 2 of the 5 women using estrone and medroxyprogesterone acetate discontinued their treatment because of side effects.

A much larger study done in 1995 (the PEPI trial) examined the effects of sex hormones on cholesterol and HDL-cholesterol as well as their effects on the endometrium. This three-year, multicenter, randomized, double-blind, placebo-controlled (the gold standard of medical research), $22 million, federally funded trial found that estrogen taken alone "significantly increased the occurrence of severe hyperplasia" in those women with an intact uterus (hyperplasia is considered to be a step along the pathway to cancer), whereas estrogen with natural progesterone or medroxyprogesterone acetate (the progestin) completely protected women from this side effect. Estrogen caused these precancerous changes in one-third of the women who took estrogen alone. However, estrogen did effectively lower total cholesterol and raise HDL-cholesterol (the "good" cholesterol), followed closely by the estrogen/natural progesterone combination, which was significantly superior to the estrogen/progestin combination. In the news items that followed the publication of this study, natural progesterone was described as "a little known 'natural' form of progesterone derived from wild yams or soybeans." From my point of view, the trial would have been even better had they included a subgroup of women using only natural progesterone.

Even though I get phone calls every day from health professionals around the world who are using progesterone with great success, we are very much in need of further clinical trials comparing progesterone therapy alone with progesterone/estrogen therapy. Since the menopausal decrease of estrogen is only 40 to 60 percent, true estrogen deficiency is a misnomer. My experience, and the experience of many of the doctors who correspond with or call me, has been that most menopausal symptoms will respond to progesterone supplementation alone. If they do not, such women may need very low-dose estrogen supplementation for several years, which can then be gradually discontinued without recurrence of the symptoms.

The Difference between Synthetic Drugs and Natural Compounds

My definition of a synthetic drug is that the substance is not found in nature. Thus, while man-made progesterone is extracted from wild yams or soybeans in a laboratory, the final result is a molecule that is identical to that found in the human body, and thus it is natural. Aspirin is an example of a drug originally made from a natural substance. It has its medicinal origins in trees of the *salix* species, most commonly known as willow and poplar. Various teas, decoctions, tinctures, and poultices of *salix* were used medicinally in America, Europe, and Asia for centuries to relieve pain, especially the pain of headaches and arthritis.

In the late 1800s laws were passed in the United States that allowed medicines to be patented only if they were *not* natural substances. If a drug company discovered a naturally occurring medicine, anyone else was free to capitalize on the discovery. Needless to say, drug companies quickly became disinterested in naturally occurring medicines. These days, when a plant with medicinal value is discovered, the "active ingredient" is isolated and transformed. This new molecule can be patented. In the case of *salix*, a chemist at the Bayer company in Germany synthesized acetylsalicyclic acid in 1897 and aspirin was born.

While there is no doubt that aspirin is a wonderful drug—Americans consume somewhere around 30 billion tablets every year—willow bark does not have aspirin's side effects. Aspirin and the whole family of nonsteroidal anti-inflammatory pain relievers (NSAIDs) have a wide range of side effects, mostly in the area of stomach inflammation, and cause in excess of 10,000 fatalities and 30,000 hospitalizations every year due to bleeding in the stomach or intestines. Acetaminophen (e.g., Tylenol) is damaging to the liver. Aspirin and acetaminophen, however, are readily available and easy to use—willow bark is neither.

The history of creating synthetic drugs consistently shows that separating the so-called active ingredient from the rest of the plant to create substances not found in nature almost always creates harmful side effects, whereas plant medicines, used properly, rarely have harmful side effects. Nature has a great wisdom that humans have not been able to duplicate in synthetic drugs. Over millions of years of evolution, our biochemistry has become integrated very specifically with the natural world. Our bodies know how to take many natural substances, use them for energy, maintenance, and repair, and then efficiently excrete them when they are used up. Conversely, when synthetic, chemically altered hormone drugs occupy cell receptors, the message they convey may be different, even contrary to the hormone they are meant to simulate. Such effects are called side effects. Further, being foreign to normal metabolic processes, they cannot be excreted as well.

Tryptophan, a naturally occurring amino acid found in the greatest abundance in milk and turkey, became very popular some 20 years ago as a sleep remedy and antidepressant. It is very effective and has minimal side effects when used sensibly. A contaminated batch of tryptophan from Japan killed a number of people and caused a debilitating disease in others, so the FDA asked manufacturers for a voluntary recall of the substance as a supplement, meaning it is effectively banned in the United States. Ironically, however, tryptophan is still used in the United States in baby formulas and tube feedings for the elderly. If it wasn't present in these substances it wouldn't be nutritionally complete! There is not a shred of evidence anywhere that *uncontaminated* tryptophan taken in prescribed doses is harmful. Coincidentally—or perhaps not so coincidentally—about the same time that tryptophan was banned, the pharmaceutical industry poured millions of dollars into advertising and public relations to introduce the antidepressant drugs known as selective serotonin reuptake inhibitors (SSRIs), including Prozac and Zoloft. These drugs work in a way similar to tryptophan but differ greatly in their risk of side effects.

Many synthetic drugs are made patentable simply by changing a few atoms of the natural substance. This may sound harmless enough, but the addition or subtraction of a few atoms of a molecule can make a big difference in their effects on the body. This holds especially true with hormones. Tiny amounts can create major effects on the body. For example, the molecular difference between testosterone and estradiol is one hydrogen atom and a couple of double bonds. Amazing! Adding or subtracting one hydrogen atom at a specific place on a molecule can make the difference between a man and a woman!

Now compare that exquisite level of biochemical specificity to what a pharmaceutical company does to a perfectly good natural hormone—they add whole chains of molecules! They do this not to make a better drug, but to make one that behaves similarly yet is different enough to be patentable.

I am reminded of a menopausal woman in Canada who sent me a 10-pound packet of her medical records from the five or six doctors she had consulted, asking for my advice. In the packet was a series of laboratory tests for serum progesterone. The patient had been put on the progestin, medroxyprogesterone acetate (Provera), and her doctor had ordered a serum progesterone level. Finding it still zero, he doubled the progestin dose and ordered a second test. This, too, was zero. He doubled the progestin dose again and ordered a third test, which again indicated zero progesterone. But on this lab report the technician had written, "Doctor, you are giving this woman Provera. You are ordering tests for serum progesterone. Provera is not progesterone!" By this time, the patient was experiencing numerous side effects from the drug, specifically loss of appetite, nausea, indigestion, fatigue, and depression. I circled the lab tech's comment in red and sent it back to the woman with an information sheet on natural progesterone. Several months later I got a very nice note from her telling me how much better she felt using natural progesterone and that she had fired all but one of her doctors.

What Is a Progestin?

A progestin is often defined as "any compound able to sustain the human secretory endometrium." This refers to the ability to keep the lining of the uterus healthy and blood-rich in preparation for pregnancy and to support the developing embryo. When a woman comes to the end of her monthly cycle and no pregnancy has occurred, the levels of her reproductive hormones drop dramatically and in response the lining of the uterus is shed in menstruation.

Throughout much of medical literature, natural progesterone is either equated with progestins, as if they were the same thing, or classed as one of the progestins, which, strictly speaking, is also incorrect. There is only one *progesterone*, the specific molecule made by the adrenal glands or by the ovary as a consequence of ovulation. (To complicate things even further, European writers refer to progestins as gestagens or progestogens.) I would define progestins as any compound *other than natural progesterone* able to sustain the human secretory endometrium.

Progesterone and Progestins: What's the Difference?

I receive frequent mail from women who say that their doctor insists that progesterone and progestins are the same. I suggest that those who still insist that progestins and progesterone are the same, or that progesterone is a generic term that also covers progestins, ponder the following questions. If progesterone and progestins are the same:

- Why do fertility doctors always use progesterone and not progestins?
- Why are progestins associated with birth defects, while progesterone is essential for a viable and healthy pregnancy?
- Why don't synthetic progestins show up in blood and saliva tests of progesterone levels? In other words, why doesn't taking a progestin raise progesterone levels in the body?

- Pregnant women are making 300 mg of progesterone daily in the last trimester. Why don't they have higher rates of breast cancer, as women do who use progestins?
- Why doesn't natural progesterone cause the side effects listed for medroxyprogesterone acetate (Provera) the most commonly used synthetic progestin for HRT?

To appreciate the scope of progestin side effects, it is instructive to review the *Physicians' Desk Reference* (PDR) pages for medroxyprogesterone acetate. An *abbreviated* list from the *Physicians' Desk Reference* (PDR) follows:

Potential Side Effects of Medroxyprogesterone Acetate (Provera)

WARNING FOR WOMEN

- There is an increased risk of minor birth defects in children whose mothers take this drug during the first 4 months of pregnancy. [Genital abnormalities, which the children might not consider "minor."]

WARNINGS

- Beagle dogs given this drug developed mammary nodules, some of which were malignant.
- The physician should be alert to the earliest manifestation of thrombotic disorders (thrombophlebitis, cerebrovascular disorders, pulmonary embolism, and retinal thrombosis).
- Discontinue this drug if there is sudden partial or complete loss of vision.
- Detectable amounts of progestin have been identified in the milk of mothers receiving the drug. The effect of this on the nursing neonate and infant has not been determined.

CONTRAINDICATIONS

- Thrombophlebitis, thromboembolic disorders, cerebral apoplexy; liver dysfunction or disease; known or suspected malignancy of breast or genital organs; undiagnosed vaginal bleeding; missed abortion; known or suspected pregnancy.

PRECAUTIONS

- Because progestogens may cause some degree of fluid retention, conditions which might be influenced by this factor, such as epilepsy, migraine, asthma, cardiac or renal dysfunction, require careful observation.
- May cause breakthrough bleeding or menstrual irregularities.
- May cause or contribute to depression.
- The effect of prolonged use of this drug on pituitary, ovarian, adrenal, hepatic, or uterine function is unknown.
- May decrease glucose tolerance; diabetic patients must be carefully monitored.
- May increase the thrombotic disorders associated with estrogens.

ADVERSE REACTIONS

- Breast tenderness and galactorrhea.
- Sensitivity reactions such as urticaria, pruritus, edema, or rash.
- Acne, alopecia, and hirsutism (excess hair growth).
- Edema, weight changes (increase or decrease).
- Cervical erosions and changes in cervical secretions.
- Cholestatic jaundice.
- Mental depression, pyrexia, nausea, insomnia, or somnolence.
- Anaphylactoid reactions and anaphylaxis (severe acute allergic reactions).

- Thrombophlebitis and pulmonary embolism.
- Breakthrough bleeding, spotting, amenorrhea, or changes in menses.
- Fatigue, backache, itching, dizziness, nervousness, loss of scalp hair.

WHEN TAKEN WITH ESTROGENS, THE FOLLOWING HAVE BEEN OBSERVED

- Rise in blood pressure, headache, dizziness, nervousness, fatigue.
- Changes in sex drive, hirsutism and loss of scalp hair, decrease in T3 uptake values.
- Premenstrual-like syndrome, changes in appetite.
- Cystitis-like syndrome (urinary tract infections).
- Erythema multiforme, erythema nodosum, hemorrhagic eruption, itching.

Most of the progestins are synthesized from progesterone or from another synthetic hormone called nortestosterone, and none of them are found in nature. They may be only a couple of atoms different from natural progesterone, but it is evident that such a seemingly slight shift can make the difference between a successful pregnancy and an unsuccessful one, for example.

Because progesterone is a natural hormone, the body is normally able to produce it, use it, and eliminate it as needed. The synthetic progestins, on the other hand, are not well processed by the body. Their activity is prolonged, creating reactions in the body that are not consistent with natural progesterone.

Progestins bind to the same receptors in the cell as progesterone, but from that point on they carry different messages to the cell. In other words, the parts of the body that need progesterone at first identify progestins as a progesterone. However, the small alterations in the progestins will then convey a different message. This undoubtedly explains the alarming array of listed warnings, contraindications, precautions, and adverse reactions to progestins, all of which are uncharacteristic of natural progesterone. To complicate matters even more, synthetic progestins generally bind to the progesterone receptor more tenaciously and thereby inhibit the action of the natural hormone. Furthermore, each variety of progestin differs from the others and carries its own unique array of side effects.

Progestins in general are similar to progesterone and estrogen in their ability to be easily absorbed into the body through the skin (transdermally). Thus some HRT regimens and oral con-

Table 2: Comparison of the Effects of Natural Progesterone and Synthetic Progestins

Conditions	Natural Progesterone	Progestin
Sodium and water into body cells		✓
Loss of mineral electrolytes from cells		✓
Intracellular edema		✓
Depression		✓
Birth defect risks		✓
More body hair, thinner scalp hair		✓
Thrombophlebitis, embolism risk		✓
Decreased glucose tolerance		✓
Allergic reactions		✓
Cholestatic jaundice risk		✓
Acne, skin rashes		✓
Protects against endometrial cancer	✓	✓
Protects against breast cancer	✓	
Normalizes libido	✓	
Less hirsutism, regrowth of scalp hair	✓	
Improves lipid profile	✓	
Improves in vitro fertilization	✓	
Improves new bone formation	✓	modestly
Improves sleep patterns	✓	

traceptives utilize a patch that gradually releases the hormones into the body.

Progestins and estrogen cause water retention, often accompanied by hypertension (high blood pressure). Natural progesterone helps balance fluid in the cells and appears to have a protective effect *against* hypertension. While progesterone has a beneficial effect of improving the ability of the body to use and eliminate fats, progestins have the opposite effect. As described in the PEPI study, the combination of estrogen and progesterone was clearly superior to estrogen and Provera in its cholesterol effects. Progestins share with natural progesterone the ability to promote new bone formation but with less success. Dr. Jerilynn Prior has found a 5 percent increase in bone mineral density using medroxyprogesterone acetate (Provera) in postmenopausal osteoporotic patients. In my experience, in women with measurable bone density loss, the typical bone mineral density increase shown with natural progesterone was 15 percent.

Table 2 indicates some of the differences between natural progesterone and the synthetic progestins.

Progestins Gave Birth to the Sexual Revolution

Given all that is known about the great difference of actions and of safety between progesterone and the synthetic progestins, why is it that progestins dominate in the role of progesterone supplementation? Aside from the obvious financial gains to be made from a patentable molecule, the answer lies in their use in contraceptive pills.

Until the late 1960s, there were two main factors holding back the sexual revolution: the fear of unwanted pregnancy and venereal disease. In industrialized cultures, the development of the automobile effectively removed the young from their usual adult chaperones. Then the advent of penicillin and the apparent easy cures for gonorrhea and syphilis removed the perceived threat of venereal disease. All that was needed for the explosion of the sexual revolution was a convenient, effective (and private) contraceptive. Thus the stage was set for progestational drugs. When progesterone became obtainable (from plant sources) in sufficient amounts for aggressive research by private biochemical industries, it did not take long for the development of oral, highly effective (for birth control), synthetic progestins.

But how does a hormone that is crucial to the survival and development of the embryo in pregnancy act as a birth control pill? During each monthly cycle, eggs mature in both ovaries until ovulation occurs in one of them, creating the corpus luteum, which is responsible for a surge of progesterone production. This surge of progesterone, as one of its effects, stops ovulation in the other ovary (which is why fraternal twins are born only once for every 300 pregnancies). If sufficient progesterone is provided prior to ovulation, neither ovary produces an egg. This inhibition of ovulation was the original mechanism of action of progestin contraception.

The advantages of progestins were (1) ease of delivery system [oral tablets], (2) consistent potency [guaranteed contraception], (3) they lasted longer in the body [inability of the body to metabolize them], and (4) a patentable [i.e., profitable] product. In those days natural progesterone supplementation required expensive, painful injections or rectal or vaginal suppositories.

The long lists of undesirable and potentially serious side effects from the progestins in birth control pills are dutifully printed in the PDR and in product information sheets, usually in type so small that only the most curious would read them. No one really wanted to know of them because of what was being offered: sex without fear of pregnancy.

Then another use was found for the progestins. As physicians began using estrogen therapy for menopausal symptoms, problems arose. During the 1970s it became obvious that postmenopausal women taking estrogen alone for menopausal symptoms had a greatly increased risk of endometrial cancer. This cancer rarely if ever occurred during one's fertile years when normal levels of estrogen and progesterone were present. Testing of postmenopausal women with combined hormone therapy (using both estrogen and a progestin) found that estrogen-induced endometrial cancer could be largely prevented. In the mid-1970s, a Mayo Clinic consensus conference concluded that estrogen should never be given to any woman with an intact uterus (any woman who hasn't had a hysterectomy) without also giving progesterone or a progestin as protection from endometrial cancer. The effect of this was to expand the market for progestins to include *all* women, whether menstruating or postmenopausal! The financial implications of this are difficult to exaggerate.

Even the threat of breast cancer has not stopped the market for estrogen/progestin hormone therapy. As early as 1989, a report by Leif Bergkvist et al. convincingly showed that supplemental estrogen (at least estradiol) when combined with a progestin "seems to be associated with a slightly *increased* risk of breast cancer, which is not prevented and may even be *increased* by the addition of the progestins" (emphasis added). This did not slow the progestin bandwagon, and in fact prescriptions for them soared until the publication of the Women's Health Initiative showed an indisputable increase in breast cancer (see page 4).

Women should be upset that the hormone "balancing" drugs being given to them use synthetic and abnormal versions of the real goods, when the natural hormones are available, safer, and more appropriate to their bodies.

Are progestins the wave of the future? We should hope not. Our goal should be that when hormone therapy is indicated, the hormones should be the natural ones used in physiologic dosages. It can be taken as a rule that among steroids, any unnatural changes in their molecular makeup will alter their effects. It should be clear that nature produces the substances that serve us best.

CHAPTER 8

SEX HORMONES AND THE BRAIN

We're all familiar with jokes about people—males and females—whose brains appear to be located below the waist instead of in their heads. In truth, brain function involves the whole body, as we shall see. The main operating systems are indeed in the head, and the sex hormones play important roles there, too.

The Basics of Brain Communication

Weighing only three pounds, the brain is composed of 8 billion nerve cells held in specific structural arrangements by filaments, as well as by smaller, specialized connective tissue cells called *glial cells*, which comprise half of the brain's weight. Each adult brain nerve cell has on average 5,000 extensions, called *synapses*, by which it communicates with other brain cells. That means the brain has 8 billion times 5,000, or 4×10^{13} connections, a number almost too large to comprehend. If we think of the brain as a computer, that number of connections is many times larger than that found in the world's largest computer.

Among mammals, brain size is less important than function. An adult elephant's brain is four times larger and a whale's seven times larger than a human's, yet their mental ability is less than an orangutan's, whose brain is only one-third as large as a human's. The number of interconnections plus the range of sensitivity and complexity make the human brain a wonder to behold.

Brain cells communicate with each other via electrochemical impulses carried between the synapses by neurotransmitters, which are substances made up of amino acids. The brain communicates with all tissues and cells of the body via neurotransmitters circulating in the bloodstream and generated by nerve extensions throughout the body.

When carried any distance, nerves are sheathed in an off-white insulating covering called *myelin*, which protects the nerves from trauma and chemical erosion and prevents short circuiting of the electric impulse along the way. All along the peripheral nerves (throughout the body) are special cells called *Schwann cells*, which continually maintain the myelin sheath. If the myelin sheath becomes eroded for any reason, nerve function is adversely affected. This is known as *peripheral neuropathy*, such as occurs in diabetic neuropathy, Guillain-Barré syndrome, and multiple sclerosis.

Guess what the ability of the Schwann cell to perform this vital function is a result of? Right—progesterone! In fact, the Schwann cell itself makes progesterone for this function. Recent research shows that anything that interferes with progesterone receptors (e.g., the "morning after" birth control pill, RU-486) in Schwann cells stops the production of protective myelin.

Within the brain, nerve cells in one part of the brain communicate with nerve cells in other parts of the brain and these nerves also need to be protected with myelin sheaths. It is not yet known, but it is likely that here, too, progesterone is needed.

Brain cells communicate with the body in other ways, too. Some brain cells make special neurotransmitters that flow through minute veins to the pituitary to tell the pituitary to make hormones that affect various organs of the body, such as the ovaries, testes, adrenal gland, and thyroid gland. Minute amounts of neurotransmitters also flow through the bloodstream and to the receptors present in all tissues, including white blood cells. There are abundant neurotransmitters in the gut, and as a result gastrointestinal disturbances can affect brain function. The brain is in touch with every part of our body at all times. Not only does the brain tell the body what to do, but it monitors the response (electrolyte balance, hormone production, oxygen levels, nutrients, inflammation, temperature, blood pressure, and so on) to determine what to do next, even during sleep. This is the biofeedback cycle essential for maintaining our optimum health. The sex hormones are major players in this ongoing cycle.

How the Inner and Outer Brains Regulate the Body

We have one brain inside another, and they are different from each other. The outer layer of the brain, which we see in pictures of whole brains, is called the *cortex*. Deep inside the brain, however, is another area of cortex called the *limbic brain*.

Both the outer and inner areas of the brain are subject to learning and conditioning, both require optimal nutrition for best performance, and the sex hormones are important in both.

The outer brain is the one we are conscious of. By means of the outer brain cortex we receive our senses of sight, hearing, and touch; we control our speech, our muscular movements, and voluntary behavior; we make our plans, ponder the future, and grapple with language, grocery bills, mathematics, other symbolic thinking, and much, much more. Different sites within the outer cortex correlate with specific functions that are more or less independent of each other. A lesion in the sight area does not affect our hearing, for example.

The inner, limbic brain is the seat of emotions, our sense of pain, our primary drives (fight, flight, feeding, and sex), involuntary reactions, and all the automatic adjustments necessary for body function, including the immune system. Whereas the outer cortex functions are separated into different anatomical sites, the limbic brain is more interrelated in the sense that all its different functions affect each other. For example, if something frightens us, our pupils will dilate, our mouth goes dry, our muscles tense, blood is diverted away from our stomach and to our muscles, our skin color pales, and we may urinate or defecate involuntarily. Our reaction to stress is a limbic brain function.

As we've already seen, the menstrual cycle occurs as the result of a feedback loop of coordinated messages from the hypothalamus (in the limbic brain), to the pituitary gland, to the ovaries, and back to the hypothalamus. Thus it is natural that stress can affect one's menstrual cycles, too. It is wise therefore to always keep in mind that menstrual irregularity may arise simply from stress.

Estrogen and the Brain

It is the experience of many women that menopause is associated with some depression and that estrogen supplementation can lift one's mood. There is a good explanation for this. Elevated mood occurs when noradrenalin, the form of adrenaline active in brain cells, is raised. This happens, for example, after fairly strenuous exercise or when some pleasant excitement happens. Noradrenalin is inactivated by the enzyme monoamine oxidase (MAO). If, for some reason, MAO is relatively high compared to noradrenalin production, a depressed mood results. Estrogen inhibits MAO and thus raises the mood. (Synthetic progestins, on the other hand, tend to stimulate MAO and thus can lead to a depressed mood.)

Excess estrogen, however, can have a negative effect on mood. This has to do with copper and zinc ratios. Copper and zinc are important cofactors for brain enzymes. Estrogen increases a blood protein, *ceruloplasmin*, which binds to copper and prevents dietary copper from finding its way into brain cells. Too much ceruloplasmin leaves too much copper in the blood, causing zinc levels to drop in the blood and the brain. The result is an imbalance that leads to exaggerated stress reactions, serious mood swings, and depression. (Sounds like PMS, doesn't it?)

Excess estrogen has several other effects that can adversely affect the brain. Estrogen tends to make blood more likely to clot. In the Nurses' Questionnaire Study, for example, the relative risk of ischemic stroke (blockage of blood vessels by clots) mortality among estrogen users compared to non-estrogen-using nurses was 46 percent greater after adjustment for age and other risk factors. That is, the risk of dying from an ischemic (more generally called thromboembolic) stroke was 46 percent higher among the estrogen-using nurses.

As a compensatory effect for its increased clotting risk, estrogen promotes blood vessel dilation. This, along with estrogen's water retention effect, explains why estrogen can induce migraine headaches in women. Cyclical migraine attacks (usually just preceding menstruation) are classic symptoms of estrogen dominance. Fortunately, progesterone promotes normal vascular tone and thus can prevent migraine. Again, hormone balance is the key.

Estrogen also tends to suppress thyroid gland function. Women who have estrogen dominance are often diagnosed with hypothyroidism despite normal levels of T3 and T4 in blood tests. The metabolic rate of all cells is dependent on thyroid hormone function, and brain cells are no exception. The impact of low thyroid on the brain is multidimensional.

One of the major brain neurotransmitters is a substance known as GABA (gamma-aminobutyric acid), the function of which is to "tune down" cell excitability. The production of GABA is related to cell metabolism; the lower the metabolic rate, the less GABA is formed. When estrogen interferes with thyroid production and slows the metabolism of brain cells, it indirectly decreases GABA production and increases brain cell excitability, a factor in epilepsy.

Further, the respiratory enzymes of cells are thyroid-dependent. When thyroid function is low, cellular oxygen is low (cellular hypoxia). Thus estrogen-induced thyroid interference contributes to less-than-optimal brain function. Cell oxygen is, fortunately, enhanced by vitamin E and progesterone. This is probably the primary explanation for the increased mental acuity in many elderly women with signs of senility when they begin using progesterone.

The makers of HRT have reported claims of sharper brain function in older women receiving hormone replacement therapy (HRT), and the presumption was made that this was due to estrogen. The more likely reason is that the women seeking HRT were of a higher socioeconomic class with better diets, more years of education, and more favorable access to medical care, with a greater likelihood of having received thyroid supplements and vitamin E than the control group.

Progesterone and the Brain

Progesterone, like other fat-soluble compounds, is found in brain cells. What is surprising is that its concentration in brain cells is 20 times higher than blood serum levels. The same is true of testosterone and DHEA. It is fair, I believe, to infer that brain cells do this for a purpose. Let's look at some of the evidence for progesterone's effect in the brain.

Progesterone and Fetal Brain Development

Progesterone appears to play a critical role in fetal brain development. During pregnancy, placental production of progesterone increases from 20 milligrams a day to over 350 milligrams a day during the last trimester. This is a phenomenal level of hormone. Progesterone promotes metabolism of maternal fat for energy and maintains stable blood glucose, both of which support fetal growth and development, especially of the brain. The brain requires approximately three times more energy than other body tissues. The brain of neonates is proportionately much larger relative to the body than it is in adults. Thus energy requirements for the brain of a neonate are especially crucial.

In this regard, Dr. Katherina Dalton has reported that babies of mothers who received natural progesterone showed greatly improved intelligence. Ray Peat, Ph.D., in his book *Progesterone in Orthomolecular Medicine*, published in 1993, reports, "Other investigators find that progesterone babies have strong, serene, independent characters." It is quite likely that, in addition to the improved cellular energy and stable glucose levels, progesterone has specific beneficial effects on brain cell maturation through mechanisms yet unknown. This in itself is not surprising. Spina bifida (incomplete closure of the lower end of the spinal cord) can be largely prevented by small but adequate doses of folic acid, and the mechanism of action is also unknown at this time.

Progesterone and Brain Injuries

Progesterone can reduce the severity of brain injuries. In an experiment by Emory University Professor Donald Stein and colleagues, deliberate laboratory-induced head trauma to rodents resulted in reduced mortality and more rapid recovery of function among females compared to males. When male animals were given estrogen, no survival or recovery advantage was found. In fact, postmortem examinations revealed that cerebral (brain) contusions and edema were killing neurons far beyond the site of the original injury. When male animals were given progesterone, however, their survival and recovery rates corresponded to that of female rats. Stein and his colleagues have begun researching the effects of progesterone on human patients coming into selected emergency rooms with brain injuries.

In other work on progesterone and the degeneration of nerves in spinal cord injury, researchers used a unique strain of mutant mice that have degeneration of the spinal cord. A 20-mg progesterone pellet implanted in some of the mice for 15 days created substantial positive change in the nervous system, both at the cell level and at the level of physical functioning, including enhanced grip strength and prolonged survival at the end of the 15-day observation period. The researchers concluded that their results "suggest a new and important role for this hormone in the prevention of spinal cord neurodegenerative disorders."

Even though rats are not necessarily the same as humans, if I suffered a head injury I hope someone would give me a good dose of natural progesterone.

Progesterone and the Elderly

"Doctor, I can think again!" I have heard this so often from patients after they have started progesterone therapy that I now regard it as routine. A writer got back to the book she was writing. Another woman resumed her painting. Others are just happy to be able to deal with letter writing and checkbook balancing. When progesterone is supplemented in anovulatory premenopausal or postmenopausal women, mental clarity and concentration ("focusing") improves. Many families have told me of elderly female relatives languishing in nursing homes. After progesterone therapy is started, the family reports being surprised at the improved mental clarity and attitudes they observed. I was paid a visit by Dr. George Moraes, a gerontologist from São Paulo, Brazil. He told me of his 91-year-old mother, who had been consigned to a nursing home because of weakness and senility. After Dr. Moraes had given her progesterone cream for her dry, fragile skin and osteoporosis, he was surprised on his next visit to see her improved cognitive, conversational, and socializing abilities—skills that had deteriorated in the preceding years.

Obviously, more research is needed. It would be interesting to test progesterone and other hormones (estrogen, testosterone, cortisol, and DHEA) levels in women with and without Alzheimer's disease. Since estrogen dominance and early follicle failure are common in the United States, it is tempting to speculate that progesterone deficiency is a factor in premature brain deterioration.

Progesterone and Libido

Libido, or sex drive, though mediated by sex hormones, is really a brain function. Specific areas of the brain have been identified in mice, rats, and hamsters as essential for sexual receptivity and mounting behavior. When one or another of these areas is experimentally destroyed, sexual behavior is lost, regardless of hormone levels. In female hamsters with their ovaries removed, estrogen alone is insufficient to restore sexual receptivity; progesterone is required. The inference is that low doses of estrogen "prime" the brain cells but progesterone "turns on" the sex drive.

In male rats, pharmacologic (large) dosages of progesterone inhibit sexual behavior but physiologic (similar to what the body would naturally produce) doses appear to have an opposite effect, stimulating male copulatory behavior. Here we learn that a hormone usually considered to be a female hormone also works in males.

Admittedly, rats and hamsters are not human, and human sexuality is modified by numerous social, behavioral, and other factors. However, the underlying primary sexual drive in all mammals surely emanates from brain centers mediated by sex hormones. The effect of progesterone on human libido has been largely ignored in mainstream medical research. The common "wisdom" is that estrogen is the primary sex drive hormone in women. The experience of my progesterone patients, however, does not bear this out. Their flagging libido returned only when progesterone was added. Testosterone also plays a role in restoring libido.

Postpartum Blues

Many women experience depression in the days (and weeks) following childbirth. Other symptoms include headache, irritability, and sleeplessness. The depression can be incapacitating and prolonged. Research by Brian Harris and colleagues in Wales found that among 120 women, those with the highest prenatal and lowest postnatal progesterone levels also scored highest on measures of postpartum depression scores.

Recall that as pregnancy advances, placental production of progesterone rises to levels of 350 to 400 milligrams a day, and the ovaries' contribution at that point is nil. With delivery, the placenta-derived progesterone is suddenly gone. The only source of progesterone at that time would be the adrenal glands. It is possible that adrenal exhaustion plays a role in a woman's inability to provide even a modicum of progesterone in the days following childbirth. Postpartum depression is notoriously difficult to treat. It would seem appropriate to measure progesterone levels a day or two after childbirth and, if found to be low, progesterone could be promptly supplemented. It is possible that this simple and safe therapy could make postpartum depression much easier to treat. For more detailed information on nutrition, hormones, and postpartum depression, please read the excellent book, *A Natural Guide to Pregnancy and Postpartum Health* (Raffelock, Roundtree, Avery, 2002).

Progesterone and Sleep Patterns

Many of my patients have volunteered that the first benefit they perceived from using natural progesterone was an improved sleep pattern. After years of unsettled sleep they now look forward to retiring each night because they know they will enjoy sound sleep and awake refreshed in the morning. This is one of the reasons I tend to recommend that progesterone cream be applied at bedtime.

Research concerning progesterone's role in brain cell function is still in its infancy. It is likely that as research progresses more discoveries of progesterone's benefits will emerge.

CHAPTER 9

WHAT ARE ANDROGENS?

Androgens are a class of hormones that include androstenedione, testosterone, and dihydrotestosterone (DHT). Although dehydroepiandrosterone (DHEA) isn't, strictly speaking, an androgen, in a woman's body it can be quickly converted to androstenedione and testosterone, so it will be included as an androgen in this chapter. Androgens are commonly thought of as the "male hormones," because they can have masculinizing effects, but they also play an important role in female health. Women make smaller amounts of androgens than men do so they don't normally have the masculine traits of baldness, whiskers on the face, or a deep voice. The androgens bring many positive effects to a woman's body, and you'll find out more about those in this chapter.

Of the androgens made in a woman's body, about half are made in the adrenal glands, and the remaining half are made in the ovaries. When a woman has a "total" hysterectomy (both her uterus and ovaries are removed), her testosterone and DHEA levels usually drop to half of what is normal. Along with progesterone, the androgens are the most neglected hormone following total hysterectomy. Most women are given only unopposed estrogens despite estrogen dominance symptoms, and clear androgen deficiency symptoms. The most common symptoms of low androgens following removal of the ovaries are low libido, depression, memory lapses, bone loss, vaginal dryness, and incontinence.

Androgens are also very important for the health of the skin. The cells of the skin (dermis), hair follicles, and sebaceous glands (glands that produce oils that lubricate the skin), contain high levels of androgen receptors. When androgens bind to them this stimulates the skin cells to divide and thicken, hair to thicken, and more oil to be produced. Because men produce more androgens, they have thicker skin, more facial and body hair, and are more prone to acne. Women who suffer from poly-cystic ovary syndrome (PCOS) produce excessive amounts of androgens and have more facial/body hair, acne, and oily skin. These women generally tend to have greater muscle mass and are stronger.

There are many conjugates, or subcategories of androgens that are intermediaries in the process of becoming one major steroid hormone or another, and although they don't have direct activity on cells, they circulate in the blood in higher amounts than testosterone does. These conjugates are one of the body's many systems designed to keep the steroid hormones in balance. Many of the androgens are conjugated in the liver, so impaired liver function (caused for example by taking multiple prescrip-tion drugs) can create an androgen imbalance.

Enzymes (referred to as aromatases), which are present in fat tissues, can convert the androgens to estrogens. This is why women with more body fat have higher estrogen levels even after menopause when the ovaries reduce their production of es-trogens. The majority of women in industrialized cultures have enough estrogen even after menopause; they have more than enough fat cells to make enough estrogen.

Androgens are important in women as intermediaries in the production of estrogen. In other words, the body makes choles-terol, which is converted to pregnenolone, which is converted to DHEA and progesterone, which are converted to androgens, which are then converted to estrogens. The estrogens are at the bottom of the steroid hormone cascade, and this makes the proper balance of androgens essential to the proper balance of estrogen.

If something biochemically interferes with the conversion of androstenedione to estrogen, it may cause symptoms of andro-gen excess, such as hair growth on the face, hair loss on the head, and acne. These symptoms also appear as a symptom of poly-cystic ovary syndrome (PCOS).

The effects of the androgens begin in the womb. All fetuses

begin life as a female, and then when the Y chromosome sends out instructions to make androgens, the development of male physiology begins to take place. There are two phases of androgen production in boys: *adrenarche*, when the adrenals begin production of DHEA, and *puberty*, when the testes begin production of testosterone. Boys and girls begin adrenarche at about the same time. Boys produce only slightly more DHEA than girls. At puberty, a boy's testicles begin to produce more testosterone and DHT, while a girl's ovaries begin the cyclic production of estrogens and progesterone. The higher androgens produced by boys promotes the characteristic male facial and body hair, thickening of whiskers, more muscle, and a deepening voice.

In girls, estrogens suppress the expression of androgen receptors in the skin, hair follicles, and sebaceous glands, preventing androgen expression so commonly seen in young boys as they transition through puberty. Progesterone produced by the ovaries also plays an important role in curbing excessive growth of facial hair and acne in young women by blocking the conversion of testosterone to DHT (dihydrotestosterone, the most potent form of a natural androgen). Testosterone must be converted to DHT directly within the cells of the skin, hair follicle, or sebaceous gland before it can activate the androgen receptor in these cells. This conversion of testosterone to DHT is carried out by the enzyme 5-alpha reductase. Progesterone occupies the testosterone binding site of 5-alpha reductase, preventing it from binding testosterone and converting it to the more potent DHT.

Androgens have what are known as anabolic effects, causing the growth of muscle, bone, and organs. The more muscle mass you have—whether you're a man or a woman—the more androgens your body will produce, and vice versa: The more androgens your body produces the more muscle mass you'll have. This is why both male and female professional athletes dose themselves with androgenic hormones, because in many sports, more muscle mass means better performance.

Women who develop symptoms of androgen dominance such as thinning hair on the head, heavier hair growth above the lip and a prominent belly, may be lacking in the enzymes or enzyme cofactors (usually vitamins and minerals) necessary to convert androstenedione to estrogen. Androgen dominance can also be caused by eating too much sugar and refined carbohydrates, which chronically raise insulin levels. This is increasingly common in teenage girls.

DHEA

Dehydroepiandrosterone (DHEA) is a steroid hormone just like estrogens and progesterone. It's made in the adrenal glands, which make over 150 different hormones. Estrogens and testosterone are made primarily from DHEA, and to a lesser extent progesterone, throughout the body. The amount of DHEA made in our bodies is greater than any other of the steroid hormones. Ninety-five percent of the body's DHEA circulates in the blood joined to sulfur molecules (DHEAS), serving as a reserve that can easily be converted back into the active form. DHEAS is the primary source of androgen precursor for testosterone and DHT, but it apparently also has an important role in maintaining a healthy immune system independent of its role as an androgen precursor. We know that DHEA is important for the maintenance of health, but we don't yet have a complete understanding of its specific actions.

Between the ages of 20 and 25, DHEA production peaks. Men produce more than women, but both sexes make about 2 percent less every year after the age of 25. By the time a woman reaches her mid to late 40s, DHEA levels can be quite low, particularly in individuals whose adrenals have been exhausted from stress.

The onset of diseases like cancer, heart disease, allergies, diabetes, and autoimmune diseases correlate with this gradual drop in DHEA levels. We don't know yet if this means that lower DHEA levels play a causal role in these diseases, or if lower DHEA levels are a biomarker for aging in the same sense that gray hair and bifocals are. We do know that in elderly people, higher levels of DHEA mean better health and longer life span.

Many feel that DHEA replacement actually takes years off their chronological ages. There is also evidence that adequate DHEA levels help protect against osteoporosis, which is likely through its conversion to estrogens and androgens, both of which are important for healthy bones.

Before taking DHEA supplements, you should first check both DHEA (or DHEAS) and cortisol levels. If cortisol is low, DHEA supplementation may not be as effective and may make an already low blood sugar (hypoglycemia caused by low cortisol) worse. If your cortisol is low, you need to consider lifestyle modifications (more sleep and laughter, less stress), better diet (more protein, less sugar), supplemental nutrients (particularly vitamins C and B5 [pantothenic acid]), and herbs (e.g., licorice), all of which help the adrenals produce more cortisol.

If your cortisol is normal, you're over 40, and you are interested in possibly supplementing DHEA, ask your doctor to do a blood or saliva test to measure your DHEA-S (the sulfur-bound form) levels. The normal blood range for women between the ages of 40 and 50 is 400 to 2,500 ng/ml; for women over 50, it falls to 200 to 1,500 ng/ml. Those are pretty big ranges. If yours fall in or below the low half of the range, and you are generally fatigued and have worked to balance your other hormones, diet, and stress levels, you might want to give DHEA a try. Please turn to Chapter 20 for more details on supplementing DHEA.

Testosterone

Women make about a tenth as much testosterone as men. The adrenal glands and the ovaries are responsible for maintaining adequate testosterone levels in women. Testosterone gradually declines with age, with the steepest decline around the time of menopause. Testosterone levels of a perimenopausal woman tend to be about half of a woman in her early 20s. However, after menopause the ovaries continue to produce both testosterone and androstenedione.

Testosterone is one of the hormones responsible for maintaining libido, or sex drive, in a woman. Falling levels of testosterone around the time of menopause may result in a falling libido, although lack of sex drive is more commonly caused by estrogen dominance and associated thyroid deficiency. Studies of hormone replacement in women have shown that adding a low dose of natural testosterone can sometimes enhance the positive effects of other hormones and restore libido. The other side of this coin is that in many cases, as the ovaries wind down, women show signs of becoming more *androgen* (male hormone) dominant rather than estrogen dominant, and testosterone will only exaggerate that process.

Higher androgen production can occur in some menopausal women due to increased production by the ovarian stroma. The ovarian follicles no longer cyclically produce estrogens and progesterone, and the ovarian stroma begins to produce androgens in response to the increased levels of LH that occur at menopause. Facial hair and male-type pattern baldness are indicative of this shift. This can happen in premenopausal, estrogen-dominant women as well, because testosterone clearance from the body is partly controlled by the balance between estrogen and progesterone. Excess estrogen decreases testosterone clearance and natural progesterone enhances it. (For those who are interested in biochemistry, this is because progesterone suppresses estrogen-induced SHBG, which would increase testosterone bioavailability, yet it also reverses androgenic changes because it blocks, via inhibition of 5-alpha reductase, testosterone conversion to the more potent DHT.)

Please see Chapter 20 for details on supplementing testosterone.

Androstenedione

This steroid hormone is a precursor to testosterone and estrogens, and it can theoretically act as a DHEA precursor. Secreted from the adrenals and the ovaries into the circulation, it has its own jobs to do before being converted into other hormones. In older women androstenedione travels from the ovaries to the fat cells, where it is converted to estrogen.

Androstenedione is a popular supplement for bodybuilders, who use it to boost their testosterone levels, increasing muscle mass and decreasing the length of time needed to recover from hard workouts. Many of the positive effects of supplemental testosterone—including enhanced energy, libido, and sense of well-being—have also been attributed to androstenedione, and this is due to its conversion to testosterone.

Androstenedione may also be involved in maintaining the strength of bones because it's converted to testosterone, which helps build muscles and bone, and to estradiol, which helps slow bone loss.

CHAPTER 10

HORMONE BALANCE AND THE MENSTRUAL CYCLE

The human menstrual cycle has been the subject of scientific investigation since the 1890s. The word *menstrual* comes from the Greek word for "month," which itself was derived from earlier roots meaning "moon," or the period of time of the waxing and waning of one new moon to the next. Despite a century of study, full understanding of the menstrual cycle eludes us. The workings of nature surpass our current levels of understanding.

Let's briefly review the menstrual cycle again. The hallmark of menstruation is the monthly vaginal flow of blood. From puberty to menopause, the female uterus prepares a specially thickened and blood-filled lining in preparation for a possible pregnancy. This lining is shed if fertilization of the egg does not occur in a timely fashion, and the preparation of the lining begins anew. The cycle of uterine preparation and shedding occurs at approximately monthly intervals. We know that this uterine cycle is under the control of ovarian-secreted hormones, namely estrogen and progesterone.

Estrogen dominates the first week or so after menstruation, starting the endometrial buildup as the ovarian follicles (the sacs that hold and mature the eggs) are stimulated to begin the development of an egg. In addition, estrogen causes an increase in vaginal mucus, making it more tolerant of male penetration during sexual activity, as well as increased secretion of the glands of the cervix, making it more hospitable to sperm.

About 12 days after the beginning of the previous menses, the rising estrogen (primarily estradiol) level peaks and then tapers off just as the follicle matures and just before ovulation.

When the egg has been released from the follicle, the follicle then becomes the corpus luteum ("yellow body" in Latin), so named because the follicle that produced the egg appears as a small yellow body on the surface of the ovary. The corpus luteum is the site of progesterone production, which dominates the second half of the menstrual month, reaching a peak of about 20 milligrams per day. Progesterone production during the luteal phase of the cycle (days 12 to 26 of the menstrual cycle) leads to the maturing or ripening phase of the development of the thickened and blood-filled uterine lining, called the secretory endometrium, in anticipation of a possible fertilized egg. In addition, progesterone influences the cervical glands, causing the secretions to change from watery to sticky, much like an uncooked egg white. (Allowing cervical mucus or saliva to dry on a glass slide will allow the appearance of a "ferning" pattern during progesterone dominance, which is not seen during the time of estrogen dominance.)

The rise of progesterone at the time of ovulation also causes a rise in body temperature of about 1 degree Fahrenheit, a finding often used to indicate ovulation. If pregnancy does not occur within 10 to 15 days after ovulation, estrogen and progesterone levels fall abruptly, triggering the shedding of the accumulated secretory endometrium and the menstrual flow of blood. If pregnancy occurs, progesterone production increases, and this shedding of endometrium is prevented, thus preserving the developing embryo. As pregnancy progresses, progesterone production is taken over by the placenta, and its secretion gradually increases to levels of 300 to 400 milligrams per day during the third trimester.

The Rise and Fall of Hormone Levels

Thus the monthly rise and fall of estrogen and progesterone levels explain the events of menstruation. But what determines the synchronous cycling of these two hormones? The answer is found in two hormones secreted by the anterior pituitary gland in the brain: the gonadotropic hormone follicle-stimulating hormone (FSH) and luteinizing hormone (LH). Simply put, FSH drives the ovary to make estrogen, promotes maturation of the follicle, and, at the same time, sensitizes the follicle receptors to LH. Meanwhile, LH rises a day or two before ovulation, triggering ovulation, and then falls dramatically as the corpus luteum starts turning out progesterone.

Now the question becomes: What determines the marvelous synchrony of FSH and LH? The answer lies in the hypothalamus within the limbic brain, a primitive but remarkably complex and sensitive control system. The hypothalamus is situated immediately above the pituitary, where it monitors not only the levels of estrogen and progesterone, but also the various body effects they are creating and, with exquisite timing, produces and sends to the pituitary (via special vein-like channels) a hormone made of ten linked amino acids called gonadotropin-releasing hormone (GnRH), which is responsible for the release of either or both of the gonadotropins, FSH and LH. At the present, it is not known how a single hypothalamic hormone can control both FSH and LH.

The reproductive hormone cycle just described is pictured in Figure 6.

Another illustration of the hormone changes during a normal menstrual cycle is depicted in Figure 7.

As might be imagined, the complete mechanism of the action of this vital nucleus within the hypothalamus is beyond present knowledge. It might help, however, to realize that the limbic brain, of which the hypothalamus is a part, is a biofeedback information and control center, with multiple neural centers sharing and integrating myriad biochemical, hormonal, immunologic, and emotional conditions. It functions as a giant analog computer complex with the capacity to formulate and send signals to the pituitary, as well as to control our autonomic nervous system balance and immunomodulators, and create for us our sense of emotions and their physiologic responses. When all this is grasped sufficiently, it is no wonder that menstruation (and a great number of other things) can be affected by emotional states of mind, stress, diet, other hormones (e.g., thyroid), illness, or drugs of all sorts.

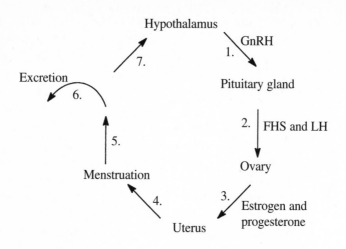

Figure 6:

1. *Low levels of estrogen and progesterone stimulate the hypothalamus to send* gonadotropin-releasing hormone *(GnRH) to the pituitary.*

2. *Stimulated by GnRH, the pituitary sends* follicle-stimulating hormone *(FSH) to the ovary, which initiates the maturation of ova in follicles and the production of estrogen. In about 10 days, the high estrogen level signals the pituitary production of* luteinizing hormone *(LH), which promotes ovulation.*

3. *The maturing ovarian follicles produce* estrogen, *which promotes proliferation of endometrial cells. After ovulation, the follicle (now the corpus luteum) produces* progesterone, *which becomes the dominant gonadal hormone during the second half of the cycle and converts the proliferative endometrium into the secretory endometrium.*

4. *If pregnancy does not occur, the corpus luteum involutes and the production of both estrogen and progesterone falls, a signal for the shedding of the endometrium, i.e., menstruation.*

5, 6. *Serum levels of estrogen and progesterone fall as they are metabolized and excreted from the body via the liver (bile) and urine.*

7. *The fall of estrogen and progesterone is detected by the hypothalamus, which then initiates another round of GnRH, starting another cycle.*

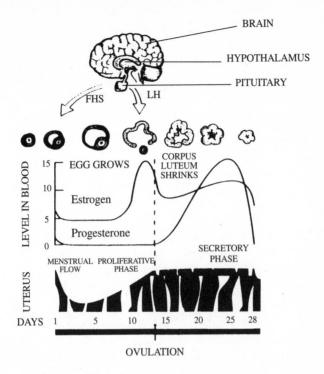

Figure 7: Normal menstrual cycle. (Reprinted with permission from Kate Neil, Balancing Hormones Naturally *[London: ION Press, 1994]).*

Clearly, this is a delicate system that is best not tampered with unless there's a good reason to do so. Yet this system is profoundly affected when synthetic progestins are prescribed in birth control pills and patches, or in conventional HRT. When the various pituitary and hypothalamic gonadal hormone receptors are filled with synthetically altered hormones, as in contraceptive pills and HRT, the net result is inhibition of one's natural hormones. In the past, some of these drugs resulted in permanent loss of ovary function (amenorrhea), with often tragic consequences for the women who had used them. The long lists of potential side effects for each and every one of the progestins does not seem to deter their use. The confusion wrought within the hypothalamus by the absence of the true hormones will reverberate throughout the province of this remarkable limbic center, with effects that are bound *not* to be recognized by one's physician. Limbic system imbalance can lead to decreased immune response, decreased adrenal response, sleep disorders, peptic ulcers, depression, anxiety, panic, rage, learning disorders, and hormone disorders.

Anovulatory Cycles

There is also the problem of anovulatory cycles, or cycles in which premenopausal women do not ovulate even though they continue to menstruate. This is known to occur in women athletes undergoing strenuous physical training, who may stop menstruating altogether. Anovulatory cycles also occur in nonexercising women, as is becoming evident through the many doctors such as myself who have tested progesterone levels in women. For example, Dr. Peter Ellison of Harvard University tested salivary hormone levels in 18 regularly cycling, sexually active women, average age 29, and found that 7 of them were not ovulating. I believe anovulatory cycles are epidemic among women in the industrialized countries. While factors such as nutrition, stress, and overexercising may be implicated, the most important factor for anovulatory cycles is most likely to be our xenoestrogen exposure. Without ovulation, no corpus luteum results, no progesterone is made, and the result is estrogen dominance. The graph in Figure 8 depicts hormone levels during anovulatory periods when no progesterone is produced.

Several problems can result from anovulatory cycles. One is the monthlong presence of unopposed estrogen with all its attendant side effects, including the syndrome known as PMS. Another is the present, generally unrecognized problem of progesterone's role in osteoporosis. Contemporary medicine is still unaware that progesterone stimulates new bone formation. A third is the interrelationship between progesterone loss and stress. Stress influences limbic brain function, including the

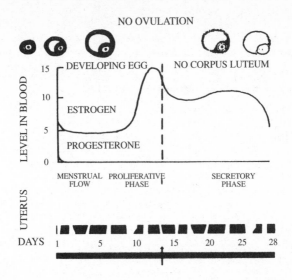

Figure 8: Hormone levels during an anovulatory menstrual cycle. (Reprinted with permission from Kate Neil, Balancing Hormones Naturally *[London: ION Press, 1994]).*

functioning of the hypothalamus. In brief, stress (and a bad diet) can also induce anovulatory cycles. The consequent lack of progesterone interferes with adrenal corticosteroid production by which one normally responds to stress. The effects of stress are therefore heightened, predisposing one to anovulatory cycles, creating the ultimate vicious cycle.

It should be obvious that hormone balance cannot be achieved if doctors continue to ignore the problem of progesterone deficiency. Since progesterone levels are rarely measured, most doctors are unaware that their menstruating patients may be deficient in progesterone. Adding estrogen and tranquilizers will not solve their problems.

An equally obvious corollary is that we must decrease our exposure to xenoestrogens. This requires several steps: (1) increased education on the dangers and sources of xenoestrogens; (2) decreased use of xenoestrogens such as petrochemical pesticides, PCB plastics, and some volatile solvents; and (3) learning to eat foods that not only have a lower load of petrochemical xe-noestrogens but are good sources of phytoestrogens, the benign, weakly acting estrogenic compounds from plants that will compete at the receptor sites, and help protect us from the more toxic petrochemical estrogenic compounds.

PART II

HORMONE BALANCE AND ILLNESS

CHAPTER 11

PROGESTERONE AND MENOPAUSE SYMPTOMS

This should have been the easiest chapter to write. After all, menopause symptoms are the defining characteristic of the menopause "problem." Yet much mystery prevails. Not all women passing through menopause have any of the usual panoply of symptoms, and the characteristic symptoms that some U.S. women and women in industrialized countries have are rare in Third World cultures. Though solid statistics are hard to validate, medical authorities teach that about 50 percent of women in the United States experience some degree of hot flashes during menopause, and only 15 percent seek medical treatment for them. Yet all women who go through menopause experience a drop in estrogen. Why do only some of them experience menopausal symptoms? Why don't menopausal women in other cultures experience these symptoms?

Early in my career, when I still felt assured of the medical education I had received and before I knew anything about natural progesterone, I was visited by a patient who first brought home to me the inadequacy of mainstream medical treatments. She was a 62-year-old lady with persistent, quite severe hot flashes despite years of estrogen replacement therapy. She could tolerate the hot flashes but, as she apologetically explained, she was worried about the loss of libido, her inability to lose weight, and the thinning of her scalp hair. She was overweight and aware that the more estrogen she took the fatter she got and the more water she retained.

My medical examination and laboratory workup found nothing abnormal. In my naïveté, I thought I would be able to help her. I put her on my favorite low-fat, low-sugar diet, added small doses of essential vitamin and mineral supplements, and tried manipulating her estrogen supplements to avoid water retention and fat buildup. Nothing I did helped her. With estrogen she had normal vaginal lubrication, but she still had hot flashes and her libido was just not there.

But failure is often a better instructor than success. Although I unfortunately wasn't much help to this patient, *she* was a help to *me*. In my attempt to unravel this knotty problem, I came to learn four important lessons:

1. Not all women with hot flashes are helped by supplemental estrogen.
2. Fat increases estrogen levels in postmenopausal women.
3. Fatter postmenopausal women generally have higher estrogen levels than thinner women.
4. Postmenopausal women with normal estrogen levels can suffer hot flashes.

Something more than estrogen deficiency is going on.

Let us look again at the symptoms associated with menopause for some women. Such a list would include:

hot flashes
vaginal dryness and atrophy
water retention
fat and weight gain, especially in the hips, thighs, and abdomen
sleep disturbances (insomnia, less REM-time sleep)
decreased libido
mood swings—depression, irritability
headaches, fatigue
short-term memory lapses, lack of concentration
dry, thin, wrinkly skin
thinning of scalp hair, some increase of facial hair
bone mineral loss (osteoporosis)
diffuse body aches and pains

The Mystery of Menopause

I know this will sound implausible, but the truth is that we don't really fully understand what happens during menopause and precisely why the menstrual cycle winds down. The prevailing medical view of menopause is that when a woman runs out of eggs, she stops menstruating and goes into menopause. Strangely enough, however, this is largely theory. The prevailing theory goes that a woman is born with all her follicles (from which eggs can be matured) already formed. Of the millions of follicles present before birth, about 300,000 are present at puberty. With every menstrual cycle, even those cycles when ovulation is suppressed by birth control hormones, hundreds of eggs vanish. When only about 1,000 eggs are left, ovulation rarely occurs, even though estrogen production may remain adequate for menstruation. Thus such women continue menstruating and are in a state of estrogen dominance. In other words, loss of fertility is due to the disappearance of follicles and their eggs rather than age per se.

The cause or causes of actual menopause are still unclear. In some women, the hypothalamus stops producing GnRH—presumably a genetically programmed change—whereas in many others, GnRH and the pituitary hormones, FSH and LH, continue being produced at regular levels and yet the ovaries do not or cannot respond. This latter situation is the one in which hot flashes are more likely to occur. The ovary is the weak link in the cycle of events. Although poor nutrition and stress have traditionally been blamed, the more likely cause is xenoestrogen-caused ovarian dysfunction, a circumstance not anticipated by Mother Nature.

Fertility is also a function of the number of mature eggs a woman produces each month. Regardless of how many times a couple has sexual intercourse, the monthly probability of a 38-year-old woman conceiving is only about one-fourth that in a woman under age 30 because she is releasing fewer eggs or none at all.

The incidence of birth defects also rises as women and men

age, although the exact mechanism of how this happens is not clearly understood.

A Brief Look at Premenopause

Menopausal symptoms may begin as much as a decade before menstruation stops altogether. This is due to the increasing numbers of women who are having anovulatory (nonovulating) cycles beginning in their mid-30s. When this happens, they may menstruate but not ovulate. As we have seen, most progesterone is produced by the corpus luteum, itself formed at the time of ovulation. If there is no ovulation, progesterone levels drop dramatically. If there is too little progesterone, then estrogen dominates the hormonal environment. Anovulatory cycles may be regular or irregular, though often a woman notices that her menstrual flow is different, usually heavier or longer.

Low premenopausal progesterone caused by anovulatory cycles may lead to estrogen dominance prior to menopause. It is interesting to note that the most common age for the initial stages of breast or uterine cancer is five years or more *before* menopause, well before estrogen levels fall, but coinciding with a drop in progesterone.

To address the many health issues that can occur in the 10 to 15 years before menopause, I have coauthored a book titled *What Your Doctor May* Not *Tell You About Premenopause* (1998, Warner Books). In it you will find detailed information about PMS, cervical hyperplasia, fibroids, endometriosis, oral contraceptives, and much more.

Falling Estrogen and Progesterone, Rising GnRH, and Hot Flashes

Around age 45 to 50, sometimes a little earlier or later, estrogen levels begin to fall. When they fall below the levels necessary to signal the uterine lining to thicken and gather blood, the menstrual flow becomes less and/or irregular, eventually stopping altogether.

Let's zero in and take a closer look at hot flashes, the hallmark of menopausal symptoms. The prevailing explanation for hot flashes is as follows: Recall that an area (which we'll call the GnRH center) in the brain's hypothalamus monitors estrogen and progesterone levels. When levels fall, this center makes GnRH, which stimulates the pituitary to make hormones (FSH and LH), which in turn result in the ovarian production of estrogen and progesterone. The rise in these hormones inhibits further production of GnRH. At menopause, estrogen levels fall and progesterone levels are usually already low. The ovaries no longer respond to the FSH and LH prompt.

When a woman's ovaries *don't* respond to the FSH and LH signals by ovulating, the hormone signaling system can go awry. In effect, the hypothalamus begins "shouting," trying to tell the pituitary to tell the ovaries to ovulate. The inability of the ovaries to respond is most likely due to a final depletion of eggs and their surrounding follicle cells. This overactivity of the hypothalamus and pituitary signal begins affecting adjacent areas of the brain, which we'll call the vasomotor center (specifically the arcuate nucleus of the hypothalamus that controls capillary dilation and sweating mechanisms), and these are the women who get hot flashes and night sweats. In addition to hot flashes, the heightened activity of the hypothalamus can cause mood swings, fatigue, feelings of being cold, and inappropriate responses to other stressors. Many women will have symptoms of hypothyroidism despite normal thyroid hormone levels.

In a nutshell:

1. The GnRH center effectively signals to increase estrogen and progesterone synthesis.
2. Elevated estrogen and progesterone inhibit GnRH release.
3. After menopause, the ovaries no longer make estrogen and progesterone.
4. Lack of estrogen and progesterone response results in increased activity of the GnRH center.

5. Heightened GnRH activity activates the vasomotor center, causing hot flashes and perspiration.

It is important to recognize that the GnRH center monitors
both estrogen and progesterone. Thus, since the postmenopausal woman continues to make estrogen in respectable
levels and makes little or no progesterone, hot flashes may well
respond to progesterone supplementation alone. Hot flashes
will also respond to much smaller doses of supplemental estrogen when progesterone is added. Even synthetic progestins like
Provera (medroxyprogesterone acetate) or Megace (megestrol
acetate) have been found effective in treating hot flashes, further
indicating that estrogen per se is not the only factor in hot
flashes.

The truth is that estrogen is only one part of the menopause
picture and is certainly not a cure-all. In fact, these days I hear
more complaints about the side effects of taking estrogen than I
do about menopausal symptoms.

Progesterone Deficiency

If so much of a woman's health depends on a consistent level of
progesterone, why does progesterone deficiency occur at
menopause in Western societies? Did Mother Nature make a
mistake? Mother Nature did not make the mistake; we did.
Many plants (over 5,000 known) make sterols that have
progestogenic effects. In nonindustrialized cultures not subjected to xenoestrogens and whose diets are rich in fresh vegetables of all sorts, progesterone deficiency is rare. Not only do the
majority of women in these cultures have healthy ovaries with
healthy follicles producing sufficient progesterone, but at
menopause their diets provide sufficient progestogenic substances to keep their sex drive high, their bones strong, and their
passage through menopause uneventful and symptom-free.

Our food supply system uses many processed foods and foods
that are picked days before being sold. Their vitamin (especially
vitamin C) content and their sterol levels fall. We do not receive

the progestogenic substances our forebears did. A *Lancet* article reported that the bone mineral density of skeletons from a church in England dating back to 1729 showed better bones at all ages compared with our skeletons of today. It is likely that both exercise and diet had something to do with that.

A drop in progesterone can cause a concurrent drop in corticosteroid production, leading to a whole other set of symptoms. As you can see in Figure 9 on page 133, progesterone is a major precursor of the important corticosteroid hormones aldosterone and cortisol, made in the adrenal cortex. These corticosteroids are not made via any other hormone pathway. They are responsible for mineral balance, sugar control, and response to stresses of all sorts, including trauma, inflammation, and emotional stress. A lack of corticosteroids can lead to fatigue, immune dysfunction, hypoglycemia, allergies, and arthritis. Not infrequently, progesterone supplementation effectively resolves these problems.

The adrenal cortex is also capable of making progesterone, principally for its precursor role in making corticosteroids, but many women are so stressed out trying to work, raise children, and be wives that by the time they're in their mid- to late 30s or early 40s their adrenal glands have nothing left to give. My guess is that when Western women stop making progesterone in their ovaries and their adrenal cortex and brain need to pick up 100 percent of that function to produce corticosteroids, there isn't much progesterone left over for other functions, such as balancing estrogen levels. The adrenals of many women in Western cultures are so depleted they can't even make enough progesterone to make the corticosteroids. This may be an important factor in chronic fatigue syndrome, which is so common in women in their mid-30s and early 40s.

Menopause and Estrogen

Remember, the prevailing myth in mainstream medicine is that menopause is an estrogen deficiency disease, but estrogen levels drop only 40 to 60 percent at menopause, while progesterone levels can drop to nearly zero.

One of the paradoxes of the delicate dance of hormones in a woman's body is that estrogen and progesterone, though mutually antagonistic in some of their effects, each sensitize receptor sites for the other. That is, the presence of estrogen makes body target tissues more sensitive to progesterone, and the presence of progesterone does the same for estrogen. Each sets the stage for the body to be more responsive to the other—an interesting example of nature's efficiency.

Progesterone has an opposing, or balancing, effect on estrogen. When progesterone levels drop to near zero, we have estrogen dominance, which causes a long list of unpleasant symptoms. Estrogen dominance does not necessarily mean a woman has too much estrogen; it simply means that estrogen levels are *relatively* higher than progesterone, creating a hormonal imbalance with its attendant estrogenic side effects.

Unopposed estrogen (i.e., lacking progesterone) carries health risks itself. Mainstream medicine acknowledges that unopposed estrogen greatly increases the risk of endometrial cancer, for instance, and probably promotes breast cancer. Not yet generally understood is that estrogen alters cell membrane function such that sodium and water influxes into body cells, while potassium and magnesium are lost from cells. This results in intracellular edema or bloating and water retention. Estrogen also promotes abnormal cellular retention of copper and loss of zinc. These important changes in intracellular electrolytes and cellular edema go a long way to explain mood swings, loss of concentration, and the aches and pains that menopausal women suffer from, even with estrogen replacement. Progesterone, on the other hand, works to protect the cell membrane from these estrogen-induced problems.

Androgens and Menopause

Androgens are hormones that have masculinizing effects. In women they are made primarily in the ovaries and adrenal glands. Androgen hormones include testosterone, dihydro-testosterone, androstanediol, androstenediol, and two weakly androgenic hormones, androstenedione and dehydroepiandro-sterone (DHEA). The precursor hormone to the androgens is pregnenolone, which then follows a pathway either through progesterone or DHEA. We'll call these the "progesterone" pathway or the "DHEA" pathway.

Figure 9 shows a simplified diagram of the two pathways.

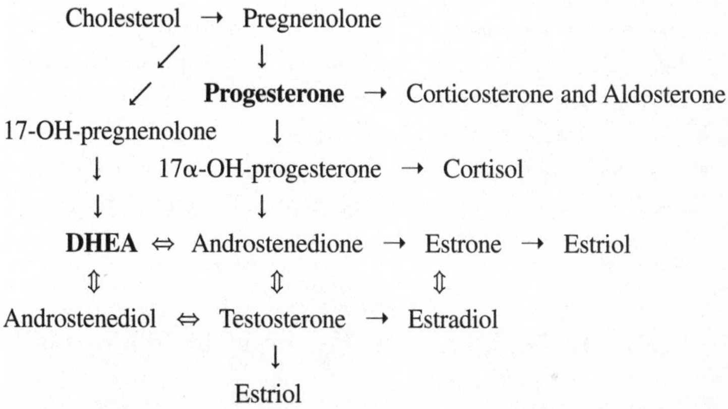

```
Cholesterol  →  Pregnenolone
         ↗           ↓
       ↗      Progesterone  →  Corticosterone and Aldosterone
17-OH-pregnenolone     ↓
     ↓       17α-OH-progesterone  →  Cortisol
     ↓                ↓
   DHEA  ⇔  Androstenedione  →  Estrone  →  Estriol
     ⇕                ⇕                ⇕
Androstenediol  ⇔  Testosterone  →  Estradiol
                     ↓
                  Estriol
```

Figure 9: The progesterone and DHEA hormone synthesis pathways.

The DHEA pathway is more active in males than females and can occur in both the testes and adrenals. In ovulating women, both pathways are operative. However, in the ovaries a highly active enzyme called *aromatase* rapidly converts androgens into estrogen, thus sparing women the masculinizing effects of the androgens. At menopause, when ovary function slows, the adrenal DHEA pathway becomes more active in women. They may experience symptoms of hair loss on the head and the growth of coarser hair on the face and arms (hirsutism), caused by a shift in hormone pathways that favors the androgens. Their body fat becomes a reservoir for the major androgens, some of which are converted into estrone, an estrogen. In women with ample body fat, significant amounts of estrone can be obtained by conversion from fat-stored androgens. Be that as it may, the fact is that after menopause, androgen/estrogen ratios shift in favor of androgens, often leading to increased facial and body hair and male pattern baldness. My clinical experience is that progesterone supplementation often results in the disappearance of facial hair and the regrowth of scalp hair. Why should this be?

The most active of the androgens is testosterone, which also is a product of the adrenal DHEA pathway. In women, about 99 percent of their testosterone is bound to other substances and thus is unavailable as an active hormone. The rate at which available testosterone is cleared from a woman's body is related to her hormone balance. Estrogen decreases testosterone clearance whereas progesterone increases it. Thus, when estrogen is dominant, testosterone clearance is decreased, increasing the effect of available testosterone. When progesterone is added, the clearance of testosterone is increased and its androgenic effects are reduced.

What Can Be Done for Menopausal Symptoms?

The common thread running through all these conditions is estrogen dominance in relationship to a relative insufficiency of progesterone. The vast majority of menopausal problems can be avoided by good nutrition, avoidance of toxins, regular exercise, and the proper supplementation, when indicated for hormone balance, of real, honest-to-God, natural progesterone and when needed, estrogen and testosterone.

CHAPTER 12

HORMONE BALANCE AND THE ADRENAL AND THYROID GLANDS

When it takes place as nature intended, menopause isn't a sudden stopping of menstrual periods. It isn't an event, like a birthday. It's a long, gradual process of lowering hormone levels. Eventually hormone levels drop below the point necessary to create a menstrual cycle. Throughout the book so far I've been alluding to the period of time in a woman's life called *premenopause*, the decade or so before menopause when a woman's reproductive functions are winding down. In agrarian, nonindustrialized cultures, this is an uneventful time. In Western, industrialized countries, it's a time when increasing numbers of women suffer from chronic fatigue, weight gain, mood swings, unstable blood sugar, and rapid aging. Women who have waited to have children may find they are infertile. What has gone awry?

Premenopause and Stress

There are clear physiological and biochemical reasons for premenopause problems, but the whole woman—including the emotional, mental, and spiritual aspects—needs to be taken into account if we are to get to the root causes. At the risk of sounding unscientific, let's first look at the female body in a way that owes much to Chinese medicine and the concepts of yin and yang. This will be a simplified explanation, but it will suffice for the purposes of illustrating my point.

In its essence the female body is yin and the male body is yang. Each contains some of the other, but yin predominates for females and yang predominates for males. Yin is dark and earthy. The yin personality would tend to be nurturing, passive, introverted, calm, intuitive, and soft.

Yang is light and abstract. The yang personality would tend to be active, outgoing, focused, aggressive, logical, and impatient.

Estrogens, the hormones responsible for female sexual development, and progesterone, the progestational, or mothering, hormone, tend to produce yin behavior. Testosterone and DHEA, two of the hormones responsible for male sexual development, tend to produce yang behavior. Although generalizations are always untrue by their very nature, women tend to "default" more on the side of yin behavior and men tend to "default" more on the side of yang behavior.

The environment of raising children naturally favors the yin or female attributes. The business world naturally favors the yang or male attributes. What happens when a woman finds herself spending her days in an environment that's very yang, as so many working women do these days? To survive and thrive, she is going to minimize her yin aspects and maximize her yang aspects. Her body will pay attention to these signals and respond accordingly. The stereotype successful woman executive is slim, trim, and muscular—yang. The stereotype mother figure is ample in breasts, hips, and thighs—yin. These differences in roles work fine when a woman's life is balanced, when she has ample time and energy to develop both sides. But take a woman who is working full-time, has a couple of kids, and a husband who also works and we have a recipe for imbalance and stress. This woman is going to be pulling on her yang attributes at the expense of her yin attributes. She's likely to be chronically exhausted, always "on," never taking time for herself. She is constantly forced to push the limits of her endurance to keep up. She rarely has time to spend quiet, nurturing time with her children or herself, not to mention her husband. In an effort just to maintain her lifestyle, her adrenal glands are constantly pumping out hormones meant to be used sparingly for "fight or flight" situations and they eventually become tired, sluggish, and depleted. Her body gets the message that survival is at stake. Blood sugar becomes constantly unstable. Digestion goes awry so she isn't absorbing nutrients properly. The ovaries respond by shutting down in favor of survival. When her ovaries shut down, progesterone production occurs only at the adrenals, but they aren't working and she's not getting enough progesterone because of her poor dietary habits, so she becomes progesterone deficient and estrogen dominant.

The estrogen dominance causes the all-too-familiar signs of fatigue, depression, little or no desire for sex, weight gain, water retention, headaches, and mood swings. By her late 30s and early 40s, she probably has fibrocystic breasts, uterine fibroids, or endometriosis. The estrogen dominance interferes with thyroid function, which increases her fatigue, so she's cold all the time and she's gaining more weight. But her doctor gives her a thyroid function test and it comes out normal; she produces the normal amount of thyroid, but it's not being used effectively. Not realizing the role of estrogen dominance, her doctor often prescribes thyroid supplements.

She diets continuously (bingeing in between on sugar, caffeine, and refined carbohydrates in a desperate attempt to get her adrenals jump-started), but it does no good because her metabolism has also gone into survival mode, which is to say it is extremely slow. Due to her sluggish adrenals, she finds it very difficult to get out of bed in the morning. Does this sound familiar? It's an all-too-common scenario. In fact I would venture to say it's epidemic among working mothers in their 30s and 40s. But premenopause problems are by no means limited to working mothers. Even without children, women who get on a career track and develop their yang attributes at the expense of their yin attributes are likely to suffer from hormone imbalances.

Another major source of hormonal stress is the xenoestrogens. As I mentioned earlier, people living in an industrialized culture are continuously exposed to environmental sources of petrochemical derivatives that convey potent "estrogenic" actions.

These sources include pesticides, herbicides, auto pollution, poly-cyclic aromatic hydrocarbons (PAHs), polychlorinated biphenyls (PCBs), and nonylphenols (alkylphenol polyethoxylates or APEs) found in many detergents. In females, the results may be enlarged ovaries, possible ovarian tumors, breast cancer, and premature "burnout" of ovarian follicles, contributing to premenopause syndrome. In males, the results include atrophy of testes, reduced sperm counts, small penises, and possibly prostate cancer.

To add insult to injury, once anovulatory cycles begin, the insidious process of osteoporosis follows. Progesterone, the bone-building hormone, is missing. Poor diet and lack of exercise are pulling calcium off the bone faster than it can be put on. Many women arrive at menopause with osteoporosis well under way, already having lost 25 to 30 percent of their bone mass.

Follicle Burnout

It's hard to say whether adrenal exhaustion or anovulatory cycles come first. Anovulatory cycles are those in which a woman does not ovulate. No egg is released into the fallopian tube for its journey to the uterus and no progesterone is produced. The anovulatory woman will still menstruate because the estrogen is still present, but her progesterone levels will be low because there is no corpus luteum present to produce it. Anovulatory cycles are becoming common in women in their mid-30s long before actual menopause. Dr. Jerilynn Prior, professor of endocrinology at the University of British Columbia in Vancouver, British Columbia, Canada, found that it was very common for women athletes (who developed osteoporosis despite normal estrogen levels) to have anovulatory periods. If they were training hard enough, eventually even their periods would stop. However, when Prior went out to find a control group of "normal" women for her studies, she discovered that anovulatory cycles among women from their mid-30s through 40s was quite common. When Drs. Ben C. Campbell and Peter T. Ellison tested menstrual variation in salivary testosterone among regularly cycling women ages 24 to 42 (average age 29), they also tested salivary progesterone during the luteal phase and found 7 of the 18 subjects were not ovulating. More and more women are truly progesterone deficient prior to menopause.

The constellation of stress, poor diet, exposure to xenoestrogens, and progesterone deficiency is very likely the cause of the spectrum of health problems endured by many premenopausal women. Furthermore, the xenoestrogens very likely contribute to endometrial, ovarian, and breast cancer.

Estrogen Excess

Not only is progesterone deficiency common during the premenopause years, but estrogen levels tend to fluctuate and become excessive. Two causes for this are higher FSH levels and a matter of energetics. When women with symptoms of premenopause syndrome arrive at a physician's office, frequently a lab test for estradiol, FSH, and LH is ordered. Because progesterone is low, FSH levels may be high. The increased FSH levels result in increased ovarian production of estrogen but not of progesterone, because of follicle depletion. The attempt of the hypothalamus to restore hormone balance is subverted by the follicle depletion and leads instead to increased estrogen dominance. Most physicians, however, are unaware of the follicle depletion and interpret the test to mean merely that the patient is not yet truly menopausal.

Other researchers such as Dr. Ellison point out another possible mechanism for this estrogen excess that characterizes premenopausal women in industrialized countries. It has been found that when energy intake is low (insufficient dietary calories) and energy requirements are high (more physical labor), women's estrogen levels fall, often to such low levels that fertility is impaired. That is, during starvation periods, birth rates fall. Conversely, when energy intake is high and energy requirements are low, estrogen levels rise. This excess estrogen frequently produces heavy irregular menstrual bleeding as well as a host of other symptoms reflecting unopposed estrogen side effects.

In my practice over the years, I found that serum estrogen

levels taken during these premenopause years reveal great variability, not only from person to person but also in any given woman when such tests are taken randomly.

A premenopausal woman called me to ask what her recently measured estrogen level might mean. When I told her of the day-to-day and week-to-week variability of estrogen levels during the premenopausal years, she talked her doctor into ordering a series of weekly estrogen levels during the weeks between her periods. She called back later to report that her serum estrogen levels varied from a low of 11 to a high of 300 picograms/milliliter, with levels of 60 and 220 in between, none of them appropriate for the time of her menstrual month. She also reported that her doctor was mystified, saying he'd never seen anything like this before. I asked if her doctor had ever done serial tests on anyone before!

Thus, among premenopausal women in industrialized countries, there exist variable inappropriate surges of estrogen, a generally higher-than-normal level of estrogen, and a generally unrecognized epidemic of progesterone deficiency. Each of these contributes to the remarkable incidence of premenopausal symptoms we see in the United States and other industrialized countries.

The following is a list of symptoms that may be suffered by premenopausal women with estrogen dominance:

fatigue

depression

weight gain

water retention

headaches

loss of sex drive

mood swings

inability to handle stress

irritability

fibrocystic breasts

uterine fibroids

endometriosis

low metabolism

symptoms of hypothyroidism
  with normal T3 and T4
  levels

unstable blood sugar

craving for caffeine, sweets,
  and carbohydrates

sluggishness in the morning

The Adrenal Glands

The adrenals are two small glands about the size and shape of a flattened prune that sit on top of the kidneys. Each adrenal gland is composed of an outer and inner part: the outer cortex and the inner medulla. Both the medulla and the cortex produce important secretions that are part of our stress reactions.

The adrenal medulla plays a role in regulating the sympathetic nervous system: It speeds up the heart rate, narrows blood vessels, and raises blood pressure and blood sugar by secreting two hormones called *epinephrine* (also called *adrenaline*) and *norepinephrine* (*noradrenaline*). You probably recognize the name epinephrine because synthetic variations of this hormone are found in over-the-counter cold and allergy remedies that work by narrowing blood vessels. Epinephrine is the hormone secreted when you're under stress, inducing Hans Selye's now famous "fight or flight" reaction in the body that our ancestors evolved to help them survive by fleeing or fighting off attackers. When epinephrine is released, many things occur simultaneously and quickly in the body: The heart speeds up; blood is sent flooding into the heart, lungs, muscles, and brain and away from the digestive system; sugar is dumped into the blood in large quantities to provide quick energy; and breathing is faster. This is a great system if you need to run from or turn and fight a saber-toothed tiger. If your boss is yelling at you, the fight or flight response still occurs, but its manifestations are suppressed by "higher" parts of your brain telling you that fleeing or physically fighting are counterproductive in that situation. Your body is flooded with contradictory messages and reactions. This in itself is a factor in disease, eventual fatigue, and physical illness.

Events that provoke a fight or flight response are called *stressors*. Stress is a household word these days—we all have it to one degree or another. We have the day-to-day stressors of hectic schedules, traffic jams, colds and flus, pressure on the job, mechanical breakdowns, and troublesome relationships. Then we have the big stressors such as the death or serious illness of a loved one, losing or gaining a job, moving, having a child, marriage and divorce. Any of these types of stressors can send the adrenal medulla into action with epinephrine.

To go back to the yin and yang metaphor, epinephrine is a very yang hormone. When we're stimulated by it we tend to be very alert, focused, and energetic. This type of energy is particularly valued in the business world. Some people will work themselves into an anger or fear response just to get a "hit" of epinephrine. The bad news is that epinephrine is not a hormone meant to be used all the time—it's designed to be used in emergencies for short bursts of intense energy. If we're always calling on our epinephrine to get us up and going, eventually we fall prey to an imbalance and our adrenal medulla becomes exhausted.

The Adrenal Cortex

The adrenal cortex secretes three classes of hormones—glucocorticoids, mineralcorticoids, and androgens—that play literally dozens of ongoing roles in regulating bodily functions. While the secretions of the adrenal medulla provide quick and short-term responses to immediate stress, the adrenal cortex hormones provide longer-term responses for stress and homeostasis, the maintenance of balance in bodily functions. The adrenal cortex hormones are often considered essential for life. Animals with their adrenal glands removed will survive for a long time if maintained in an environment providing proper nutrition and freedom from stress. However, if put to any significant stress such as infection, trauma, hunger, or fatigue, they will quickly die. Adrenal cortical hormones are essential for life because life as we know it is stressful. Let us take a closer look at the three adrenal cortex hormones.

The most important glucocorticoids are cortisol and hydrocortisone, which play a role in regulating blood sugar; how carbohydrates, proteins, and fats are moved in and out of cells; inflammation; and muscle function. If too many cortisols are present (as from adrenal cortical tumors or pharmaceutical dosages of cortisol medication), the symptoms are weight gain (especially around the midsection), blood sugar imbalances, thinning skin, muscle wasting, and other signs of aging. Women whose glucocorticoid pathways are not functioning properly or who are deficient in the cortisols (as from adrenal exhaustion or lack of adrenal reserve after overly prolonged stress or malnutrition) may have fatigue, low blood sugar, and sometimes weight loss and menstrual dysfunction.

The mineralcorticoids, especially aldosterone, regulate the balance of minerals in the cells, mainly sodium and potassium, but magnesium is also affected. Stress triggers the release of aldosterone, which raises blood pressure by its action on body cells to hold on to sodium and lose potassium and magnesium. Long-term release of stress-level mineralcorticoids can cause a potassium deficiency and a magnesium imbalance as well as chronic water retention and high blood pressure. Magnesium loss is an exceedingly important factor in our overall health, being the most common cofactor for optimal enzyme function, but magnesium deficiency is not commonly recognized by standard blood tests. Since it is predominantly an intracellular mineral, standard serum (the watery, noncellular part of blood) tests do not adequately measure magnesium. A red blood cell magnesium level test is better.

The adrenal cortex also makes all of the sex hormones, but in very small amounts. One cortical hormone, DHEA, which is weakly androgenic, is made in relatively large amounts in both men and women; its production is greater than that of any of the other corticosteroids. Its full range of functions is yet to be understood. The sex hormones, as you have discovered in reading about estrogen and progesterone, play a part in regulating many bodily functions and are inextricably bound up with the balance of the adrenal hormones.

As you can see from Figure 9 on page 133, cholesterol is a precursor to all of the adrenal cortex and sex hormones, and progesterone is a precursor to aldosterone, the mineralcorticoid that regulates fluids in your cells, and cortisol. This means that aldosterone and cortisol are made from progesterone. Now that you know how important aldosterone and cortisol are to bodily functions, you can imagine what havoc a deficiency of progesterone can wreak on hormone balance and bodily functions. It's no wonder that progesterone-deficient women are suffering from so many illnesses.

You can also now understand how chronic stress can cause hormone imbalances and may even contribute to a deficiency of progesterone, as it is used for "survival," meaning the production of adrenal hormones, rather than contributing to all the hormone pathways, in particular balancing and opposing estrogen.

Nutritional Adrenal Support

Not surprisingly, nutrition is as important to the adrenal glands as it is to all tissues of the body. But in the case of adrenal glands, vitamin C is uniquely important: Cells of adrenal glands use vitamin C at a higher rate than any other cells. Their use of vitamin C varies with their need, and their need rises when the body is required to respond to stress of any sort. It follows that vitamin C deficiency adversely impacts on adrenal gland performance. Chronic stress will more likely lead to adrenal exhaustion or lack of reserve ("lazy" adrenal gland function) if vitamin C levels are lower than optimal. The RDA (recommended daily allowance) of 60 milligrams per day for vitamin C intake is predicated on vitamin C need in healthy young adults without metabolic stress; this RDA is *not* appropriate for people under such stress as illness, infection, surgery, trauma, fatigue, or any metabolic or even psychological stress.

The vast majority of animals make their own vitamin C as needed. When put under stress, their vitamin C production increases. Humans are one of the few animals (along with Rhesus monkeys, guinea pigs, rind-eating bats of India, and parakeets) who do not make their own vitamin C and must therefore obtain it from diet or supplements. The typical animal with a metabolic rate similar to humans makes about 4 grams (⅛ of an ounce or 4,000 milligrams) daily per 100 pounds of body weight. During stress, their production can rise to 12 grams daily per 100 pounds of body weight. Since humans are part of the animal kingdom, it is likely that our vitamin C intake should approximate at least 4 grams per day to avoid stress-induced exhaustion of our adrenal glands. Even without undue stress, one's vitamin C intake should be 1 to 2 grams a day to maintain optimal levels. This is not easy to do through diet alone. An orange provides 60 milligrams of vitamin C. To achieve an intake of 1 gram (1,000 milligrams) of vitamin C, one would have to eat approximately 18 oranges; thus the need for vitamin C supplements.

Metabolic stress from oxidation reactions is unavoidable. Numerous studies show the benefits of natural antioxidants. Our diet selections should include optimal antioxidants such as are found in unprocessed fruit and vegetables of all sorts.

A middle-aged woman came to me with a problem of advanced osteoporosis caused by 10 or more years of cortisone medication taken for chronic asthma. She had shrunk about eight inches in height. Every attempt to wean her off cortisone had resulted in symptoms of Addison's disease—severe weakness as a result of adrenal gland failure—and a return of her asthma. Her adrenal cortex was so suppressed by the long-term use of cortisone medication that it could not return to function on its own. She had been told that the cause of her allergic asthma was aspirin (acetyl-salicylate), which she strictly avoided. Nobody had told her of the salicylates found naturally in food. I provided her with a list of salicylate-containing foods to avoid and recommended vitamin C in divided doses to 4 grams total a day, plus progesterone cream for its important role as a precursor in cortisone synthesis. Then I instructed her to slowly reduce her cortisone medication dosage. Two months later she returned feeling well and off medication for the first time in 10 years. With continued use of progesterone, her cortisone-induced bone loss abated and eventually her bones became stronger again, greatly reducing her risk of fracture.

Several lessons can be learned by examples such as this. Treating the disease's cause is better than treating its symptoms. The knowledge and application of nutrition is important to the health of all cells. Aiding normal health-giving mechanisms is better than suppressing normal functions. Our natural ability to heal and be well is far too great an asset to ignore (or inhibit).

INTERVIEW

How Cortisol Levels Affect Thyroid Function, Hormone Balance, and Aging

David Zava, Ph.D., is a biochemist, breast cancer researcher, a much-published author of professional research papers, and the laboratory director of ZRT Laboratory in Portland, Oregon, which does state-of-the-art saliva hormone assay and blood spot testing. He is also the coauthor of What Your Doctor May *Not* Tell You About Breast Cancer, *and a sought-after speaker on the topic of hormones and saliva hormone testing. This was an interview with Dr. Zava published in the March 2003 issue of the* John R. Lee, M.D., Medical Letter.

JLML: Cortisol is needed for nearly all dynamic processes in the body, from blood pressure regulation and kidney function, to glucose levels and fat building, muscle building, protein synthesis, and immune function. You've been specifically studying the effects of cortisol on thyroid function.

DTZ: Yes, one of cortisol's more important functions is to act in concert or synergy with thyroid hormone at the receptor-gene level. Cortisol makes thyroid work more efficiently. A physiologic amount of cortisol—not too high and not too low—is very important for normal thyroid function, which is why a lot of people who have an imbalance in adrenal cortisol levels usually have thyroid-like symptoms but normal thyroid hormone levels.

JLML: Would you explain this thyroid-cortisol relationship in more detail?

DTZ: One way to understand the synergy of cortisol and thyroid is to think of trying to turn on a big round valve with one hand, as opposed to two hands where you can really grip it and turn it on. Both thyroid and cortisol have to be there in the cells, bound to their respective receptors at normal levels, to efficiently turn the valve on and get gene expression. So, when cortisol levels are low, caused by adrenal exhaustion, thyroid is less efficient at doing its job of increasing energy and metabolic activity. Every cell in the body has receptors for both cortisol and thyroid and nearly every cellular process requires optimal functioning of thyroid.

JLML: And what happens when cortisol levels get too high?

DTZ: Too much cortisol, again caused by the adrenal glands' response to excessive stressors, causes the tissues to no longer respond to the thyroid hormone signal. It creates a condition of thyroid resistance, meaning that thyroid hormone levels can be normal, but tissues fail to respond as efficiently to the thyroid signal. This resistance to the thyroid hormone signal caused by high cortisol is not just restricted to thyroid hormone but applies to all other hormones such as insulin, progesterone, estrogens, testosterone, and even cortisol itself. When cortisol gets too high, you start getting resistance from the hormone receptors, and it requires more hormones to create the same effect. That's why chronic stress, which elevates cortisol levels, makes you feel so rotten—none of the hormones are allowed to work at optimal levels.

Insulin resistance is a classic example. It takes more insulin to drive glucose into the cells when cortisol is high. High cortisol and high insulin, resulting in insulin resistance, is going to cause you to gain weight around the waist because your body will store fat there rather than burn it.

JLML: This would certainly be a significant effect when it comes to creating balanced hormone levels.

DTZ: When cortisol is high the brain also is less sensitive to estrogens. That's why you can have a post-menopausal woman with reasonable amounts of estrogen, but when you put her under a stressor and her cortisol rises, she'll get hot flashes, which are a symptom of estrogen deficiency. She really doesn't have an estrogen deficiency, the brain sensors have just been altered. If you then drive the estrogen levels up with supplementation to treat the hot flashes, she'll start getting symptoms of estrogen dominance like weight gain in the hips, water retention, and moodiness. And the hot flashes usually don't go away.

This is why you often can't effectively treat someone with hormonal imbalance symptoms such as hot flashes by simply adding what seems to be the missing hormone, be it thyroid, progesterone, estrogen, or testosterone. If your cortisol is chronically high you'll have overall resistance to your hormones.

JLML: What percentage of the saliva tests for cortisol are high?

DTZ: I'd say it's as high as ten to twenty percent, but you have to remember that the population that's sending in saliva hormone tests tends to have health problems. It also depends on the time of year and what's happening in the world. I saw a lot of high cortisol in the saliva samples that came in after 9/11. Around the winter holidays, cortisol skyrockets, and then after the holidays it takes a nosedive. The adrenals were keeping pace with the holiday stressors and then they collapse because they're exhausted. That's a very common pattern. It's no different with other stressors like exams or war. Most of us can remember how we made it through the stress of exams only to get sick shortly thereafter. Adequate levels of cortisol are necessary to acutely activate the immune system when we are exposed to viruses, and when the adrenals are just too tired to make any more cortisol we are vulnerable to viral infections.

Stress is what both high and low cortisol have in common. Stress hits the adrenals and in response they either collapse in fatigue and do not produce enough stress hormones, resulting in a functional thyroid deficiency, or they can go in the other direction where they're pouring out cortisol and it's causing overall hormone resistance, including thyroid resistance. Either way, low or high cortisol, and thyroid hormones become inefficient.

JLML: Let's talk more about the good and bad aspects of cortisol.

DTZ: Most people with cortisol problems, high or low, are in the gray zone, meaning that they are outside of a normal physiological range necessary for optimal health. Cortisol helps maintain blood glucose levels by activating gluconeogenesis, the breakdown of tissue protein to amino acids and then to glucose. That's a good thing, but not in excess. Too much cortisol, caused by stressors, over a prolonged period of time, results in excessive breakdown of all structural tissues of the body including muscle, bone, skin and brain, causing accelerated aging.

In bones, high cortisol activates nearly every biochemical pathway involved in bone resorption. Cortisol specifically inhibits osteoblast activity, or bone building; it suppresses the production of androgens [male hormones] in the gonads [androgens build bone]; it activates osteoclasts which causes bone to be resorbed faster; it decreases mineral absorption in the gut, so you won't be absorbing the calcium and magnesium you need to build bone; and it increases renal [kidney] tubule spilling of calcium. Calcium supplementation and alendronate-type drugs used to inhibit bone resorption, such as Fosamax, will always fight a losing battle to high cortisol. I frequently see women reporting continued bone loss, despite use of pharmaceutical bone resorption inhibitors, when salivary cortisol levels are very high.

With saliva testing we see that when people have very high cortisol and low androgens they tend to have bone loss even when their progesterone and estrogen are normal. I see the most bone loss in women who have had a total hysterectomy.

JLML: What is the relationship between cortisol and melatonin, yet another hormone?

DTZ: Cortisol is released from the adrenal glands in a rhythmic pattern throughout the day. It's high in the morning, which energizes you. If you don't have enough cortisol in the morning you have a hard time getting out of bed. It's at its lowest levels at 2 A.M. when melatonin is high. Melatonin and cortisol are inversely related, so when cortisol is down and melatonin is up you're regenerating your body.

When your cortisol stays high you also won't produce enough growth hormone or thyroid-stimulating hormone, which are important anabolic [tissue building] hormones. This is why a good sleep is so important. People with high salivary night cortisol levels are usually complaining of sleep problems.

JLML: What are normal saliva cortisol levels for a perimenopausal woman?

DTZ: At ZRT Laboratory a normal morning saliva hormone level for cortisol for a perimenopausal woman is 3 to 8 ng/mL, and by 10 at night it's 0.5 to 1.5 ng/mL, which is a big drop. Very early in the morning when you're in a deep sleep it goes even lower, so if you're not sleeping properly and resting, your cortisol rhythms will be thrown out of balance. This is where progesterone plays an important role because it's the only natural hormone that actually competes with cortisol for the glucocorticoid receptors. It can counter the stimulating effects of cortisol at night when you need to be sleeping.

Progesterone and Thyroid Hormone

Though each hormone is unique, hormone balance involves a complex harmonious blend of all hormones. I tend to think of hormones as instruments in an orchestra—the harmony we seek is the proper contribution of all the instruments together not only in pitch but also in volume and rhythm. The same is true of sex hormones and thyroid hormone. Let's take a quick look at the interaction of thyroid with progesterone.

In my medical practice, I was impressed with the much greater number of women taking thyroid supplements for hypothyroidism (low thyroid) than men. Thyroid is the hormone that regulates metabolic rate. Low thyroid tends to cause low energy levels, cold intolerance, and weight gain. Excess thyroid causes higher energy levels, feeling too warm, and weight loss.

What difference should gender make to the incidence of hypothyroidism? As I became aware of estrogen dominance, I noticed that the taking of thyroid supplements was especially common in women with this condition. When I attempted to correct their estrogen dominance by adding progesterone, it was common to see that their need for thyroid supplements decreased and could often be successfully eliminated. Thus I became aware that estrogen, progesterone, and thyroid hormones are interrelated.

Many of these women had come to me from other doctors' offices for PMS or osteoporosis prevention and/or treatment. On reviewing the laboratory studies that had led to their presumed diagnosis of hypothyroidism, I often found that their T3 and T4 levels had been normal and their TSH levels only slightly elevated. Their thyroid supplement had been prescribed on the basis of hypothyroid-like symptoms such as feeling tired or sluggish, a little cold intolerance, and thinning hair, for example. While the thyroid medication had improved their tiredness a bit, it had not corrected the symptoms I had learned to associate with estrogen dominance such as fat and water retention, breast swelling, headaches, and loss of libido. When their hormones were balanced, meaning progesterone deficiency was adequately treated, not only did their estrogen dominance symptoms decrease or disappear but so did their presumed hypothyroidism!

Another common thyroid dysfunction is Hashimoto's thyroiditis, which is an autoimmune inflammatory process of the thyroid gland. That means the body is creating antibodies against the cells that make up the thyroid gland. The exact cause of this disease is unknown. However, inhibitory antibodies bind to TSH receptors, displacing TSH, and this may be at least one of the mechanisms by which this disorder results in inefficient production of thyroid hormone. As the disease progresses, cells of the thyroid gland are destroyed and inflammation occurs, along with fibrous deterioration of the entire gland.

Autoimmune disorders in general are thought to be triggered by transient viruses in susceptible people; the virus triggers antibodies against some protein component of the virus. By some probably minor fluke, the antibodies attack similar proteins in certain body tissues, in this case the thyroid. Corticosteroids block this attack by one's own antibodies. Diagnosis is made by detecting the presence and serum levels of the particular antibody. In some people, Hashimoto's thyroiditis also causes leakage of excess T3 and T4 into the serum, resulting in a hyperthyroid state (thyroidtoxicosis) usually of short duration. The usual treatment of Hashimoto's thyroiditis is suppression of gland function by full doses of thyroid medication, such as thyroxine and/or triiodothyronine.

It has been my experience in practice that when a woman with Hashimoto's thyroiditis is given progesterone for osteoporosis, for example, there results a gradual diminution in the severity and sometimes a complete resolution of the thyroiditis problem. One can hypothesize that estrogen dominance may have had a hand in triggering the errant antibodies and thus correcting the estrogen dominance leads to gradual correction of the problem. Progesterone is also the main precursor of corticosteroids and in progesterone-deficient women, restoration of normal progesterone levels may enhance normal corticosteroid production, thus suppressing the autoimmune attack.

CHAPTER 13

HORMONE BALANCE, NUTRITION, AND OSTEOPOROSIS

As my family practice got older, so did my patients. After 30 years, my 30-year-old patients were 60 and my 50-year-old patients were 80. The many women coming to my office debilitated from osteoporosis was one of my biggest inspirations to begin researching ways to prevent and reverse this distressing disease. I noticed that while calcium supplements, estrogen, and exercise seemed to make the disease less severe, they didn't prevent or reverse it. My research confirmed this observation.

I treated a woman who broke her arm lifting a grocery bag and another who broke a rib coughing. I watched helplessly as straight spines became hunchbacks and formerly active women shuffled along on walkers and canes. I saw evidence on X rays of the vertebrae in the spine crumbling and attended the funerals of women who had been killed by the inactivity forced on them by a hip fracture.

Osteoporosis is the disease American women are most likely to develop as they age. It is the most common metabolic bone disease in the United States: Over 45 percent of white women age 50 or more have bone mineral density over two standard deviations (SD) below the mean of normal young women. The lifetime risk of fracturing a hip, spine, or forearm is 40 percent for white women in the United States. Osteoporosis annually causes over 1.5 million fractures at an estimated cost of over $10 billion. The personal cost in quality and quantity of life is incalculable. Twenty percent of the women who fracture their hip die within a year. Unfortunately, proper treatment of this dangerous and (as it turns out) easily preventable disease has been drowned in a flood of misinformation brought to you by your friendly pharmaceutical companies. Let's debunk three osteoporosis myths right away, and I'll explain them in detail later in the chapter.

Debunking the Osteoporosis Myths

Osteoporosis Myth 1

OSTEOPOROSIS IS A CALCIUM DEFICIENCY DISEASE

Most women with osteoporosis are getting plenty of calcium in their diet. It is quite easy to get the minimum daily requirement of calcium in even a relatively poor diet. The truth is that osteoporosis is a disease of excess calcium *loss* caused by many factors. In osteoporosis, calcium is being lost from the bones faster than it is being added, regardless of how much calcium a woman consumes.

Osteoporosis Myth 2

OSTEOPOROSIS IS AN ESTROGEN DEFICIENCY DISEASE

Not even basic medical texts agree with this—it is a fabrication of the pharmaceutical industry with no scientific evidence to support it. Osteoporosis begins long before estrogen levels fall and accelerates for a few years at menopause. Taking estrogen can *slow* bone loss for those few years, but its effect wears off within a few years after menopause. Estrogen cannot rebuild new bone.

Osteoporosis Myth 3

OSTEOPOROSIS IS A DISEASE OF MENOPAUSE

This is at least a decade short of the truth. Osteoporosis begins anywhere from 5 to 20 years prior to menopause, when estrogen levels are still high. Osteoporosis accelerates at menopause, or when a woman's ovaries are surgically removed or become nonfunctional, such as can happen after hysterectomy. I shudder to think how many thousands or even millions of women have been doomed to a crippled old age and early death because their uterus and/or ovaries were unnecessarily removed before menopause and progesterone replacement was ignored.

What Is Osteoporosis?

Osteoporosis is a progressive disease with many factors contributing to its cause. It is a disease of bone loss exceeding new bone formation, resulting in decreased bone density. That is, over time there is less bone, and what is left is lighter and more porous. The danger in osteoporosis is an increased risk of bone fractures, which can be painful and debilitating enough to lead to premature death.

The most common fractures occurring as a result of osteoporosis are of the spinal vertebrae, forearm, hip, shoulder (humerus), and ribs, with hip fracture the most costly and most likely to be disabling. Osteoporosis occurs earlier and with greater severity in white women of Northern European extraction who are relatively thin. It is also more common among those who smoke cigarettes, are underexercised, deficient in vitamin D, calcium, or magnesium, and in those whose diet contains excessive sugar and meat and not enough vegetables and whole grains. Alcoholism is also a potent risk factor.

A Bit About How Bones Are Built

Bones are living tissue and, unlike teeth, they can grow as the body grows, mend when broken, and continually renew themselves throughout life. Bone can be thought of as mineralized cartilage. The skeleton begins developing early in fetal life and grows under the influence of pituitary growth hormone until puberty, when the gonadal (sex) hormones come into play. Our bones allow us to operate in gravity by supporting our weight. Muscles attached to bone allow movement by imposing the force of torsion when we lift heavy objects or move against resistance. Thus bones are designed for compression strength (weight/force) and tensile strength (lengthwise pressure and force).

There are two types of bone cells important to the process of osteoporosis: osteo*clasts* and osteo*blasts*. Osteoclast cells continually travel through bone tissue looking for older bone in need of renewal. They dissolve (resorb) the old bone, leaving tiny, unfilled spaces behind. Osteoblasts then move into these spaces and produce new bone. This astounding process of continual resorption (by osteoclasts) and new bone formation (by osteoblasts), called *remodeling*, is the mechanism for the remarkable repair abilities and the continuing strength of our bones.

At any stage in life, our bone status is a product of the balance between these two functions of bone resorption and new bone formation. If the two processes are in balance, bone mass and bone strength remain constant. During the years of our major skeletal growth, new bone formation dominates. After puberty, the processes are usually balanced.

Osteoporosis is bone loss as the result of relative osteoclast dominance: More bone is being resorbed than is being made anew. Decreased bone mass may also result from deficiency of a variety of other essential factors, such as calcium, vitamin D, and magnesium, and is given the generic name *osteopenia* or, in the case of vitamin D deficiency in the young, *rickets*.

The rate at which bone tissues renew themselves (called *turnover* rate) is quite remarkable. Our long bones, such as our arm bones and leg bones, are very dense and their structure provides great tensile strength for activities such as running, jumping, hammering, and pushing. The turnover time for 100 percent renewal in these long, dense bones (called *cortical* bones) is about 10 to 12 years.

Other less dense bone (called *trabecular*, meaning "little

beams"), needing only compression strength, is constructed as an open meshwork of little struts, and is found mostly at the ends of long bones, in the heel bone, and in vertebral bones. The 100 percent turnover time for these bones may be only two to three years. Thus osteoporosis will show itself earlier in trabecular bone than in cortical bone. Likewise, the progression of (or the recovery from) osteoporosis will be revealed earlier in trabecular bone. This is why I suggest that bone density tests be done on trabecular bone.

Osteoporosis and Estrogen

Bone mass in women is highest during their early or mid-30s, after which there occurs a gradual decline until menopause, when the loss rate accelerates for three to five years and then typically continues at the rate of 1.0 to 1.5 percent per year. The menopausal acceleration of bone loss suggests that the decline in sex hormones is a causative factor. In the mid-1970s, estrogen replacement after oophorectomy (removal of the ovaries) was found to lessen the loss of bone mass when compared with untreated oophorectomized control patients. Estrogen's role in osteoporosis was further supported by population studies demonstrating that women treated with estrogen sustained fewer fractures than did untreated women. These studies do point to estrogen's role in bone loss, but, as a number of scientists have pointed out, the earlier studies suffer from a number of defects, including inadequate sample size, insufficient duration, and lack of precise bone density measurement technology. In addition, these studies tended to include a disproportionate number of otherwise healthy women who had undergone oophorectomy (which means loss of progesterone and testosterone, also) or had experienced hot flashes. It is now generally agreed, however, that estrogen therapy temporarily retards osteoporosis progression, but does not truly prevent or reverse it.

About the same time that studies were showing that estrogen could temporarily slow bone loss in osteoporotic women, it became evident that estrogen replacement therapy was not without risk. Estrogen unopposed by progesterone was found to cause salt and water retention, increase blood clotting, promote fat synthesis, oppose thyroxin (a thyroid hormone), promote uterine fibroids, promote mastodynia (breast pain) and fibrocystic breasts, increase the risk of gallstones and liver dysfunction, and, more ominously, increase the risk of endometrial cancer, pituitary tumors (prolactinoma), and probably breast cancer. It was further found that the bone benefits of estrogen replacement after menopause wane after three to five years.

Mainstream medicine strangely persists in the single-minded belief that estrogen is the mainstay of osteoporosis treatment for women. This is exceedingly odd because even the most authoritative medical textbooks do not support it, as the following examples illustrate:

- *Cecil's Textbook of Medicine*, 18th edition, 1988: "Estrogen is more effective than calcium but has significant side effects."

- *Harrison's Principles of Internal Medicine*, 12th edition, 1991: "Estrogens may decrease the rate of bone resorption, but bone formation usually does not increase and eventually decreases" and "estrogens retard bone loss . . . although restoration of bone mass is minimal."

- *Scientific American*'s updated medicine text, 1991: "Estrogens decrease bone resorption" but "associated with the decrease in bone resorption is a decrease in bone formation. Therefore, estrogens should not be expected to increase bone mass." The authors also discuss estrogen side effects, including the risk of endometrial cancer, which "is increased six-fold in women who receive estrogen therapy for up to five years; the risk is increased 15-fold in long-term users."

If one pursues the supporting references for these lukewarm endorsements of estrogen replacement therapy, the evidence favoring estrogen's alleged bone benefits becomes even more clouded. None of the studies using estrogen alone showed any increase of bone mass. The modest increase of bone mass reported by Claus Christiansen et al. in *Lancet* occurred in post-menopausal women given estrogen *and* a progestin (northin-drone acetate). This particular progestin tends to have more androgenic (male hormone) properties than the others.

A few years ago I attended a National Osteoporosis Founda-tion (NOF) symposium in Seattle, where Professor Christiansen himself presented his material on estrogen and osteoporosis, in-cluding the paper referenced above. During the question period after his talk, I pointed out to him that he had given his patients both estrogen and progestin and asked him how he had con-cluded the benefit observed resulted solely from estrogen. After looking again at his chart he pondered a bit and then, as I recall, said, "Oh, yes, I see what you mean. That was not part of the grant protocol. But if someone would give me a grant to do such a study, I think I could find the answer." I reminded him I had done such a study, giving osteoporosis patients progesterone without estrogen, and found better bone results than his. The lesson I learned from this little exchange was that the protocols for much of the research we see published, and which parts of the outcome are emphasized and publicized as well, are deter-mined by the grantor of the money for the research.

Since the mid-1970s, when the estrogen/endometrial cancer link was noted, all but a couple of studies of hormone supple-mentation in postmenopausal women for osteoporosis have included a progestin along with the estrogen. The potential con-founding effect of progestins has simply never been considered.

Present evidence suggests that estrogen's actions regarding bone are only related to bone resorption. A study by Stavros C. Manolagas et al. in *Science* reported that the *lack* of estrogen stimulates production of a substance called interleukin-6, which stimulates growth of osteoclasts, thus increasing bone loss. This effect of estrogen lack causing increased bone loss is most no-ticeable in the five years immediately following menopause. After that period, continued use of estrogen is relatively ineffective, with bone loss proceeding at the same rate as in those not on estrogen. I would take this as an indication that, after a period of a few years, the body adjusts to the lower estrogen levels. In cultures where overall estrogen levels are much lower, and thus the drop at menopause is much less, women are less likely to suffer from osteoporosis.

A 1995 issue of *The New England Journal of Medicine* reported on a major study, "Risk factors for hip fracture in white women," which was supported by no less than five different grants from the Public Health Service, involved over 9,500 women in various areas of the United States, and was eight years in the making. One of its major findings was that current estrogen use by these women over age 65 was found to have *no benefit in preventing hip fracture!* The authors, however, argue that women who had used estrogen earlier in life had fewer fractures when arriving at age 65, and thus they support the current view that estrogen protects against fracture. This very likely reflects socioeconomic differences between those who were prescribed estrogen and those who weren't, and the acknowledged benefit of using estrogen during the three- to five-year interval around menopause time when acceleration of bone resorption *can* be slowed in United States women by estrogen supplementation. They do not comment on the fact that bone resorption after this particular time period is no longer affected by estrogen. This study showed that by seven years after menopause, the ongoing decline in bone mineral density (BMD) was the same in estrogen-treated and non-estrogen-treated women. This shows that estrogen treatment has a bone benefit only during the few years around menopause time. However, since the estrogen-treated women lost less bone during those seven menopausal years, they had a higher BMD in the subsequent years, when their yearly bone loss was unaffected by continuing estrogen treatment. The last sentence of the study's abstract (which was curiously ignored by the mainstream newspapers and magazines) says it all: "Women should take estrogen for at least seven years after menopause. Even this duration of therapy may have little residual effect on

BMD among women 75 years of age or older, who have the highest risk of fracture."

These studies do not take into account the possibility of new bone formation sufficient to balance the ongoing bone loss. That is where progesterone comes in. Despite the menopausal acceleration of bone loss due to estrogen decrease, progesterone-induced new bone formation is sufficient to prevent BMD loss. In fact, women more than seven years postmenopausal will gain new bone and higher BMD from progesterone therapy whether or not they take estrogen.

The Bottom Line

The majority of women do not need supplemental estrogen in order to have strong bones. Women who are slim (they don't have a lot of fat cells making estrogen postmenopausally), and women who have had a hysterectomy (and thus do not have functioning ovaries), may very well need a little bit of estrogen to achieve over-all hormone balance and maintain bone density. See Chapter 20 for recommendations on using supplemental estrogen.

Osteoporosis and Progesterone

For decades, the makers of Premarin and other estrogen manu-facturers would have had us all believing that estrogen loss is the major hormonal factor in osteoporosis in women. Fortunately that myth is beginning to change. We know that significant bone loss occurs during the 10 to 15 years before menopause, when estrogen levels are still normal. In the United States, peak bone mass in women occurs in their mid-30s, and a good per-centage of women arrive at menopause with osteoporosis well under way. The more important factor in osteoporosis is the lack of progesterone, which causes a decrease in new bone for-mation. In women with low bone density, adding progesterone can actively increase bone mass and density and may *reverse* os-teoporosis.

Several examples illustrate progesterone's bone benefits. In 1982, a 72-year-old woman came to see me after she had fractured her arm lifting her ill husband, and had been found to have severe osteoporosis. Until then she had followed a good diet and had considered herself in good health. Her doctor had recommended a fluoride treatment, but she refused and came to me to try the progesterone skin cream therapy. After the first six months, her bone tests showed no improvement. She had been using Tagamet (a drug that suppresses secretion of gastric acid) and liquid antacids for chronic indigestion. Suspecting that her indigestion was actually due to lack of gastric acid and knowing that gastric acid is essential for calcium absorption, I had her discontinue her medications and continue with the progesterone. Soon after, she noted that her indigestion was gone (the Tagamet and antacids were no longer suppressing gastric acid secretion) and the persistent pain in her "healed" fractured arm disappeared. Subsequent bone mineral density results are pictured in Figure 10.

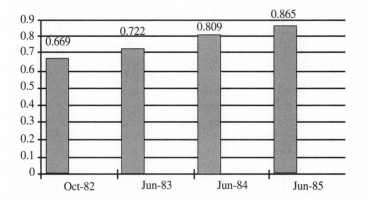

Figure 10: Serial lumbar BMD (gm/cm^2) of patient, age 72, treated with transdermal progesterone

This represents a 29 percent increase in bone mineral density in less than three years of progesterone therapy. This is not at all unusual. When I originally wrote about this in my first book, this woman was 85 years old and continued to do well using progesterone cream. She recently died at home in her mid-90s.

More recently, I received a phone call from a 72-year-old woman from Pennsylvania who had developed a very painful back due to a spinal fracture. Bone density measurements showed she had advanced osteoporosis. I had met this woman on a previous occasion at a health conference and knew she prided herself on her youthful looks, good diet, and other good health practices. She was appalled that despite all her good habits she had developed such severe osteoporosis. She had heard of my work with natural progesterone and was asking my advice. Her husband and son were both physicians. They and her own doctor told her that my ideas about progesterone and bone building were totally unsubstantiated. I sent her a copy of my treatment protocol and suggested she give it a try, under the care of her physician. Sixteen months later she sent me copies of her bone mineral density tests, performed initially after 8 months and again after 16 months. They showed a progressive BMD increase of 23 percent in 16 months. Of course, she was very pleased and was happy to report that her husband, her son, her own doctor, and the radiologist were amazed, and they were all now using natural progesterone in their own practices.

Figure 11 shows her serial bone mineral density test results.

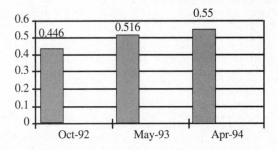

Figure 11: Serial lumbar BMD (gm/cm²) of patient, age 71, treated with transdermal progesterone

In preventing bone loss, we have to look as far back as a woman's early 30s. Dr. Jerilynn Prior at the University of British Columbia in Vancouver, British Columbia, Canada, measured estrogen and progesterone levels in female marathon runners who were developing osteoporosis. She found that they developed osteoporosis when their estrogen was still high. But they had stopped ovulating, a common syndrome in female athletes, and their progesterone levels had fallen. It was the lack of progesterone that brought on the osteoporosis. These women were estrogen dominant and progesterone deficient. Dr. Prior then tested nonathletic women and found a similar syndrome: In their mid-30s, their progesterone levels fell. This falling off of progesterone levels due to anovulatory cycles occurs in all the industrialized countries and is epidemic in North America and Western Europe, where it is no doubt contributing to the alarming rise in infertility among women in their 30s. As noted above, osteoporosis in women typically starts in their mid-30s, often 15 years before menopause, with a bone loss rate of about 1.0 to 1.5 percent per year. With menopause, bone loss accelerates to 3.0 to 5.0 percent per year for five years or so, after which bone loss continues at the rate of about 1.5 percent per year. If the estrogen hypothesis of osteoporosis were true, there would be no reason for the premenopausal bone mass loss when estrogen levels remain high. Clearly there is something wrong with the estrogen hypothesis. The more important hormone is progesterone. It is during the years prior to menopause that *progesterone* levels fall due to anovulatory periods.

The accelerated loss of bone as a consequence of menopause suggests the additional effect of estrogen loss. Recall, however, that this stage of accelerated loss lasts for only four to five years, and then resumes the more typical loss rate of 1.0 to 1.5 percent per year, suggesting that the estrogen effect is subject to adaptive adjustment by bone cells. Figure 12 depicts typical bone mineral densities relative to a woman's age.

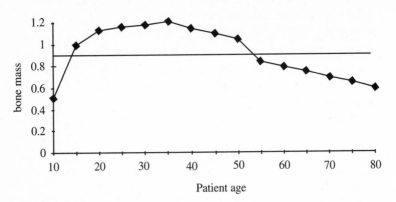

Figure 12: Schematic graph of bone mass relative to age, with menopause at age 50. Bone mass below horizontal line represents level of increased fracture risk. Note the more rapid decrease in bone mass during years around age 50—the average menopause age. Note also that bone mass loss starts a number of years before actual menopause.

On the other hand, Jerilynn Prior, M.D., has presented the evidence that progesterone does have receptors in osteoblasts, and is therefore more likely to affect new bone formation. Several small studies have further shown modest bone benefit (though less than that from natural progesterone) from the use of synthetic progestins. From the available evidence, several deductions can be made:

- Estrogen retards osteoclast-mediated bone resorption.
- Natural progesterone stimulates osteoblast-mediated new bone formation.
- Some progestins may also stimulate new bone formation to a lesser degree.

Since it is clear that estrogen can retard but not reverse osteoporosis and estrogen cannot protect against osteoporosis when progesterone is absent, the addition of natural progesterone should be used in preventing or treating postmenopausal osteoporosis. Further, since some estrogen is produced by fat cells, muscle cells, and skin in postmenopausal women, it is pos-

sible that progesterone alone is sufficient to prevent and/or reverse osteoporosis.

Between 1980 and 1989, I treated postmenopausal osteoporosis with a program of diet, mineral and vitamin supplements, modest exercise, and natural progesterone cream, which

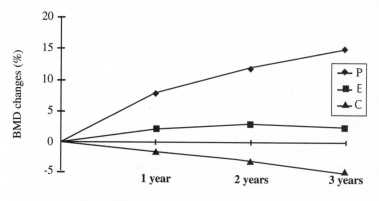

Typical BMD changes with progesterone (P),
estrogen only (E), or control (C)

*Figure 13: Typical three-year bone mineral density (BMD) changes in patients
using progesterone, estrogen, and controls (i.e., without hormone therapy). In
this graph, it can be seen that the untreated postmenopausal patient with osteoporosis will lose 1.5 percent bone mass per year. Estrogen supplementation
will tend to maintain bone mass, but only the addition of natural progesterone
will increase bone mass, thus reversing the osteoporotic process.*

resulted in the true reversal of osteoporosis even in patients who
did not use estrogen supplements. (See Figure 13.)

A minority of the patients using transdermal natural progesterone were also given low-dose estrogen for treatment of vaginal
dryness, while the majority used no estrogen. Approximately 40
percent of the progesterone-treated patients in my study had been
on estrogen supplements prior to starting progesterone, and most
discontinued their estrogen if not needed for vaginal dryness.
Those with the lowest bone density readings at the beginning
showed the greatest response to progesterone. In addition, a comparison of patients younger than 70 years of age with those over

70 showed no difference in their bone response to progesterone. Further, patients who are now well up in their 80s continue to enjoy strong bones without evident bone loss while continuing their use of natural progesterone. I get regular letters and phone calls from these women telling me how well they're doing.

For example, Mary was a slim, active 70 years old when she contacted me about her osteoporosis concern. One of her great joys in life was to go skiing each winter in the Sierras with a university group in which she enjoyed being one of the oldest members. Her doctor had measured her BMD and, finding it to be low in her spine, told her she should no longer go skiing. She wisely stopped skiing and started on my osteoporosis program, including using a natural progesterone cream. In two years her BMD had improved significantly (0.800 to 0.864 gm/cm), and she decided it was time to start skiing again! When I last heard from her she had enjoyed three injury-free ski seasons. Age is not the cause of osteoporosis; poor nutrition, lack of exercise, and progesterone deficiency are the major factors.

In 1989, when I retired from active practice, I took the opportunity to review the charts of 100 patients presently using transdermal progesterone under my care for osteoporosis prevention and/or treatment. Of these, 63 had followed through with serial bone mineral density (BMD) testing, and 62 of them had been on natural progesterone for at least three years. One patient who had gained 15 percent in BMD in less than two years was excluded because she had not yet completed three years on the program. From these records I was able to record their initial lumbar BMD results and results after three years of natural progesterone. About 40 percent of them were also using low-dose estrogen orally (Premarin, 0.3 to 0.625 milligrams daily for three weeks a month) or intravaginally for vaginal dryness. This dosage has been found in numerous studies never to reverse osteoporosis. The ages at which they had started natural progesterone ranged from 38 to 83 years, with the average (mean) age at the time of entry into the progesterone program at 65.2 years. The average time from menopause was 16 years. The majority had already experienced height loss, some by as much as five inches. Table 3 shows the results of this collation of data.

Table 3: Three-year treatment results relative to initial lumbar BMD (in gm/cm²)

Lumbar BMD gm/cm²		Initial[f]	3-yr[f]	net gain	% gain
0.5–0.8	12*	0.745	0.911	0.166	23.4
0.8–0.9	12*	0.838	0.992	0.154	18.1
0.9–1.0	18*	0.957	1.122	0.165	17.1
1.0–1.1	9*	1.026	1.134	0.108	10.5
1.1–1.2	8*	1.152	1.215	0.063	5.5
1.2–1.3	3*	1.256	1.289	0.033	2.6

* indicates number of patients
f indicates arithmetic mean (average)

As can be seen in Figure 14, women with the lowest bone densities experienced the greatest relative improvement. Those with good initial BMD either retained their good levels or improved only slightly. In these women, neither age nor time from menopause was an apparent factor. The improvement of those patients over 70 years of age was equal to those less than 70 years.

As the reader might anticipate, with experiences such as these in patient after patient over a 10-year period, I cannot doubt that natural progesterone, along with a program of diet, a few vitamin and mineral supplements, and modest exercise will effectively, inexpensively, and safely reverse osteoporosis in women. Since bone cells are not inherently different between the sexes, I would predict that the same benefits would occur in men lacking testosterone. Men with a lack of testosterone, such as men castrated either surgically or chemically, will experience accelerated osteoporosis within two to three years. Such a condition happens, for instance, in the treatment of prostate cancer. Since there is no evidence that progesterone is a risk for men with

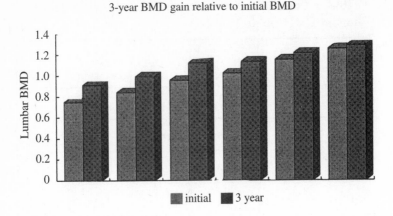

Figure 14: This graph represents the three-year improvement relative to initial BMD in the patients in Table 3.

prostate cancer, I would hope that a clinical trial of progesterone would be offered to protect their bones in conditions of testosterone deficiency.

A Progesterone Cream and Bone Density Study

One short-term study has been done on the effects of progesterone cream on bone density, and it didn't show bone-building effects. Why did my study show bone-building effects and this one didn't? In my study, the patients were, on average, 65 years old, 15 years or so after menopause, and I followed their bone mineral density (BMD) for 3 years. Dr. Leonetti, who led the other study, chose subjects who were perimenopausal (entering menopause or just through it) and followed them for only one year.

During the three to five years around menopause, BMD usually decreases by as much as 5 percent per year, a loss not easily overcome by new bone formation. I do not expect progesterone to change that in just one year, or even two years. Three to five years after menopause, bone loss slows considerably, at which time progesterone's effect of building bone can catch up and show increased BMD. Given the slow rate at which bones renew themselves, I wouldn't expect to see a progesterone benefit in women of this age until after at least two to four years. In fact, it is quite remarkable that none of the women in the study lost significant amounts of bone, and this is likely due to Dr. Leonetti's program of diet, exercise, and nutritional supplementation.

The second point is that if your bone density is normal, progesterone will not increase it. None of the women in the study started out with significantly low bone density.

I have hundreds of letters and BMD reports from women showing how their bone density increased after they began using progesterone cream, and I regularly hear the same thing from clinicians around the world. Dr. Leonetti's study is a good one but, like everything else in life, it must be taken in context.

Other Osteoporosis Treatments

The pharmaceutical industry has come up with a variety of drugs to treat osteoporosis, which predictably have limited effectiveness and unpleasant side effects.

The Phosphonates (Fosamax, etc.)

Fosamax (alendronate), Actonel (risedronate), Didronel (etidronate), and other bi- (or di-) phosphonates are drugs that slow bone loss, leading to gradual (in two years or so of use) retention of old bone and an apparent modest increase in bone mass. The accumulated old bone is, however, not good bone and results in an *increase* in hip fracture incidence by the third or fourth year of use. Bone resorption and new bone formation are linked in the sense that a decrease of bone resorption is associated with a decrease in new bone formation. Fosamax and its cousins, in my opinion, are of very questionable value and have potentially harmful side effects. Fosamax is billed as the only nonhormonal drug approved to treat osteoporosis, but studies of this drug were stopped at four to six years. This is just the point at which the fracture rate for women taking similar drugs such as Didronel began to rise. These types of drugs temporarily create denser-looking bones in bone density tests because they block the resorption of old bone. But old bone is constantly resorbed and replaced because it's weak and needs to be replaced, and it can't be replaced if it isn't resorbed. In people who take Fosamax, the old bone may remain in place and over time begin to crumble, and eventually this is likely to cause the fracture rate to sharply increase. Until there are Fosamax studies that go on for at least eight years and show a reduced fracture rate, I recommend avoiding this drug and others like it.

According to recent studies, Fosamax may also cause severe, permanent damage to the esophagus and stomach, which may require hospitalization, especially if you lie down after taking it. This drug may also be hard on the kidneys, and may cause diarrhea, flatulence, rash, headache, and muscular pain. Some rats given high doses of these drugs have developed thyroid and adrenal tumors. Fosamax may also cause deficiencies of calcium, magnesium, and vitamin D, all essential to the bone-building process.

In addition, bi-phosphonates are complicated to use, expensive, and their long-term toxicity is presently unknown. Despite several requests by pharmaceutical interests, FDA approval of etidronate for osteoporosis has not been granted.

Calcitonin-salmon (Calcimar) is another so-called osteoporosis drug. In humans, calcitonin is a hormone made by the thyroid gland. However, osteoporosis is not a disease of calcitonin deficiency. The drug Calcimar is extracted from salmon pituitary glands. When injected into humans, there is a brief period of new bone formation. With further sets of injections, the bone response becomes progressively less. When discontinued, the benefits gained are quickly lost.

SERMs (Evista)

Evista (raloxifene) is a SERM (selective estrogen receptor modulator) similar to tamoxifen. It's a synthetic estrogen prescribed to women with osteoporosis. Even before FDA approval, media blitzes advertised raloxifene for osteoporosis treatment, claiming improvement in bone mineral density (BMD) and prevention of fracture without estrogen's usual risk of endometrial and breast cancer. The bone benefits of raloxifene were said to be superior to any other treatment and did not increase the risk of endometrial cancer as tamoxifen does.

Ads for raloxifene claimed that it reduces compression fractures in the spine (vertebral fractures) by 55 percent. Little compression fractures can be painful, but in the spine they do not often put patients in a nursing home. The ad doesn't mention hip fractures, which are far more serious, because the three-year study they were referring to showed no effect on the incidence of hip fractures compared to placebo. Raloxifene's effects on bone are certainly not as good as those of Premarin, for example.

If you get out your magnifying glass and read the fine print in the patient information sheet on this drug, you'll find that it increases the risk of blood clots (like in the lung and brain) by 300 percent compared to placebo. These are referred to as VTEs, for venous thromboembolic events. Also, the incidence of hot flashes was considerably higher (27.8 percent) compared to regular hormone replacement therapy (HRT) (3.1 percent). Under "infection" as an adverse reaction, the incidence for Evista was 11 percent compared to 0 percent for regular HRT.

Another large study of the drug, published in the *Journal of the American Medical Association* (JAMA) (August 18, 1999) showed that by the second year of taking the drug, femoral neck (where the thigh bone meets the hip bone) bone mineral density (BMD) among raloxifene users increased a little over 2 percent compared to placebo. At three years, the femoral neck BMD *decreased* 1 percent in both raloxifene users and in controls. Vertebral (spine) BMD at three years increased 3 percent compared to placebo controls. A more important outcome measurement is the incidence of new fractures. At three years, the incidence of new nonvertebral fractures among raloxifene users was *no different* from that among placebo controls. The only fracture prevention finding involved the incidence of new vertebral compression fractures, which was about 5 percent less among raloxifene users than in the placebo group. Newer, longer studies have shown comparably modest benefits.

Again, while raloxifene was not associated with enlargement of the uterus or with cancer, it was associated with a statistically significant higher (though slight) incidence of influenza syndrome, hot flashes, leg cramps, peripheral edema, and endometrial cavity fluid, as well as a much higher risk of venous blood clots.

As with estrogen, the BMD gain with raloxifene represents a modest accumulation of older bone that may delay minor vertebral compression fractures but has little or no benefit in bones subject to torsion stress, such as femoral neck (hip) fractures that clinically are far more important. Raloxifene apparently shares with natural estrogens their well-known proclivity to cause venous thromboemboli (blood clots in the veins). This side effect of unopposed estrogen should not be taken lightly: pulmonary emboli (blood clots in the lungs) can be life threatening.

Keeping Your Bones Strong

Progesterone is not a magic bullet for curing osteoporosis. Successfully preventing and treating this disease requires proper diet, weight-bearing exercise, and some vitamin and mineral supplements as a safety factor. Some women, especially those who have had a hysterectomy, may need a little estrogen and testosterone. Bone building should be considered as a chain of linked factors, each of which must be strong for the chain to be strong.

Because calcium is the predominant mineral in bone building, it is helpful to follow the chain of events that facilitate its bone use from ingestion to incorporation into bone:

Ingested calcium   <u>Facilitating factors</u>

         ↓   gastric hydrochloric acid (HCl) and
                  vitamin D

Absorbed calcium

                exercise, progesterone (stimulates
                osteoblasts), estrogen (restrains
         ↓   osteoclasts), magnesium, micronutrients.
                Avoid excess protein, phosphorus,
                diuretics, antibiotics, fluoride, and
                metabolic acidosis.

Bone incorporation

Testosterone

Testosterone is an anabolic or tissue-building hormone, and it plays a role in bone building in women. In most menopausal women the ovaries are still making small amounts of androgens (male hormones), and the adrenal glands contribute to androgen production as well. Some of the androgens are converted to estrogen in the fat cells, while some remain androgens and contribute their anabolic effects, including bone building.

Women who have had a hysterectomy frequently benefit from some supplemental testosterone for bone building, muscle building, and increased metabolism. Only 0.5 to 1.0 mg of testosterone daily is needed. For details on testosterone supplementation, please turn to Chapter 20.

Calcium

The role of calcium in bone building is widely known. Approximately 98 to 99 percent of body calcium is in bones, where it is used in bone mineralization and as a reservoir from which calcium can be taken to satisfy other demands, such as blood serum calcium levels, a process primarily facilitated by *parathyroid* hormone. When health and nutrition are in balance, one's total daily intake of calcium should be about 0.6 to 0.8 grams or 600 to 800 milligrams. It is not difficult to eat a diet that provides this amount of calcium. Therefore, many people do not need supplemental calcium. If one's diet is low in calcium, it is possible that he or she might benefit from an additional 300 mg per day. I can find no study that supports the notion that 1,200 to 1,500 mg of supplemental calcium promotes stronger bones.

The source of all calcium is from earth's soil or the sea (seashells and coral), and our best edible source is plants (broad leaf vegetables especially) that incorporate calcium into their structure along with other minerals, vitamins, and energy-rich compounds that facilitate its absorption. To be absorbed, calcium requires *both* stomach acid and vitamin D. Older folks (usually over 70) often lack sufficient gastric acid for good absorption. This can be corrected by taking betaine hydrochloride supplements with meals. The common perception, sponsored by the dairy association, is that dairy products are the primary source of calcium. Missing from this amusing perception is the fact that well over 70 percent of the people on earth live in the equatorial zone (between the tropic of Cancer and the tropic of Capricorn), where food plants grow year-round and cows' milk is not used. These people have better bones than we in the more northern industrialized areas have. Also missing from the dairy perception is the fact that cows get the calcium for their bones and milk from plants they eat. Milk contains very little magnesium, which is as important to bones as is calcium. (See the magnesium section that follows the phosphorus section below.)

Other factors being equal, vegetarians uniformly have better mineralized bone than people who include meat in their diet. This isn't just because vegetarians are getting lots of high-quality calcium in their diet. Meat is high in protein, and too much protein in the diet creates an excess of acidity in the body. The kidneys need to buffer the acidic protein waste products before they can be excreted in the urine. This buffering is accomplished with calcium, and if there's not enough in the bloodstream to buffer the acidic protein waste products, it will be pulled off the bone. This excessive loss of calcium creates a *negative calcium balance.* It is true that some people can adapt to high-meat diets by ingesting and absorbing more calcium to balance this urinary calcium loss, but this strategy is unnecessary if one's diet is primarily vegetarian. In the United States, contemporary medicine advocates supplementing 1,200 to 1,500 milligrams of calcium per day for osteoporosis prevention.

To be incorporated into bone, calcium requires enzymes, which require magnesium and vitamin B6 as cocatalysts. If magnesium and vitamin B6 are deficient, calcium is less likely to become bone and is more likely to appear as calcification of tissues and joints, leading to tendonitis, bursitis, arthritis, and bone spurs. Good bone building thus requires not only calcium but adequate magnesium and vitamin B6, in which our typical diet is deficient.

Phosphorus

After calcium, phosphorus is the second most prevalent mineral in bones. Bone experts regard an ideal phosphorus/calcium intake ratio to be below 1.5:1. Excess phosphorus intake causes an imbalance of this ratio, leading to *decrease* in bone calcium.

Parathyroid hormone (PTH) primarily controls calcium levels in the blood. Low calcium levels trigger the release of PTH, which acts in a complex manner on three main organs (intestine, bone, and kidney) to restore calcium levels. PTH causes calcium release from bone, inhibits absorption of inorganic phosphorus by the kidneys, and, with vitamin D, increases absorption of calcium.

In bone formation, the proper ratio of phosphorus and calcium is important. If phosphorus is high relative to calcium, PTH causes osteoclasts to increase in size, number, and activity, leading to enhanced osteoclast activity and bone resorption (i.e., you lose bone). This action is dependent on nearby osteoblasts, which are the primary targets for PTH, as osteoclasts contain no PTH receptors. PTH triggers osteoblasts to release local effectors (possibly interleukin 1 or a prostaglandin), which serve to stimulate osteoclasts to resorb bone. Thus, even though phosphorus is needed by bones, an excess of phosphorus relative to calcium can actually lead to bone loss. Since the typical U.S. diet is in fact high in phosphorus, its supplementation is not indicated. Sodas—any artificially carbonated beverages—are high in phosphorus, as is red meat, and both should be restricted.

Magnesium

Magnesium, the third most prevalent mineral in bones, not only *increases* calcium absorption but facilitates its role in bone mineralization. Magnesium deficiency is common in the United States, due to our food-growing techniques, our food processing, and our diet choices. In fact, I believe that magnesium deficiency is a much greater nutritional problem than calcium deficiency. Magnesium's role in metabolism is primarily as an intracellular enzyme. Its serum level (the usual blood test) is an unreliable indicator of magnesium sufficiency or deficiency since it does not test the level of magnesium within cells. Your doctor can order a red blood cell magnesium level; this is a much better indicator of one's magnesium level.

This important mineral is normally abundant in nuts, seeds, whole grains, and vegetables of all sorts. Our grains, originally high in magnesium, are "refined," a process that removes the outer fibrous coat along with its magnesium, zinc, and other minerals. We eat more meat (low in magnesium) and dairy products (with a poor magnesium to calcium ratio). Our use of fertilizer that contains nitrogen, phosphorus, and large amounts of potassium, a magnesium antagonist, results in foods lower in magnesium than ever before. Further, sugar and alcohol consumption will both increase urinary excretion of magnesium, leading to magnesium deficiency. Interestingly, chocolate is high in magnesium. Chocolate craving can be a sign of magnesium deficiency, and this craving will often fade when magnesium intake is raised to adequate levels.

As just described, magnesium deficiency impairs utilization of calcium for bone building and results in calcium deposits in soft tissue rather than bone. In magnesium deficiency, calcium deficiency develops despite supposedly adequate supplementation. When adequate magnesium is supplied, calcium levels also rise, even without calcium supplementation. Thus proper dietary choices and adequate magnesium supplementation are vital to healthy bones. A magnesium supplement of 400 to 1,000 mg daily can increase your bone density by up to 11 percent in one year. A maintenance dose is 300 to 400 mg daily. (Like progesterone, this effect presumably occurs in women who already have measurably low bone density.) A common supplement dose of magnesium is 300 to 400 mg per day. Magnesium should be taken in a buffered form, such as magnesium gluconate or citrate, to avoid the side effect of diarrhea, and it is often combined with calcium in one tablet.

Other Bone-Building Minerals

Zinc is essential as a cocatalyst for numerous enzymes, including those that convert beta-carotene to vitamin A within cells. This is especially important in building the collagen matrix of cartilage and bone. As with magnesium, zinc is one of the minerals lost in the "refining" of grain. As a result, the typical U.S. diet is deficient in zinc, and modest supplementation (15 to 30 milligrams a day) is recommended.

Manganese, boron, strontium, silicon, and copper are also involved in building healthy bones. A diet of whole, unprocessed foods is usually sufficient in providing these minerals.

Vitamin D

Vitamin D is essential for bone building. It facilitates calcium and phosphorus transport from the intestine into the blood plasma; it decreases excretion of calcium and phosphate from the kidneys, and it facilitates mineralization of bones. Supplemental vitamin D has been shown to reduce hip fracture risk among elderly women when combined with supplemental calcium. In one study of 3,270 healthy women, mean age 84, 1,634 received 1.2 g of calcium and 800 international units (IU) of vitamin D3, while the other 1,636 received placebo. During the 18-month study, the supplemented group experienced 43 percent fewer hip fractures, 32 percent fewer nonvertebral fractures, and a 2.7 percent increase in bone density of the proximal femur (upper thigh) versus the 4.6 percent bone density *decrease* seen in the placebo group.

If vitamin D is deficient in young children, bones are incompletely mineralized, resulting in enlarged wrists, ankles, and bowed legs—a condition named rickets. Although rickets was first described in 1650 by Professor Glisson of Cambridge, not until the early part of this century was rickets learned to be limited to populations that lacked either fish oils or sufficient skin exposure to sunlight.

The missing factor came to be called vitamin D, the fourth vitamin to be discovered (after A, B, and C). The same disease in adults is called osteomalacia (soft bones), or included in the more generic term, osteopenia (bone deficiency).

If vitamin D were discovered today, it probably would have been called an essential hormone. It is unusual in that its synthesis in the skin requires ultraviolet light, a good reason to get a little sunscreen-free sunshine every day. Vitamin D deficiency is common during winter months (when more of the skin is covered by clothing) and is common among the elderly. Although vitamin D isn't found in quantity in very many foods, it is acquired in small amounts from foods such as egg yolks, butter, cod liver oil, and from cold-water fish such as salmon, herring, and mackerel.

In an extensive research and review paper on vitamin D published in the *American Journal of Clinical Nutrition* by University of Toronto researcher Reinhold Vieth, he maintains that recommended daily doses and toxic doses for vitamin D were arbitrarily created and are inaccurate. According to his research, total body exposure to the sun easily provides the equivalent of 10,000 IU a day. It takes about 20 minutes of sun exposure to produce this amount, although in the elderly the skin is less able to create vitamin D. Vieth maintains that elderly people who don't get much sunlight will benefit from as much as 1,000 IU daily in supplement form, especially during the winter months. This is also the dose he recommends for preventing osteoporosis in those at risk. Vitamin D can accumulate in the body and become toxic, creating calcium deposition in soft tissues such as synovial membranes (leading to arthritis), the kidneys, the myocardium, the pancreas, and the uterus. However, Vieth points out that the studies showing these effects were using the equivalent of 40,000 IU daily. If you get plenty of sunshine and have normal bone density, 400 IU of vitamin D3 (cholecalciferol) should be sufficient. If you're elderly and sun-deprived, take up to 1,000 IU daily; if you're somewhere in-between, select an in-between dose.

Vitamin A

Vitamin A is important in the synthesis of connective tissue and the collagen matrix of cartilage and bone. It is normally produced within the cells via its precursor, beta-carotene, found in yellow and deep green vegetables such as carrots, peppers, yams, sweet potatoes, string beans, leafy greens, and many other vegetables and fruits. The metabolic conversion of beta-carotene is inefficient if insufficient zinc is present to serve as an enzyme co-catalyst. The typical U.S. diet is deficient in zinc, due primarily to the common use of refined grain. Thus it is wise to recommend a combination of beta-carotene and zinc: 15,000 to 25,000 IU of beta-carotene and 5 to 15 milligrams of zinc.

Vitamin C (ascorbic acid)

This vitamin is essential to the synthesis and repair of all collagen, including cartilage and the matrix of bone. Throughout the animal kingdom, vitamin C is synthesized by all but a very few species—at a daily rate of about 4 grams (4,000 milligrams) per 100 pounds of animal. Most of the non-vitamin-C-producing animals choose (if free to do so) a diet that provides them with that amount of vitamin C. The typical U.S. diet provides only about 60 milligrams of vitamin C, or 1/70 of the animal standard. Generally, an adequate supplement of vitamin C should be 1 to 2 grams (1,000 to 2,000 milligrams) per day.

Vitamin K

This valuable vitamin, necessary for normal blood clotting, is also a beneficial factor in bone building. Studies indicate vitamin K will reduce calcium excretion and will facilitate binding of osteocalcin (an important bone protein) to hydroxyapatite crystal. Fortunately for most of us, our colon bacteria synthesize sufficient quantities daily under normal circumstances. Prolonged use of broad-spectrum antibiotics, however, may reduce intestinal flora such that vitamin K production is deficient. Such people may need supplemental vitamin K not only for maintaining normal blood clotting, but also for its benefit to bone and the prevention of osteoporosis.

Vitamin B6 (pyridoxine)

Pyridoxal-5'-phosphate, the active form of vitamin B6, is a co-catalyst along with magnesium for a large number of enzymes. As such, it is a facilitator in the production of progesterone and reduces inflammatory reactions in connective tissue and collagen repair. Several studies have found low B6 levels in osteoporosis patients relative to same-age controls. Since this vitamin is inexpensive and remarkably safe at effective levels (50 milligrams once or twice a day), it is wise to supplement it.

Exercise

Bone building responds to exercise. Immobilizing an arm in a sling for a prolonged period will result in bone mass loss in that arm. Immobilization in bed will result in bone loss throughout the skeleton. Astronauts in a so-called gravity-free (actually, gravity balanced by centrifugal force) environment will begin losing calcium within a couple of days. Mineralized bone (hydroxyapatite) is a crystalline structure and, as such, will respond to physical stress just as other crystalline structures do. In particular, any force tending to distort the crystalline arrangement generates an electric voltage, called the piezoelectric effect, producing a small electric current (discovered by Pierre Curie in 1883). This also happens in mineralized bone, and may explain the wondrous ability of osteoclast and osteoblast action in constructing and reinforcing bone trabeculae along lines best suited for maximum strength and physical efficiency. When viewed microscopically, trabeculae remind one of the vaulted chambers and flying buttresses of the best Gothic cathedrals.

Our modern-day, laborsaving devices and engine-powered travel have greatly reduced the exercise previously experienced in everyday living. This lack of exercise diminishes the stimuli that promote bone strength. This, along with nutritional deficiencies, is probably the primary reason for the decrease in bone mineralization now evident. When bone mineral density is compared between present-day skeletons and those buried two centuries ago, as reported recently in *Lancet*, the "ancient" bones showed better BMD results than "modern" bones.

The specific form of exercise to benefit bone is relatively unimportant as long as it imposes some exercise against resistance. Exercise such as walking, bicycle riding, tennis, and weight lifting works well to build bone. Swimming is not an exercise that would build bone if done in a "lazy" fashion, but it does result in bone building if done strenuously. In otherwise healthy postmenopausal women, 22 months of weight-bearing exercise increased the density of the lumbar spine by 6.1 percent, whereas women not exercising lost bone. Bone building simply does not occur in the absence of physical stress on bones. In advanced osteoporosis, however, some care must be given to avoid excessive force that could increase the risk of fracture.

Lack of exercise and a diet of junk food are the primary reasons that teenage girls lose bone. Girls who *over*exercise or who have anorexia/bulimia also lose bone because their ovaries shut down, their periods stop, and so they aren't making any bone-building hormones.

How Bones Are Depleted

Just as attention must be paid to factors that promote good bones, so one must pay attention to factors that are deleterious to bone.

Excess Protein

Protein is essential for tissue growth and repair, and for enzyme synthesis, nucleic acids, neurotransmitters, and some hormones (e.g., insulin). For many years, science endorsed the concept of eating large amounts (120 to 185 grams a day) of protein, based on the theory of Liebig in the early 19th century that muscle protein is actually consumed by activity and must be constantly replaced. The fact that a large intake of protein is unnecessary was first suggested by Chittenden in 1905. However, it is only recently that science has agreed that protein requirements for adults are generally only about 40 to 60 grams (or 1.5 to 2.0 ounces) per day. Red meat, for example, is about 25 percent protein. Thus a 6-ounce, low-fat hamburger provides 1.5 ounces of protein, meeting your recommended daily allowance. Any additional protein eaten that day may result in calcium loss. Eating meat daily in larger quantities is sure to result in calcium loss from bones and increase one's risk of osteoporosis.

If one eats more protein than required for nutritional purposes, it is not stored by the body (as fat is, for example) but must be excreted. Excess protein waste products are excreted in the urine. As we discussed earlier, the excretion of protein waste products through the kidneys increases the urinary excretion of calcium. The ratio between calcium ingested and calcium lost in urine is called the *calcium balance*. A high intake of protein creates a negative calcium balance (i.e., more is lost than was ingested). A negative calcium balance will cause it to be pulled from the bones.

In calculating protein intake, it is important to consider the protein content of various dietary components. The following list may be helpful:

Most meats	approximately 25 percent protein
Chicken, turkey, cheese, and fish	25 to 30 percent protein
Beans, peas, and nuts	approximately 10 to 12 percent protein

| Other vegetables | range from 3.5 to 10 percent protein |
| One egg (egg white) | 0.22 ounces protein; same as one bagel |

Diuretics

Diuretics increase urine volume and are used extensively in medicine to treat edema, congestive heart disease, high blood pressure, or water retention from any cause. The use of diuretics correlates with increased fracture risk. A number of diuretics cause increased urinary excretion of minerals. Furosemide (Lasix) promotes the greatest loss of calcium, and thus is a potential cause of osteoporosis. Other diuretics (e.g., thiazides) retain calcium, but tend also to increase one's fracture risk by causing nocturnal urination, which, among the elderly, increases the risk of accidental falls in the bathroom at night.

A better approach to water retention problems is by diet (avoid salty foods and sodium bicarbonate), if possible. If diuretics must be used, it is wise to choose those that do not increase calcium loss.

Antibiotics

Broad-spectrum antibiotics kill friendly intestinal bacteria that make vitamin K for us. Vitamin K is a bone-building factor. Long-term or frequent courses of antibiotics result in low vitamin K levels, and thereby interfere with bone building. Since body stores of vitamin K are small, a deficiency can develop in as little as one week. If antibiotics must be used long-term or frequently, it is wise to supplement vitamin K and replenish friendly colon bacteria such as *L. acidophilus*. Take both as long as you are taking antibiotics and for two to four weeks afterward.

Fluoride

For some years, fluoride enthusiasts claimed fluoride is good for bones. The fact is that fluoride may slightly increase the X-ray appearance of bone mass, but the resultant bone is of inferior quality and the risk of hip fracture is actually increased. This is found not only in fluoride doses used in osteoporosis "therapy" (i.e., 15 to 20 milligrams a day) but also in doses obtained in fluoridated communities (i.e., 3 to 5 milligrams a day). Fluoride is a potent enzyme inhibitor and causes pathologic changes in bone, leading to increased risk of fracture.

More recent research shows us that fluoride is also toxic to bone collagen (the nonmineralized matrix of bone). Poor bone collagen reduces bone strength, but is not measured by BMD. Fluoride affects not only the quantity but also the quality of the collagen. In the presence of fluoride, the micro-architecture of collagen fibers is disordered, leading to a lack of tensile strength. After 30-plus years of studying the effects of fluoride on humans, I believe that this is the main cause of the increased incidence of hip fracture in communities with fluoridated water. Collagen fragmentation due to fluoride also leads to the inflammation and eventual destruction of cartilage, and the loss of "cushioning" effect in the event of falls.

The concentration level at which waterborne fluoride increases hip fracture risk is of great concern, because the U.S. Public Health system continues to press for fluoridation of all drinking water at a level of about 1 mg/L (ppm). This ambition of the U.S. Public Health system is not only outmoded but ill-advised, in every sense of the word. There are now eight good studies (and no good contrary ones) showing that fluoridation is associated with increased incidence of hip fractures. A recent report in JAMA found that hip fracture incidence among white women 65 years and older increased significantly in those communities in France with water fluoride levels over 0.11 mg/L (ppm). Throughout the world, water fluoride levels are generally less than 0.10 mg/L unless artificially raised. It would appear that humans can tolerate this low level of fluoride, but are adversely affected by drinking water with more fluoride in it.

Interestingly, it is now generally acknowledged by scientists that the supposed dental benefits of higher fluoride levels to children's teeth has been an illusion fostered by incompetent earlier fluoride studies and the misplaced zeal of fluoride promoters. The overall decrease in the rate of cavities in children is the same in nonfluoridated communities as it is in fluoridated communities, indicating that the change is probably due to better hygiene and nutrition. The fluoride used in water fluoridation is a toxic by-product of industry, particularly the phosphate fertilizer and aluminum industries, who wish to dispose of it by trickling it away in our drinking water supplies.

Fluoride in all forms, including toothpastes, should be avoided by everyone.

Metabolic Acidosis

Metabolic acidosis refers to an increase in the acidity (lower pH) of blood. It is necessary for the body to maintain blood pH within very narrow limits. As we saw in the example of excessive dietary protein (page 184), when acidity is too high, the body uses calcium to bring it back into balance. Cigarette smokers, for example, develop emphysema, or chronic obstructive pulmonary disease, leading to retained lung carbon dioxide and increased serum carbonic acid. One of the body's responses to the acidosis threat is to buffer the excess acid with calcium, usually taken from bone for the purpose.

Alcohol Abuse

Whether from specific alcohol toxicity to bone, magnesium loss, or other nutritional deficiency, osteoporosis is rampant among alcoholics. A history of more-than-modest alcohol use is a potent risk factor for osteoporosis.

Hyperthyroidism

Hyperthyroidism (excessive thyroid hormone), especially that resulting from excessive L-thyroxin supplementation, accelerates bone resorption and thus promotes osteoporosis, presumably by stimulating osteoclast activity. Persons receiving L-thyroxin supplements should routinely be checked with thyroid tests to prevent this risk of bone loss.

Cortisone

From a molecular point of view all glucocorticoids are remarkably similar to progesterone so it is not surprising that they share some common receptor sites. In fact, progesterone and glucocorticoids compete for receptor sites in osteoblasts, the bone-building molecules. The "message" brought to the molecule by each of the two hormones is, however, quite different. The message of progesterone to the osteoblast is to stimulate new bone formation, whereas the message of glucocorticoids is to suppress that action. When glucocorticoids exceed normal production, as in Cushing's disease, osteoporosis results. Further, people placed on long-term use of large (pharmacologic) dosages of glucocorticoids will develop osteoporosis. In his book *The Safe Uses of Cortisone*, Dr. William Jefferies did not report osteoporosis as a risk when physiologic dosages (the small amounts needed by the body for normal functioning) of cortisol or hydrocortisone were given to patients for over twenty years. The patentable synthetic analogs of cortisone now in vogue (e.g., prednisone, prednisolone, triamcinolone, methyl prednisolone, and dexamethasone) are considerably more potent and generally used in pharmacologic dosages: People taking these drugs over a long period of time all develop osteoporosis. It would be interesting to see whether larger doses of progesterone could prevent or reverse the osteoporosis caused by these drugs.

Stress can cause progesterone deficiency (as in anovulatory cycles) but also raises cortisol levels, and both factors lead to osteoporosis.

Asthma Inhalers Containing Steroids

Asthma incidence is increasing exponentially in the United States, and inhaled glucocorticoids are the most commonly used medication for it. A three-year study published in the NEJM shows that even small, inhaled doses of synthetic glucocorticoids can deplete bone. Inhaled triamcinolone acetonide in premenopausal women aged 18 to 45 caused a dose-related decline in bone density, especially at the total hip and the head of the thigh bone. Serum and urinary markers of bone turnover or adrenal function did not predict the degree of bone loss.

Depo Provera

Although bone loss caused by Depo Provera (an injectible contraceptive using a progestin) is not likely to be an issue for a menopausal woman, it may be an issue for the daughters and granddaughters of menopausal women! A number of studies show that Depo Provera can cause bone loss in adolescents. One study, published in the journal *Obstetrics and Gynecology* in 1999 showed that young women who use Depo Provera lose bone mass at a time in their lives when they should still be building it. The bone loss was especially steep (around 10 percent) in younger women aged 18 to 21.

According to a study published in the journal *Epidemiology*, researchers from the University of Washington, Seattle, compared bone density in women who had been exposed to Depo Provera with those who had not. The women were aged 18 to 39 years, and their bone density was measured every six months for three years. The women using Depo Provera experienced 0.87 percent *loss* of bone density in the spine and 1.12 percent loss in the hip, compared to a *gain* of 0.4 percent and 0.05 percent, respectively, among those not using Depo Provera.

The good news is that when the Depo Provera injection wore off, bone density rapidly increased. Other side effects of Depo Provera include an increased risk of blood clots (some leading to stroke), weight gain, headaches, dizziness, abdominal pain, nausea, nervousness, fatigue, and back pain.

I hope this information will put to rest the common but misguided practice of prescribing birth control pills to help adolescents build bone. There is no evidence that birth control pills of any kind build bone, which makes sense since the progestins would block the normal bone-building action of progesterone. I recommend against the use of all progestin-based contraceptives, especially Depo Provera.

In a Nutshell

Having summarized the various factors required for healthy, strong bones and the factors deleterious to bones, it is important that the central thesis of this chapter be restated: *Postmenopausal osteoporosis is a disease of excess bone loss relative to new bone formation caused by a progesterone deficiency and secondarily a poor diet, estrogen deficiency, and lack of exercise. Progesterone restores bone mass. Natural progesterone hormone is an essential factor in the prevention and proper treatment of osteoporosis.*

When all the right factors are present, bone building continues throughout life. Whenever I see a woman bent over from osteoporosis, I wish she could have been given the benefit of natural progesterone. I receive letters regularly from women with success stories. The following letters were written to me on three consecutive Christmas cards by a woman who was 81 years old at the time of writing the first letter:

Dear Dr. Lee,

Since I first wrote you [about 2½ years ago], I have been using the progesterone cream every day. I found that my benefits did not peak at four months of using the cream but continued on a cumulative basis.

I can get into and out of bed without taking a few breaths to settle down and feel comfortable—I feel comfortable immediately. In the morning, I do not have to sit on the edge of the bed to adjust; I am adjusted at once. I can shift my position in bed without supporting myself at my hips.

I can walk without feeling that my back will collapse, and I can walk at a good clip! In driving I no longer need to hold myself rigid to keep from feeling that my spine is slipping at a turn, and I no longer dread any normal unevenness in the road surface.

I am able to hold saucepans of soup and carry them across the kitchen. (Previously, I had to carry an empty saucepan to the stove and then fill it cup by cup.) I can fill a quart bottle and carry it easily across the room. I can stand free and take a picture with my camera—I used to have to brace myself by leaning against a wall. I used to have to hold on to my bureau to dress and undress; now I only have to hold on for clothes I have to step into. Over the head clothes I can stand free. I can brush my teeth without having to lean on the counter.

I feel so wonderful and am so very grateful for your consideration in my regard.

One year later:

Dear Dr. Lee,

I continue to get better and better. Now I can turn my head around to back out of a parking lot. When I last wrote you my back had improved driving on turns, but now it is even more solid and I don't even think about it anymore.

Last July I flew to Boston to be with my families in five different locations with many long car trips riding with my daughter or granddaughter. I had no problem with my back and slept comfortably in five beds!

It is miraculous to have a solid back. The enclosed picture is of me and my sister, whose caretaker I am. She has considerable dementia and aphasia, but we are doing very well. I keep her as active as possible.

By the way, I can now pick things up off the floor, although I am exceedingly careful in doing so.

Sincerely and gratefully,

One year later:

Dear Dr. Lee,

All the improvements I told you about continue and more so. I can lift a ten-inch iron frying pan with one hand from the bottom shelf, and easily load and unload the dishwasher. It is wonderful to be strong and I have no pain!

Thank you! Thank you! Thank you!

What Your Doctor May Not Know About Bone Density Measurement (BMD)

Contrary to what you'd expect, BMD has not been found to be a good predictor of future fractures. This was clearly shown in a nine-year study done in France, of 7,575 women aged 75 or older, with no history of hip fracture. The results of the study show that poor balance, reduced vision, lack of muscle strength, and lack of coordination were as important as bone density in predicting hip fractures. A similar study done in the United States and published in the *New England Journal of Medicine* (NEJM) in 1995 had very similar results. This means that even if your bone density is good, you need the additional protection of staying strong and coordinated, and if you're strong and co-ordinated your risk of fracture will be reduced even if your bone density is low.

Other important causes of fractures in women include:

- taking drugs that cause dizziness, such as sleeping pills.
- taking drugs that lower blood pressure.
- taking drugs that deplete bone, such as cortisone.

To complicate matters further, BMD testing doesn't account for differences in bone size. Thus, Ronnie, a petite, 105-pound, 45-year-old woman wrote me in alarm after her doctor told her she had osteoporosis. Her lumbar (spine) bone density test had measured low, and her doctor wanted her to take Fosamax. I assured her that, for her petite size, her bone mineral density (BMD) was just fine and she could stick to her good diet and plenty of exercise.

Conversely, Peggy, a rather large woman with a BMD in the "normal" range, asked me why she had several compression fractures on her spine. She had been told she did not have osteoporosis. I explained that, for her size, her bone BMD should be higher, and that she needed osteoporosis treatment. This type of confusion is created by the limitations of the BMD tests themselves.

Testing techniques include dual-energy X-ray absorptiometry (DEXA), dual photon absorptiometry (DPA), quantified CT scan (QCT), and, more recently, quantitative ultrasound (QUS) or broadband ultrasound attenuation (BUA), which are still experimental. Each technique measures slightly different bone characteristics and provides slightly different results. This means that if you want to compare your BMD results over time (serial testing), you should use the same technique each time.

Let's talk about DEXA and DPA, the most common techniques. An X ray or photon (light) beam is directed at a body site such as the hip or lumbar spine, and the energy of the beam as it exits the body is measured. As the beam passes through the body, some of it is deflected or absorbed by striking minerals. Only the particles that don't hit a mineral will pass through the tissue and can be measured as they exit. The more minerals in the path of the beam, the greater the loss of beam energy. From this drop in beam energy, a computer calculates the mass of bone minerals encountered by the beam in its passage through the body. This is then reported as bone mineral density (BMD).

What Does Bone Density Really Mean?

The use of the word *density* in BMD creates some confusion, because you would think that two women with the same amount of minerals in, say, a postage stamp–sized section of bone would have the same BMD. But this is not true because BMD levels vary depending on the size of a woman's bones, as well as on the concentration of minerals in that bone. Because a larger person generally has larger bones than a smaller person does, the energy beam going through a large person's bones will encounter more minerals than it would if it traversed a smaller person's smaller bones of the same density. This means that even if the true densities of both bones are identical, the result of DEXA or DPA tests will indicate a higher "density" in the larger person's larger bones.

Thus there are no BMD levels that are "high," "low," or "normal" for everyone: What is normal for one woman may be low or high for another, and what is low for another woman may be perfectly fine for a third.

Use BMD Measure for Treatment

Despite the shortcomings of BMD testing, it is still valuable as an index of the effectiveness of any osteoporosis therapy you may be receiving: In other words you can compare your own readings for progress. BMD is not accurate, however, in two cases. Anti-resorptive drugs such as the bisphosphonates (etidronate/Didronel and alendronate/Fosamax) inhibit resorption of old bone, leading to a rise in BMD even though the skeleton will be composed of older bone of less tensile strength. Also, elevated fluoride levels in the body, usually due to fluoridated water, result in bone that is denser but of poorer quality, but which will also yield a higher BMD reading.

Excluding these two exceptions, a rise in BMD while on osteoporosis therapy is a sign of bone improvement. I receive a lot of mail from women who are panicked by a diagnosis of osteoporosis based on one BMD reading, and the majority of them are petite. Please *do* use BMD as a tool to analyze your bone health, but please *don't* panic at one low reading. It may or may not be entirely accurate, it isn't necessarily predictive of a fracture, and as you've discovered in this chapter, there's plenty you can do to improve your bone density. You can start on a bone-building program and measure your bones again in six months, and that will give you a comparison. You'll get even more information if you wait for a year.

I recommend that women get a baseline BMD in their mid-40s, and then measure BMD every two to three years thereafter.

Use Height as a Baseline

Aside from bone density measurements, one of the first indicators of osteoporosis is a loss of height. Women should accurately measure their height when they are 30 and then have it measured every year thereafter. Any decrease in height caused by a deterioration of the spinal bones is most likely an indicator of osteoporosis.

TECHNIQUES FOR MEASURING BONE MINERAL DENSITY

Photon absorptiometry measures the decrease in energy in a photon beam passing through tissue. Photons pass easily through skin and fat, but are deflected by the minerals in bone. If you hold a flashlight up to your hand in a dark room, you can see a similar effect: Your bones make a dark shadow due to their mineral density. This method works well for the dense cortical bone found in the arms and legs.

Dual photon absorptiometry (DPA) uses photons of a slightly different absorption spectra, and is 96 to 98 percent accurate for the less dense trabecular bone found in the hips and spinal column.

Dual energy X-ray absorptiometry (DEXA) is 96 to 98 percent accurate but uses low-dose X rays.

The QCT technique, a modification of the CT or CAT scans, is also very accurate, but uses much more X ray and is more expensive. I don't recommend it.

Urinary excretion of pyridinium, while not a specific test for osteoporosis, can indicate rapid bone turnover rate. When bone undergoes resorption (bone loss), very specific types of pyridinum, called *pyridinoline* and *deoxypyridinoline*, are excreted in the urine. By measuring the ratio of these substances in the urine, the rate of bone turnover can be measured. Higher ratios indicate greater turnover, such as occurs in more rapid bone resorption. Since urinary excretion of the pyridiniums is also higher in cases of Paget's disease, primary hyperparathyroidism, arthritis, osteomalacia, metabolic bone disease such as hyperthyroidism, bone cancer, and alcoholic bone disease, all of these must be ruled out first. This test could be used to find osteoporosis under way earlier than BMD tests would indicate it, and would also be useful for monitoring the effect of osteoporosis treatment.

I prefer DPA or DEXA because they use much less X ray and are less expensive than QCT.

In Short

From the foregoing discussion in this chapter, I hope it is clear that the more authoritative medical references find only minor or no bone benefit from estrogen, except for the five years or so around menopause when it can slow accelerated bone loss. I believe that estrogen supplementation can also help women who are slim, as well as women who have had a hysterectomy. During the five-year interval around menopause, however, the use of estrogen may be of benefit in women who experience a sharp drop in hormone levels, to prevent accelerated bone loss, so that they become postmenopausal with better bones. In particular, estrogen does nothing for new bone formation. That is a function of progesterone and/or testosterone.

Since osteoporosis is a function of the relative balance between "old bone" resorption and new bone formation, the accelerated menopausal time loss of old bone can be balanced by new bone formation if progesterone is supplemented during the premenopausal phase when progesterone deficiency is common. Further studies are needed to evaluate the full protective effect of progesterone treatment during the four to five years around menopause. It is very clear that progesterone can be of great benefit to older women with measurable bone loss. In most such cases, progesterone alone will rapidly and impressively build bone.

Finally, I wish to emphasize that osteoporosis is a multifactorial disease and that progesterone without proper diet, nutrients, and exercise is not sufficient in and of itself to prevent or reverse osteoporosis. All factors come into play. It is entirely likely that not all factors are known at this time and that future research will lead to new treatments. But at the present time, in my opinion, progesterone is the most important factor that is missing in the standard, mainstream approach to this most important disorder facing most women in industrialized countries today.

CHAPTER 14

WOMEN AND CARDIOVASCULAR DISEASE

The rate of death from heart disease in the United States has gradually declined over the past 20 years, but that decline has been much steeper for men than for women, and from 1992–1995, death rates from heart attacks in women *increased*. Until a few years ago, many doctors didn't take heart disease symptoms in women very seriously—one out of three of them didn't even know it is the leading cause of death in women, more than all other causes of death combined. Eventually, with age, approximately 50 percent of women die of heart disease.

Women are more likely to die of a first heart attack, and two-thirds of them have no previous symptoms, compared to only half of men who have no previous symptoms. Some people guess that the women *do* have previous symptoms, but either don't go to the doctor for them, or the doctor doesn't take them seriously. It is also possible that the cause or mechanism of women's heart problems is different in some way to that of men. One year after a heart attack, 44 percent of women have died, as compared to only 27 percent of men. Although women tend to live about seven years longer than men, they spend twice as many years disabled before they die.

We do know that a hysterectomy, total or otherwise, greatly increases the risk of heart attack in a menopausal woman; now, thanks to the Women's Health Initiative, we know that conventional HRT increases the risk of heart disease in general and strokes in particular.

Estrogen and Heart Disease

For nearly 20 years, estrogen was touted by mainstream medicine as a great preventer of cardiovascular disease in women. The argument was that heart deaths in women are very uncommon prior to menopause, that after menopause heart deaths in women adopt the male pattern, and that the difference is due to estrogen lack after menopause. This benefit of estrogen, it was claimed, resulted from estrogen's ability to improve a woman's lipid profile (lower total serum cholesterol and higher HDL cholesterol levels). HDL cholesterol is known to protect against coronary heart disease. This neat argument had women clamoring for estrogen supplementation, but it wasn't true.

Estrogen does have cardiovascular benefits. It is necessary to maintain progesterone receptors, and a true estrogen deficiency may compromise the ability of blood vessels to relax and thus help protect against a heart attack. Conversely, when estrogen levels are too high its protective value in heart disease is reversed as the risk of blood clots and fluid imbalances rises. Thus, the question is, how much estradiol is necessary for cardiovascular benefits and how do we know which women need it. We know that 66 percent of women aged 65 to 80 make plenty of estradiol for all known needs short of preparing the uterus for a pregnancy.

It is known that progesterone deficiency down-regulates estrogen receptors, and sufficient progesterone up-regulates estrogen receptors, resulting in more estrogen action without changing the amount of estrogen already present. We see that demonstrated when a woman develops temporary symptoms of estrogen dominance when progesterone is added.

Estrogen supplementation should be given only to women in whom saliva tests demonstrate a deficiency in bioavailable estradiol that persists after giving physiologic doses of progesterone. Physiological doses (considerably less than standard HRT doses) of estradiol are safe when accompanied by physiologic doses of progesterone.

Progesterone and Heart Disease

What about progesterone? We now know that anovulatory cycles and lowered progesterone levels occur prior to menopause, and progesterone levels after menopause are close to zero. Estrogen, on the other hand, falls only 40 to 60 percent with menopause. A woman's passage through menopause results in a greater loss of progesterone than of estrogen. Perhaps the increase in heart disease risk after menopause is due more to progesterone deficiency than to estrogen deficiency. In my clinical experience, lipid profiles improve when progesterone is supplemented. In the PEPI study, lipid profiles in women on combined HRT were considerably better in women receiving natural progesterone than in those receiving the progestin medroxyprogesterone acetate.

Progesterone increases the burning of fats for energy and, in addition, has anti-inflammatory effects. Both of these actions would be protective against coronary heart disease. Progesterone protects the integrity and function of cell membranes, whereas estrogen allows an influx of sodium and water while allowing loss of potassium and magnesium. Progesterone, a natural diuretic, promotes better sleep patterns and helps one deal with stress. When one reviews the known actions of progesterone, it is clear that many of its actions are also beneficial to the heart. The time has come to study the heart history of the many women now who are using natural hormones during their postmenopausal years. It is my firm belief that they will have less cardiovascular disease.

Only Half of Heart Attack Deaths in Women Are Caused by Blocked Arteries

Only 50 percent of coronary artery disease (CAD) deaths in women are associated with major occlusive disease (blocked arteries). That is, in half the cases of death from CAD, the coronary arteries are not obstructed by plaque sufficient to stop blood flow, leading to heart attack or death. Something else causes the heart attack in those instances.

This becomes clearer when one looks at heart attack deaths in males versus females. It is well recognized that males are more prone to coronary artery occlusion. In U.S. males, the accumulation of plaque in arteries starts early in life (early teens) and becomes clinically significant in early- to mid-adulthood. It is not uncommon to find more than 90 percent occlusion in the coronary arteries of males only 45 years old. Surgical treatment at this stage may prolong life of those so afflicted, but so far it has done little to stem the tide of CAD in aging American males.

Among females, cardiac mortality presents a different picture. It is rare that a premenopausal woman dies of a heart attack. Heart attack deaths in women occur sometime after menopause. The incidence of cardiac mortality among older women eventually matches or exceeds that of males. Autopsies show, however, that the degree of occlusion in females is considerably less than that of males, most often only 20 to 30 percent occlusion and not sufficient to cause their deaths. Then what is causing the heart attacks? Experts believe it is spasms of the arteries and/or the heart muscle. A 20 to 30 percent coronary artery occlusion by plaque can be converted to a 100 percent occlusion if the artery undergoes inappropriate and serious spasm. Cardiovascular spasm can be the result of any number of factors, including prostaglandin imbalances caused by eating "bad" fats and oils, electrolyte imbalances often caused by low magnesium levels, and high levels of stress. There is also compelling evidence that conventional HRT causes vasospasm in postmenopausal women, and it's the medroxyprogesterone acetate (Provera) that appears to be the culprit.

Researchers at the Oregnon Primate Research Center led by Kent Hermsmeyer set out to study the effect of hormones on coronary artery spasm. They removed the ovaries from 12 rhesus monkeys to simulate menopause. Then six of the monkeys were put on estradiol and natural progesterone, and six were put on estradiol and the synthetic progestin medroxyprogesterone acetate or MPA (Provera). Four weeks later the monkeys were injected with a combination of serotonin plus a platelet extract (thromboxane A_2) known to stimulate coronary artery spasm. The monkeys that were on MPA and estrogen suffered from an unrelenting spasm that would have caused death had they not been injected with a drug that reversed the spasm. The monkeys that had been treated with estradiol and natural progesterone showed very little coronary artery spasm.

These findings are echoed by work done at Wake Forest University's Bowman School of Medicine in Winston-Salem, North Carolina, led by J. Koudy Williams. Their research with monkeys, heart disease, and hormones has shown that medroxyprogesterone "can obliterate the beneficial effect of estrogen therapy on the progression of coronary artery atherosclerosis," which is clogging of the arteries.

At London's National Heart and Lung Institute, in a study led by Peter Collins, women on different combinations of hormone replacement therapy were put on a treadmill. Once again, those who were using natural progesterone with estrogen could exercise significantly longer than those who took medroxyprogesterone.

My hypothesis is that the increased risk of cardiovascular disease now associated with menopause may not be due to relatively minor cholesterol plaque or to hormone deficiency per se, but to increased risk of coronary vasospasm caused by synthetic progestins such as medroxyprogesterone acetate used in HRT.

The conclusion of these studies was that MPA greatly increased the risk of coronary artery spasm while progesterone protected against it. In the light of this, one must ask why synthetic progestins such as Provera continue to be prescribed when progesterone is so superior and so much safer. MPA and estrogen drugs are massive moneymakers for the pharmaceutical industry. Profit from their sales exceeds that of any other class of drugs including H-2 blockers, tranquilizers, antibiotics, and antidepressants.

Insulin and Heart Disease

Obesity and high insulin levels are the root cause of the leading chronic degenerative diseases of our time, including heart disease and diabetes. Having said that, the normal weight gain that all of us experience as we age does not cause heart disease! Becoming fat-phobic and overly thin can be just as harmful to the health as obesity, and we know for a fact that yo-yo dieting increases the risk of heart disease.

Let's take a closer look at food and obesity. Fat makes you fat, right? And calories are calories, regardless of where they come from. If only it were that simple. In truth, your body does very different things with fats, sugars, other carbohydrates, and proteins. It also responds differently depending on how you combine food groups. For example, a combination of fat, carbohydrate, and sugar (think pastries and cookies) can create blood sugar havoc, while fat, complex carbohydrates, and protein (think meat and whole grain rice) can create blood sugar stability. Stable blood sugar is one of the foundations of maintaining a healthy weight and healthy blood vessels.

However, everything I'm about to say comes with one big caveat: moderation. If you eat enormous amounts of food you're going to become enormous regardless of what diet you're on. If you eat mostly white, doughy foods, your body is going to be white and doughy. You can eat in ways that encourage your body to put on fat, or you can eat in ways that encourage your body to burn fat.

Food Basics

Three basic kinds of foods are converted into fuel: proteins, fats, and carbohydrates. Proteins, such as dairy products, meats, fish, and eggs, are broken down into amino acids. Fats such as butter, cream, bacon, and oils are broken down into fatty acids. Carbohydrates—whether from cakes, candy, fruits, potatoes, grains, or starchy vegetables—are broken down into simple sugars. Misuse and abuse of sugars is where most Americans get their fat and their chronic disease.

Sugar enters the bloodstream in a form called *glucose*, the main source of fuel for the body, and especially the brain. The cells that ultimately use the glucose for fuel do not care whether it originally came from ice cream or the carbohydrates in broccoli. What does dramatically affect your body is how fast the glucose enters the bloodstream. Ice cream will cause a quick, large surge in glucose, while broccoli will cause only the slightest rise over time. Excess glucose is toxic to the kidneys and other organs, and this is where insulin comes in. In response to rising glucose, the pancreas secretes the hormone insulin into the bloodstream. Insulin's job is to transport glucose out of the bloodstream and into your cells, which is why a big surge of glucose causes a big release of insulin. However, too much insulin is also toxic, so your body works hard to maintain balance. Researchers estimate that there are as many as 20,000 insulin receptors or more per cell.

As your glucose level gradually falls after a meal or snack, the amount of insulin in the blood also falls. At any given time the blood can carry about an hour's supply of glucose. Any glucose that is not needed for immediate energy is converted into glycogen and stored in the liver and muscles. When it is required for energy, the liver turns the glycogen back into glucose. The body can store only enough glycogen to last for several hours of moderate activity. Finally, when its glycogen is used up, the body turns to stored fat for fuel. When glucose levels rise, your body stops using stored fat. Thus, you can understand why someone who drinks Cokes all day long isn't losing weight—their body has no need to burn its fat because it's constantly being fed instant glucose!

Insulin Resistance

Inside the insulin receptor is an enzyme called *tyrosine kinase* (TK). Once activated by insulin this enzyme triggers a cascade of events that open channels through which glucose can enter the cells to be stored or used for energy. When cells become insulin resistant, the channels do not open and the glucose fails to gain entry into the cells. Insulin resistance causes glucose to build up in the bloodstream, which in turn signals the pancreas to make more insulin. The end result is higher-than-normal levels of both insulin and glucose in the bloodstream, which promotes the formation of fat and causes abnormal cholesterol, high triglycerides, high blood pressure, and—eventually—clogged arteries. In fact, when you're insulin resistant, the only cells in the body that benefit from excess sugar are cancer cells, which happily use it for energy and growth.

Researchers in the Framingham Study estimate that as much as 60 percent of heart disease in women is caused by insulin resistance. The constellation of symptoms caused by insulin resistance has come to be known as Syndrome X, a term coined by Gerald Reaven, M.D., a Stanford University researcher. Over time, insulin resistance will cause muscle cells to weaken due to lack of fuel, and thus begins a vicious cycle of less exercise, more weight gain, and more insulin resistance. As fat increases and muscle decreases, the body loses more and more of its ability to burn fuel efficiently and metabolism slows to a crawl. Insulin resistance is often the precursor to type 2 diabetes. Clearly, eating sugars and simple carbohydrates when you're insulin resistant will only make it worse.

We don't understand the exact mechanisms that cause insulin resistance, but we do know that insulin resistance, abdominal obesity, and stress tend to go hand-in-hand. The high cortisol levels caused by stress tend to cause abdominal obesity, which in turn is one of the hallmarks of insulin resistance. So if you tend to head for the ice cream, pastries, and cookies when you're stressed, it may be time to look for a different coping mechanism.

And by the way, you can be slim and still be insulin resistant, with all of the fatigue and other damage still occurring in the body. My guess is that chronic stress combined with genetic predisposition and a sugar-laden diet are the common threads of insulin resistance.

Slowing the Glucose Train

Clearly, big surges of glucose are the foundation of obesity and heart disease. So how do we slow the glucose train? The most obvious answer is to not eat sugar and refined carbohydrates. But getting enough protein and eating some fat can also help, and that's why diets which shun protein or fat can cause weight gain and fatigue.

Whole grains, fiber, protein, and fat can all help slow things down. Complex carbohydrates, such as those found in whole grains, fresh vegetables, nuts, seeds, and beans, tend to break down slowly in the gut and cause a very gradual rise in blood sugar. Complex carbohydrates tend to be higher in fiber, which also slows down the digestive process. The body breaks proteins down into amino acids, some of which are stored in the liver for the manufacture of glucagon, which is what allows the release of glycogen, which you'll remember is the body's backup system when glucose levels start to fall after a meal. No protein means no glycogen, which means no backup glucose, which means intense sugar/carbohydrate cravings as the body signals for more glucose—fast!

This is why the vegetarian who eats a bagel for breakfast (a simple carbohydrate that breaks down quickly into glucose); a banana (fruit sugar); a salad with bread, and so forth (more simple carbohydrates); a protein bar (they're all loaded with sugar); or trail mix (raisins are very sweet); and more carbohydrates with dinner, but very little protein throughout the day, is gaining weight and feeling tired. She'd be better off having a piece of whole grain toast with butter and an egg for breakfast; tofu with her salad for lunch, and fish for dinner, for example. When I talk about fats as good foods, I'm not talking about the trans fatty acids (hydrogenated oils) found in almost all processed foods—please avoid those.

Fat slows the glucose train for a number of reasons. As fat hits the taste buds, it sends signals to the rest of the gastrointestinal system that rich fuel and calories are coming, and that creates "I'm satisfied" or satiety signals. Fats—and especially saturated fats—are easy to digest, are burned for fuel quickly and efficiently, and tend to speed up metabolism in general while slowing the digestion of sugars. As long as you're moderate in your fat consumption, your body is very good at ridding itself of excess fats, including cholesterol.

Always keep in mind that we're each unique in our genetic makeup and biochemistry, and what works well for one person may not work for another. One person may thrive on meat and vegetables, while another may thrive on fish and rice, and yet another may need a minimum of protein and more carbohydrates. If you keep the above principles in mind, you can eat in a way that's very satisfying and yet doesn't keep increasing your weight. If you're having trouble finding the right "food tune" for your body, I would recommend that you get Dr. Harold Kristal's book, *The Nutrition Solution: A Guide to Your Metabolic Type*.

What About Cholesterol?

You'd never know it by watching the advertising on TV, but most cardiology researchers agree that serum cholesterol levels after age 65 are not predictive of subsequent coronary artery disease or death. In fact, the research clearly shows that forcibly lowering cholesterol with drugs after the age 65 does more harm than good. How about elevated cholesterol under age 65?

As you learned in an earlier chapter, cholesterol is a fat-soluble steroid from which all of the steroid hormones are made. Cholesterol is also very important to brain function, being a component of the myelin sheath that protects nerves and nerve impulse propagation. Both your hormone balance and your brain function suffer when cholesterol is excessively low.

Eating food with cholesterol in it does not in and of itself cause chronically high cholesterol levels. In humans, 80 to 85 percent of our cholesterol is synthesized in the liver from sugars, and only 15 to 20 percent is synthesized from dietary fats. Any excess that comes through the diet is excreted.

Cholesterol in your bloodstream is attached to one of several different molecules. Those that have received the most attention in Western medicine are high density lipoproteins (HDL), and low density lipoproteins (LDL). The problem with LDL-cholesterol is not so much its mere presence or quantity in the blood, but the fact that it is easily oxidized or made rancid, and this sets up the conditions for the arterial plaque that clogs arteries. Once we know this, the key question is, "What causes LDL to become oxidized?"

The key answer is that the right nutrients are our first hedge against oxidation. The antioxidants such as vitamins C, A, E, the carotenes, and the bioflavonoids protect us from oxidation. All of these are found in fresh fruits and vegetables—the single food group most lacking in the American diet. HDL cholesterol helps protect LDL from being oxidized and again, what keeps HDL high, first and foremost is a good, wholesome diet. The B vitamins, and particularly niacin, found in abundance in high-quality protein such as meat, fish, and eggs, lower LDL levels and raise HDL levels.

Foods that can significantly help in healing heart disease and improving cholesterol profiles include garlic, onions, and fiber-rich foods such as vegetables. A glass of red wine with dinner has also been shown to keep cholesterol healthy, but this holds true only if you drink in moderation.

High Blood Pressure

Hypertension, or high blood pressure, undoubtedly has many causes. Estrogen dominance is one of them. Estrogen and progestins adversely affect cell membranes, resulting in sodium and water influx into cells (causing intracellular edema or water retention) and loss of potassium and magnesium. The net result is often hypertension. Dr. Milton G. Crane has extensively studied the effects of estrogen, progestins, and progesterone on cell membranes, plasma renin activity, high blood pressure, and aldosterone excretion rates. He has concluded that estrogen dominance and oral contraceptive agents are a major cause of hypertension in women.

This was borne out in my practice. The water retention caused by estrogen is the culprit. Since the extra water is contained within body cells and is not loose in the extracellular spaces, it is not effectively reduced by diuretics. In women not on contraceptive pills, estrogen dominance is synonymous with progesterone deficiency. When progesterone is resupplied, weight goes down (excess water is excreted) and blood pressure returns to normal. If you are on diuretics or other antihypertensive drugs and using progesterone, it is wise to monitor your blood pressure and reduce or eliminate your antihypertension drugs gradually as needed to prevent low blood pressure (hypotension).

Low blood pressure can be just as much of a problem as high blood pressure, and many women have it. Unfortunately, when they visit the doctor's office and their blood pressure is measured, they get pats on the back for it! Low blood pressure can lead to fatigue and dizziness when standing, which can cause falls that lead to broken bones. Low blood pressure in women is most often associated with adrenal exhaustion. (See Chapter 12 for more on adrenal exhaustion.)

Iron Overload

It used to be conventional medical wisdom that iron was an important part of a daily multivitamin. Now we know that excess iron can be very harmful, and that very few people should supplement it: Women who are pregnant may need it, and perimenopausal women who are bleeding heavily month after month may become anemic and need it. In fact, it's thought that people who are regular blood donors—men in particular—benefit from the blood loss involved because it lowers their iron levels. Having said this, it's also true that iron deficiency is one of the most common nutrient deficiencies in Western cultures, primarily due to poor diet among those living at poverty levels. What is it about iron that makes it so essential to health, and yet dangerous in excess?

Iron Is Uniquely Essential

Among the various metallic elements that are essential to humans, iron is unique in a number of ways. The total quantity of iron in the adult human body is quite small, only 4 grams, about the amount found in a 3-inch nail. Its primary role is as a component of hemoglobin (in red blood cells) and myoglobin (in muscle cells), but it is also essential in small amounts for iron-containing proteins, such as in cytochromes, which are vital for normal cellular functions.

Iron is a very reactive mineral, perpetually in a dynamic state in the body, moving rapidly from one molecule to another. This reactive quality is what makes it useful in the transport of oxygen, but it's also what makes it dangerous in excess. Iron exists in two primary forms in the body, either as ferrous iron or ferric iron. Ferrous iron is more active and available for use, while ferric iron tends to be a storage form. Excessive oxidation (from free radicals, for example) changes the iron to the ferric form, which will not function as an oxygen carrier.

The majority of your body's iron is found in hemoglobin, the part of red blood cells that carries oxygen for delivery to your cells. Hemoglobin is a highly complex molecule that has one atom of iron at its center. That one atom is what gives blood its red coloring.

After your bone marrow makes red blood cells they circulate in the blood for about 120 days, at which time they grow old and are destroyed. Thus, each day, nearly 1 percent of our red blood cells are destroyed and 25 mg of iron is released from their hemoglobin. However, the majority of this iron is conserved and reused. This is a bit odd since our environment provides abundant iron, leading some experts to theorize that at an earlier evolutionary epoch, iron may have been scarce.

Unlike other essential minerals, iron is not excreted in the urine, which serves to conserve it even further. However, iron is lost from the body by bleeding (including menstrual flow), from the gastrointestinal tract, in bile that is eliminated in feces, and in the shedding of mucosal and skin cells, and in hair. In males and nonmenstruating females, the daily loss of iron is approximately 1.0 mg. Iron loss in menstruating females runs from 1.4 to 3.2 mg per day, depending on the blood volume of the menstrual flow. To remain healthy, the daily loss of iron, however slight it may seem, must be made up by a sufficient daily dietary intake. On the other hand, iron levels can build in postmenopausal women just as they can in men. This does not mean you should avoid iron-containing foods, but it does mean it's important not to take a vitamin that contains iron unless you're sure you need it.

The liver and spleen are the normal storage sites for excess iron. Excess iron leads to a number of undesirable conditions such as enlarged liver and cirrhosis, diabetes, hypogonadism and atrophy of the testes, joint degeneration, heart disease, dusty brown skin pigmentation, and death usually due to cancer of the colon or liver. Excess iron is toxic to cells and creates oxidation reactions, often stimulating the growth of cancers due to other causes.

The body's ability to maintain proper iron levels is quite amazing. Iron absorption varies relative to iron stores in the body. When iron stores are low, absorption is greater than when iron stores are high. The mechanism for this control of iron absorption is quite unique.

In the mucosal cells of the intestine, iron is transferred to a small iron-binding protein, which is then transferred to the plasma (the watery part of the blood) where it is bound to an iron transport protein called *transferrin*, or to an iron storage protein called *ferritin*. Since the life span of intestinal mucosal cells is only three to five days, the iron that is bound to ferritin is constantly lost with the degraded cells in the feces. This process acts as a buffer to prevent iron overload. Iron transported in blood by transferrin is always in the ferric form. Once released into body tissues, the iron is changed (reduced) to the more active ferrous form. Iron that is bound to ferritin, on the other hand, is transported primarily to the main storage sites, the liver and the spleen. This plays an important role as a protection against excessive iron intake and as a reservoir for future use in times of low iron intake.

The concentration of transferrin-bound iron can be used to evaluate one's iron status. When anemic, the iron concentration of transferrin is low, and, in the case of iron overload, the concentration is high, to the point that the iron-binding sites of the transferrin are fully saturated with iron. This concentration can be tested (serum ferritin), and is especially helpful as an indicator of iron deficiency or iron overload.

It's important to eat a wholesome diet that includes a variety of iron-containing foods so that you can maintain your body's iron levels. It's equally important to avoid iron supplements unless you've tested deficient and are sure you need it. It's a good idea for perimenopausal women, or women who bleed heavily during menstruation, to have their iron levels tested at least once a year to check for iron deficiency anemia. If you do have your iron levels tested, be sure that your doctor is doing the tests that will determine the underlying cause of the deficiency.

Homocysteine

After you eat a steak, your body breaks down the rich protein content into its building blocks, the amino acids. One of the amino acids is methionine, one of the 22 amino acids that make proteins, muscle, connective tissue, and enzymes in the body. Methionine is metabolized (chemically broken down) to homocysteine, which is quickly changed to cysteine for excretion in urine. If the homocysteine is not quickly changed to cysteine for excretion, it is toxic to blood vessels and causes an inflammation of the lining of the arteries, leading to damage and the onset of plaque that clogs arteries.

More than 30 years ago, Dr. Kilmer McCully at Harvard found that adding vitamins B6, B12, and folic acid to patients with elevated homocysteine levels reduced their risk of cardiovascular disease. For this he was relegated to the basement of the lab where he worked at Harvard. Since that time, Dr. McCully has been vindicated and as of this writing is still alive to enjoy that fact. Conventional medicine (aka the pharmaceutical companies) have tried to ignore this important treatment since it uses inexpensive vitamins rather than expensive patent medicines.

The breaking down of methionine to cysteine for excretion requires good enzyme functioning. If this enzyme is not working, homocysteine levels rise resulting in heart attacks and strokes. The cofactor for this enzyme is vitamin B6. Therefore, it is wise to ensure good intake of vitamin B6 (50 mg/day is fine).

Another enzyme converts the homocysteine back into methionine to make it safe. The cofactor for that enzyme is vitamin B12. Therefore, it is wise to ensure good B12 levels (1,000 to 2,000 mcg daily).

Folic acid (a B vitamin) adds methyl groups ($-CH_3$) to the homocysteine molecule to make it innocuous to us. Therefore it is also wise to ensure good folic acid (also called folate) intake to protect against homocysteine damage (400 mcg daily).

In the past few years, interest in homocysteine has skyrocketed, and research makes it clear that elevated levels of this amino acid are an important risk factor for heart disease, causing an estimated 30 percent of heart attacks.

Although red meat is rich in methionine, a well-nourished body should have no problem excreting it. A body that's deficient in vitamins B6, B12, and folic acid will accumulate homocysteine. Thus, it's not eating the red meat, per se, that's the cause of the clogged arteries, it's the lack of other vitamins.

Homocysteine also appears to play a role in causing Alzheimer's disease. A study in the *New England Journal of Medicine* (NEJM) confirmed that an elevated total plasma homocysteine level is an independent predictor of the development of Alzheimer's disease. In this study from the Boston University of Medicine and Tufts University in Boston, homocysteine levels were measured in 1,092 healthy women and men (mean age 76). Over the next 8 years, 111 subjects developed Alzheimer's disease. It was found that an elevated homocysteine level (14 micromol/L) at baseline almost doubled the risk of dementia and Alzheimer's disease during these years. The actual mechanism for the action of homocysteine in increasing one's risk of Alzheimer's disease is as yet unknown.

Interestingly, the serum levels of B6, B12, and folate did not correlate well with the risk of dementia. This does not mean that vitamin supplementation would be ineffective. Individuals differ in their vitamin requirements, and scientists may be measuring them in a way that doesn't show disruptions in their function. It may also be possible that some individuals, particularly the elderly, aren't absorbing their nutrients efficiently, in which case digestive aids such as betaine hydrochloride or digestive enzymes can be used.

C-Reactive Protein (CRP)

C-reactive protein (CRP) is a protein made in the liver in response to any type of infection or inflammation in the body. Elevated CRP can indicate an acute event, such as a cold or a sprained ankle. Repeated high readings, however, are an indication that there is chronic inflammation in the body, most likely to be specifically in the arteries. High CRP levels are an excellent predictor of a heart attack, especially when combined with a poor LDL ("bad") to HDL ("good") cholesterol ratio. Since more than half of all heart attack patients have normal cholesterol and blood pressure levels, the CRP test takes on even more significance.

About 85 percent of sudden heart attack and stroke deaths are due to rupture of vulnerable, noncalcified arterial plaque and subsequent clot formation. What this means in plain English is that arteries become inflamed or damaged, and in response the body creates plaque to patch things up. However, "vulnerable" plaque, which is invisible to conventional angiography, has the potential to suddenly dislodge or break up, spewing its contents into the blood and creating a cascade of blood clots, pieces of plaque, and thickened blood, that can block an artery. In the heart this can initiate a heart attack, and in the brain it can initiate a stroke.

The chronic inflammation that can lead to arterial damage may be caused by chronic infection, autoimmune disease, and low cortisol levels. It's worthwhile to have your CRP levels tested when you have a physical exam.

Nutrition and Lifestyle

We know a great deal about how to prevent cardiovascular disease with nutrition and lifestyle changes. Although this subject will be covered in detail at the end of the book, let's briefly review what we know: We must eat moderate amounts of red meat and dairy products and more fish; we must choose a diet high in fresh, unprocessed plant foods of all sorts (legumes, whole grains, leafy vegetables, and fruits); and we must restrict our vegetable oils to those with less processing and more linoleic acid and alpha-linoleic acids (like olive oil) and avoid those with hydrogenated oils (such as most of the others arrayed on our supermarket shelves). Contrary to common perception, eggs are not correlated with increased heart disease risk and are in fact highly nutritious.

Getting some regular, moderate, and enjoyable exercise, and some regular, undisturbed sleep in a dark room are two other foundations of optimal heart health.

Vitamins

We would be wise to supplement our diet with more antioxidants, such as vitamin E, vitamin A, vitamin C, beta-carotene, zinc, selenium, bioflavonoids, and magnesium. It is well established that the protective level of these nutrients exceeds that which can be attained through normal dietary intake alone. Such supplements are safe to take and offer at least as great a benefit as that advertised for estrogen.

In the Nurses' Questionnaire Study and the Harvard Men's Study, those whose intake of vitamin E equaled at least 100 iu experienced 35 to 50 percent fewer heart attacks, and a more recent study from Great Britain showed as much as a 70 percent reduced risk. Vitamin E is especially effective because it is fat-soluble and thus more likely to supply oxidation protection to fatty compounds such as cholesterol. In considering the potential benefit of water-soluble vitamin and mineral antioxidants it is probably wise to include vitamin C and selenium, also. For details on vitamin supplementation, please turn to Chapter 21.

A deficiency of the mineral *magnesium* can greatly increase the chance of a coronary vasospasm, and it is also implicated in mitral valve prolapse. Magnesium deficiency is common but generally unrecognized in the United States, and yet cardiovascular survival correlates with magnesium concentrations, and higher cardiovascular disease mortality correlates with magnesium-depleting factors such as diuretic usage, diabetes, digoxin therapy, alcohol, age, congestive heart failure, diarrhea, and dietary deficiency.

A daily supplement of 300 to 400 mg of magnesium is good preventive medicine. It should be taken with no more than twice the amount of calcium for optimal absorption.

Homocysteine is a waste product of methionine that is normally converted into a safer compound for excretion in urine. If it isn't converted, it accumulates and contributes to heart disease. The B vitamins B6, B12, and folic acid play key roles in the conversion of homocysteine, and deficiency can cause high homocysteine levels. A good daily multivitamin will contain 50 mg of vitamin B6, 400 mcg of folic acid, and 1,000 mcg of vitamin B12.

What About Aspirin?

It's been about 20 years since I became a participant in the Harvard Physicians' Questionnaire Study in which aspirin was a major variable under study. Half of the 22,000 physicians received aspirin and the other half received placebo. About four years into the study, we were advised that the placebo was being eliminated and all 22,000 of us would receive aspirin since the aspirin users had been found to have significantly fewer heart attacks. Shortly after that the aspirin data were sent to us. The data showed that 18 heart attack deaths had occurred in the placebo group versus 12 among the aspirin group. However, hemorrhagic (burst blood vessel) stroke deaths were 44 in the aspirin group versus 38 in the placebo group.

I wrote a letter to the Study director pointing out that the total deaths from both heart attack and hemorrhagic stroke were equal in the two groups—the six heart attack deaths "saved" by aspirin equaled the six extra deaths from hemorrhagic stroke in the aspirin group. I could not see that aspirin saved any lives. Furthermore, a difference of 6 heart deaths among the 11,000 physicians using aspirin over a four-year period (1.5 deaths per year among 11,000 men = 0.014 percent difference) did not seem significant to me. He wrote back saying that six (heart deaths) compared with 18 is 33 percent different and that was statistically significant, whereas 6 of 44 (stroke deaths) was not considered statistically significant.

I wrote him again suggesting that statistical significance is not the same as clinical significance, adding that I would continue as a participant in the study but I refused to take the aspirin. The director thanked me for my candor and for continuing in the study, which continues to this day.

Through the subsequent years, the aspirin hypothesis has been generally accepted, the operative hypothesis being inhibition of platelet aggregation (blood clots). With the advent of nonsteroidal anti-inflammatory drugs (NSAIDs), the claim has been made that some of these drugs (like naproxen and ibuprofen) also protect against heart attacks since they, too, inhibit thromboxane, an action that is purported to prevent platelet aggregation and therefore prevent what are called "cardiovascular events," the new euphemism for heart attack. However, research has not borne this out, and, like aspirin, NSAIDs cause considerable illness and death due to their side effects of dyspepsia (indigestion), gastrointestinal hemorrhage (intestinal bleeding), renal (kidney) dysfunction, hypertension problems, and precipitation of heart failure. More recently, the cyclooxygenase-1 inhibitors (COX-1 inhibitors) are touted as being cardiovascular protectors for the same reasons as aspirin and NSAIDs. Cyclooxygenase-2 inhibitors (COX-2 inhibitors) have jumped on the bandwagon since they inhibit prostacyclin in the vascular walls. But they do not inhibit platelet thromboxane production and thus have no effect on platelet aggregation. Further, these drugs also have significant harmful side effects.

Because of my experience with the Harvard Physicians' Questionnaire Study, I am a bit skeptical about all these claims. An article in the *Lancet* reinforced my skepticism. A major study from Vanderbilt University School of Medicine and the Nashville Veterans Affairs Medical Center compared the risk of serious coronary heart disease events (heart attack or death) among users of nonaspirin NSAIDs and nonusers over a five-year period. They found no difference in the incidence of serious heart disease and concluded that NSAIDs had no protective effect against heart attacks or heart death.

In an accompanying editorial, Dr. John G. F. Cleland, cardiologist at Hull University in England, reviewed not only this study but also all available meta-analyses on the cardio-protective effect of aspirin, NSAIDs, and COX-1 and -2 inhibiting drugs. He agreed that aspirin "may" be an effective agent for the management of acute myocardial infarction, but there is little evidence to support its use beyond the first six weeks after a heart attack. He found that the evidence of cardio-protective benefit from long-term use of aspirin, NSAIDs, or COX-1 or -2 inhibitors is scant, whereas the evidence for undesirable side effects from these drugs is quite solid. He warns that reliance on these ineffective modalities may hinder research in finding better ways to prevent heart attacks.

Of course one of the primary factors commonly causing blood clots in menopausal women has been excess estrogen. Fortunately the trend in medicine is toward lower doses of estrogen, and again, as with heart attacks in women caused by arterial spasm, I suspect heart attacks caused by blood clots will drop dramatically as fewer and fewer women opt for high-dose estrogen regimens.

Strokes and Hormone Balance

Strokes don't get nearly the attention that heart attacks do, so I want to give you some sobering statistics that I hope will encourage you to pay better attention to your stroke risks. Strokes are the second-leading cause of death after heart attacks in women, and the third-leading cause of death after heart attacks and cancer in men. Though men are more likely to have a stroke, women are more likely to die from one. Women have a one-in-five chance of dying from a stroke, and they are more likely to have a stroke than a heart attack before the age of 45.

What Exactly Is a Stroke?

Strokes are sudden, often catastrophic, brain-damaging events due to either the sudden blockage or breaking of a blood vessel in the brain. An *ischemic (blood-flow stopping) stroke* occurs when a blood clot blocks a blood vessel. It may originate in the brain (a thrombus) or arrive there from elsewhere in the vascular system, such as the legs (an embolus). Ischemic events account for about 80 percent of strokes.

Hemorrhagic strokes originate as a rupture in a blood vessel within the brain, often at the site of a preexisting aneurysm (the thinning and/or ballooning of a blood vessel). In either case, blood flow is interrupted to brain tissue downstream of the clot or hemorrhage. When blood is ejected out of the blood vessel anywhere in or adjacent to the brain, it is inflammatory and causes swelling that magnifies the extent of the damage. If the patient survives the acute phase of the stroke, much of this damage eventually resolves and brain function recovers. Hemorrhagic strokes account for about 20 percent of all strokes but cause a much higher percentage of stroke deaths.

What Causes a Stroke?

The underlying causes of strokes are said to be hypertension (high blood pressure), atherosclerosis (clogging of the arteries), bleeding disorders (especially iatrogenic—doctor-caused—due to the prescribing of warfarin or other anticoagulants), head trauma, malformations of the veins or arteries, and deterioration of blood vessels in the brain. A small percentage of strokes are due to the unpredictable rupture of undiagnosed aneurysms, usually in people aged 40 to 50, and usually with disastrous consequences.

The brain damage from strokes depends on the size of the blood vessel involved and its location in the brain. Strokes may be minor, major, or instantly lethal. Some minor ischemic strokes are so small that they cause only a fainting spell, or a sudden dizzy spell of relatively short duration. That is, the neurological defect is brief and reversible. This is called a transient ischemic attack (TIA), which can be predictive of stroke: one-third of those who have a TIA will go on to have a larger stroke.

Interruption of blood flow in a larger blood vessel will, of course, cause a larger stroke. Some blood vessels nourish more "important" brain areas than other strokes. When these vessels hemorrhage or are obstructed, the resulting brain defect can be devastating: speech or vision may be lost, an arm or leg paralyzed, recall or thinking impaired, and the personality may change. Such strokes often lead to permanent neurological deficits. The nature of the neurological deficit helps to identify the location of the stroke. CAT and MRI scans (but not skull X rays) are particularly useful in visualizing stroke areas.

The Underlying Causes of Strokes

Prior to the 1970s, stroke incidence and deaths were more common in men than in women. In the last two decades, however, the incidence of fatal strokes in women has increased and now exceeds that of men, accounting for approximately 25 percent of all female deaths. Stroke deaths are relatively uncommon in young women but triple in incidence during ages 55 to 64, and rise dramatically after age 65. Though this great increase in stroke incidence with age is commonly thought to be due simply to aging, it is a mistake to ignore the effect of the sex hormone changes that come with age.

It should be obvious that the underlying health of our circulatory system includes factors of how the blood clots, how "thin" and "smooth" it is, whether plaque has accumulated on artery walls, how smoothly the heart is pumping, and the vitality of cells that make up blood vessel structure. High blood pressure alone will not rupture a healthy artery; it will rupture an artery weakened by degenerative changes.

How Hormone Balance Affects Your Stroke Risk

One of the most important things a woman can do to prevent strokes is to maintain normal physiological levels of progesterone. In regard to overall steroid hormone effects (estrogen, testosterone, cortisol, androstenedione, DHEA), balance is the key. Excess estrogen, for example, is known to increase the risk of blood clots. An analysis of six pertinent references by Grady et al. in 1997 concluded that ERT (estrogen replacement therapy) increased the risk of venous blood clots by 200 to 360 percent, compared to non-estrogen users. The more recent Women's Health Initiative showed a 41 percent increase in strokes in PremPro users.

Increased risk of stroke is also a recognized side effect of oral contraceptives (birth control pills), which contain synthetic estrogens and progestins. It was once thought that lowering the estrogen dose of oral contraceptives or adding various synthetic progestins would decrease the risk of stroke. Recent studies reported in the medical journal *Lancet* have shown, however, that the second- and third-generation oral contraceptives are just as likely to cause strokes as the earlier versions. I believe that this is because the synthetic progestins in oral contraceptives block not only the production of progesterone but also block progesterone from its receptors throughout the body, and thus block its beneficial antiestrogen effects.

In men, low testosterone levels bring an increased risk of stroke.

Preventing Strokes

To prevent strokes, then, you should focus on keeping your blood and blood vessels healthy. This, as we know, requires:

- a good diet (avoiding foods that damage the arteries such as rancid oils);
- good hydration (drink plenty of clean water);
- exercise, which creates good blood flow and larger caliber blood vessels;
- antioxidants to prevent LDL-cholesterol oxidation that damages arteries; and
- proper balance between estrogen and progesterone.

Conventional medicine generally ignores the progesterone factor. Even worse, it favors synthetic progestins when natural progesterone is indicated, such as in HRT prescriptions.

Until their doctors learn about estrogen/progesterone balance, women must take steps to maintain it themselves. In premenopausal women, you can correct estrogen dominance with appropriate supplements of natural progesterone (preferably in transdermal cream). Postmenopausal women on HRT can best treat estrogen dominance by reducing their estrogen supplement dosage and restoring normal physiologic levels of progesterone.

Similarly, low testosterone levels, which occur with aging, increase the risk of stroke in men, so it's also important that men over the age of 50 get a saliva hormone level test every few years and supplement with low-dose, natural testosterone if needed.

Preventing a stroke requires many of the same lifestyle changes that preventing a heart attack requires. But for women, hormone balance is equally important. If American women were creating hormone balance with lifestyle changes and small, physiologic doses of natural hormones, the rate of stroke would drop considerably.

WHAT INCREASES STROKE RISK

smoking
diabetes
obesity
irregular heartbeat (atrial fibrillation)
high blood pressure
excessive estrogen/estrogen dominance (men and women)
progesterone deficiency
low testosterone in men
birth control pills
high homocysteine levels
poor diet
lack of exercise
lack of antioxidants
heavy alcohol consumption
rancid oils and hydrogenated oils

What Prevents Strokes

hormone balance (men and women)
adequate exercise (not excessive)
adequate levels of magnesium and potassium
adequate fiber in the diet
eating fish regularly
drinking tea, especially green tea
adequate antioxidant levels, especially vitamins A and E
more fruits and vegetables in the diet, which lowers the risk
   of stroke
a glass of wine with dinner (more is not better)
bioflavonoids found in fruits strengthen blood vessels
eating plenty of garlic and onions, which keep the blood
   "thin" and "slippery"

The Bottom Line

Even though hormone balance created *with natural hormones in physiologic doses* is an important part of preventing heart disease, it's likely that conventional HRT with its excess estrogen and progestins has been responsible a great deal of the heart disease in women in the United States.

Equally if not more important is the role that obesity and high insulin have in creating cardiovascular disease, and the role that good nutrition and exercise have in preventing it.

CHAPTER 15

HORMONE BALANCE AND CANCER

The incidence of breast cancer (how many women are getting it) is steadily rising, and the numbers are appalling: In the year 2000, approximately 182,800 women were diagnosed with breast cancer. Since 1950, breast cancer incidence has risen by 60 percent. Some will argue that this is due to better and earlier detection. But even for women over 80 years of age, where this early detection issue is doubtful, the incidence of breast cancer has risen the past 30 years from 1 in 30 women to 1 in 8 women. About 15 percent of women who die of cancer are dying of breast cancer. Those are statistics for the United States, but it's even more sobering to realize that worldwide about 1,670,000 women have breast cancer.

The mortality (death rate) from breast cancer is also staggering. If you combine mortality rates from the United States and Canada (which have the highest rates of breast cancer in the world), in North America a woman dies of breast cancer every 12 minutes.

The incidence of breast cancer rises with age, but is also increasing in younger, premenopausal women as well as in postmenopausal women. The incidence increases with age such that the risk of breast cancer is now about 1 in 10 for women over 75 years of age. Experts agree that environmental risk factors, such as diet and toxin exposure, account for about 80 percent of breast cancers, and genetic factors account for about 20 percent.

I believe the use of natural progesterone by women who need it could greatly reduce the epidemic of breast cancer in Western industrialized countries. Breast cancer and endometrial (uterine) cancer both occur in tissues sensitive to hormones made by the ovaries (estrogens and progesterone). Unopposed estrogens are the only known cause of endometrial cancer, though there may well be other factors involved. One or more of the estrogens are known to contribute to breast cancer incidence. Given the strong associations between estrogens and these cancers, it will become apparent as this chapter unfolds that progesterone may have a balancing or opposing role to estrogens in cancer. This chapter provides a general overview of hormones and cancer. If you would like much more detailed information about hormones and cancer, and more specifically hormones and breast cancer, please read *What Your Doctor May* Not *Tell You About Breast Cancer* (Warner Books, 2002), which I wrote with coauthors David Zava, Ph.D., and Virginia Hopkins.

Reestablishing Cellular Communication

In general, cancer is the abnormal growth of cells in our bodies sufficient to kill us if left untreated. If we look at the big picture, cancer comes about from an imbalance in the body. Correct the imbalance and the cancer often goes away. When we focus in on the specific mechanisms of cancer, the picture becomes fuzzier. The truth is, even after the billions of dollars spent on research over many decades, we still don't understand exactly what cancer is.

The average person thinks of cancer as a foreign growth that has to be cut out, burned out, or destroyed by chemicals. This is a misguided approach. All cancer originates as a minor change in one of your own cells. Something has gone out of balance and the cell is multiplying at a slightly increased rate; it isn't differentiating into the type of cell it was designed to be. A cancer cell *increases* its rate of multiplication and *loses* its ability to differentiate. Cells normally replicate themselves continually as needed for normal growth and repair. Each cell (with the exception of ova and sperm) contains a full complement of chromosomes, yet each develops in a manner specific for its purpose in the body. When it becomes a cancer cell, it multiplies faster than it should and loses normal differentiation. In that sense it becomes a more primitive cell, growing at its own "undisciplined" rate. These cell changes are symptoms of disease, symptoms of an imbalance. In an article in *Lancet*, Dr. Alan B. Astrow states that after a 25-year war on cancer, with a growing assortment of anticancer drugs, ever-more radical treatment strategies, spectacular advances in our understanding of the molecular mechanism, and so on, more and more people are dying from cancer in the United States. We are losing the war on cancer using chemicals, radiation, and surgery. Astrow says a new view has to be generated. Far from being foreign invaders, cancer cells are an intimate part of ourselves, essentially normal cells in which proportionately small changes in genes have led to changes in their behavior. The treatment strategy should be to reestablish intracellular communication, the restoration of order that begins with the establishment of communication mechanisms within the cell—a rebalancing.

How Cancer Develops

The actual mechanisms by which cancer begins are still speculative. There are two competing but not mutually exclusive theories. One *genetic* theory proposes that cancer is the product of chromosomal DNA damage induced by radiation, viruses, or toxins. The body combats this damage with chromosomal repair mechanisms, but as one's life progresses, the accumulated bits of damage increase over time. Thus the incidence of cancer increases with age. Factors that interfere with or impede repair mechanisms, such as toxins and stress, will predispose one to cancer.

A more recent *epigenetic* (meaning "the action of the environment") theory holds that toxic environments within the cell can stimulate an otherwise undamaged chromosome to switch to a more primitive mode of survival in response to the toxic threat. The more primitive survival mode includes an increased rate of multiplication. The epigenetic theory suggests that maintaining a healthy intracellular environment will prevent cancer,

and that correcting a toxic intracellular environment may lead
to successful nontoxic treatment for cancer. Evidence against the
genetic theory and/or favoring the epigenetic theory includes
the following:

- Under the same risk exposure, only some people develop
  cancer.
- Under similar exposure to known carcinogens, different
  individuals develop cancer at different tissue sites.
- In humans and other animals exposed to known carcinogens, cancer can be prevented by eating foods rich in beta
  carotene, vitamin C, and other antioxidants that aid in the
  repair and maintenance of cells.
- In cell culture tests, cancer induced by known carcinogens
  can be reversed and eliminated by improving the nutrient
  quality of the cell culture.
- In humans with advanced cancer, survival time can often
  be increased by high-dose vitamin C.
- Changes in patient attitude seem to extend survival time.
  We now know without a doubt that a negative state of
  mind can adversely affect the body down to the cellular
  level.
- In humans, "spontaneous" remissions and apparent cures
  can result from dietary changes or a combination of a positive attitude and diet.

It is common in cancer circles to separate cancer causation
into two phases: initiator and promoter. It is agreed that under
normal, healthy conditions, the chromosomes (DNA) of cells
that divide are blessed with gene segments (genomes) that repair
DNA damage as it occurs. DNA damage can result from ioniz-
ing radiation, viral attack, or chemical toxins, or it may occur at
the time of early embryo formation. These are all initiators. The
defect may lie dormant for years. As time proceeds, our cells
may be exposed to chemical or biological agents that act to promote cell division and abnormal proliferation. Such agents may
damage cell membranes, activate cell receptors, inactivate receptors that moderate cell division, or may affect previously dam-

aged chromosomes directly. All of these factors can promote cell multiplication out of synchrony with similar unaffected cells. These agents would be called promoters. The risk of exposure to both initiators and promoters increases as we age. Thus the appearance or manifestation of cancer generally increases with age. Cells that do not routinely multiply (muscle and nerve cells) rarely become cancerous.

The DES (diethylstilbestrol) scenario is illustrative. When a woman takes DES during pregnancy, it can cause damage to the DNA of the developing embryo/fetus, particularly the tissues of the urogenital tract. Early in embryo life, both sexes have a common, undifferentiated urogenital tract. As the embryo grows, this tract develops (differentiates) into male and female forms, becoming the ovaries, uterus, fallopian tubes, and vagina in the female; and the testes, scrotum, and penis in the male. During this time of differentiation, the cells of the urogenital tract are particularly sensitive to the potent DES hormone, and latent damage can result. Later in life, this damage may show up as organ deformities of the uterus and an increased susceptibility to cancer of the cervix and vagina. In males it can lead to undescended testes (cryptorchidism), lower sperm counts, abnormalities of the penis, and/or an increased susceptibility to prostate cancer. Some of these effects may not manifest until late in life. The damage wrought by DES (a xenoestrogen) is not evident until late in the generation following the one exposed to DES.

From this example, we see that the timing of the exposure to an initiator can be very important, and that damaging results may not become evident for years or even until the next generation. In this regard, it is interesting to note that EPA and FDA toxicity tests look at actual toxicity and congenital defects, but do not routinely look for such late effects.

Estrogen Stimulates Cell Growth

There's little if any debate left in the scientific community about whether estrogen plays a primary role in causing breast and endometrial cancer—it does. But what the conventional medical community is not entirely clear about yet is whether the excessive doses of estrogen and the progestins in conventional HRT are among the possible causes of many breast cancers in the United States. The Women's Health Initiative, with its 29 percent higher rate of breast cancer among women using PremPro, made this point clearly, but it's a bitter pill for conventional medicine to swallow, and there is still much resistance to the evidence. It is not hormone replacement per se, but conventional medicine's specific way of prescribing it that creates estrogen dominance.

Let's take a look at some of the evidence that shows excess or deficient hormones can create cancer:

• Breast cancer is more likely to occur in premenopausal women with normal or high estrogen levels and low progesterone levels. This situation may occur in early adult life in a few women but is quite common after age 35 or so, when anovulatory periods tend to occur.

• Among premenopausal women, breast cancer recurrence or late metastases after mastectomy for breast cancer is more common when surgery had been performed during the first half of the menstrual cycle (when estrogen is the dominant hormone) than when surgery had been performed during the latter half of the menstrual cycle (when progesterone is dominant). The research on this is plentiful and makes one wonder why all breast cancer surgery isn't scheduled during the luteal phase of the menstrual cycle when progesterone is high. Or, doctors could prescribe the application of transdermal progesterone prior to surgery.

• Tamoxifen (a weak estrogenic compound that competes with natural estrogen at receptor sites) is commonly prescribed to women after breast cancer surgery for the purpose of preventing recurrence of their cancer.

• Pregnancy occurring before age 30 is known to have a protective effect. Progesterone is the dominant hormone during pregnancy.

• Only the first, full-term, early pregnancy conveys protection. Women having their first pregnancies before age 18 have approximately one-third the risk of women bearing the first child after age 35. Interrupted pregnancies (induced or spontaneous abortions) do not afford protection.

• Women without children are at a higher risk than those with one or more children.

• Women subjected to oophorectomy (removal of both ovaries) prior to age 40 have a significantly reduced risk of breast cancer.

• The protective effects of early oophorectomy are negated by the administration of estrogen.

• Treatment of males with estrogen (for prostatic cancer or after transsexual surgery) is associated with an increased risk of breast cancer.

• Recently, industrial pollutants having potent estrogenic effects, called *xenoestrogens*, are being recognized as a pervasive environmental threat, likely to be a contributing factor in the incidence of breast cancer. Such correlations strongly suggest that estrogen, especially if unopposed by progesterone, is somehow related to the development of breast cancer.

• And, of course, breast, ovarian, and endometrial cancer is more likely to occur in women that are made estrogen dominant by receiving "hormone replacement therapy," referring to ERT and to HRT that combines estrogen with a synthetic progestin.

Estrogen's job in the uterus is to cause proliferation of the cells. During a menstrual cycle, uterine cells multiply faster under the influence of estrogen, and then progesterone normally comes on the scene with ovulation and stops the cells from multiplying. Progesterone causes the cells to mature and enter into a secretory phase that causes the maturing of the uterine lining, which is now ready to receive a possible fertilized egg. An analogy would be the growth of an apple: When it's finished growing, it begins to ripen. Estrogen is the hormone that stimulates cell proliferation, or the growing phase. Progesterone is the hormone that stops growth and stimulates ripening. Some researchers have claimed that progesterone stimulates cell growth in breast tissue, but that is a misunderstanding of its role. Progesterone very temporarily stimulates tissue growth toward and into differentiation—differentiated cells are not cancerous. Promoting differentiation is one way that progesterone protects against cancer.

Three studies in particular have shown progesterone's effect on breast cells. One, by Foidart et al. and published in the journal *Fertility and Sterility*, in 1998, concluded, "Exposure to progesterone for 14 days reduced the estradiol-induced proliferation of normal breast epithelial cells in vivo." The other, by Malet et al. and published in the *Journal of Steroid Biochemistry and Molecular Biology*, in 2000, concluded, "Cells exhibited a proliferative appearance after E2 [estradiol] treatment, and returned to a quiescent appearance when P[rogesterone] was added to E2. P[rogesterone] appear(s) predominantly to inhibit cell growth, both in the presence and absence of E2."

Perhaps the most thorough study demonstrating the action of estradiol and progesterone on cell multiplication (proliferation) in breast cells was beautifully demonstrated in an important 1995 study by Chang et al. It tested the effects of transdermal (via the skin) hormone applications on normal human breast duct cells, from which cancer is known to rise, in healthy young women planning to undergo minor breast surgery for benign breast disease.

In this study, the women were divided into four groups and began using one of the creams on their breasts 10 to 13 days before breast surgery:

- Group A applied estradiol cream (1.5 mg) daily.
- Group B applied progesterone cream (25 mg) daily.
- Group C applied a combination of estradiol and progesterone (half doses each) daily.
- Group D applied a placebo cream.

At surgery, biopsies were obtained for measuring estradiol and progesterone concentrations, and for tests of cell proliferation rates. In addition, blood plasma hormone levels were measured. Following surgery the breast tissue, about the size of a marble, was divided in half and one part was sent to a pathology laboratory for viewing under a microscope to determine how the hormones affected the growth rate of the breast cells. The remainder of the breast tissue was sent to an endocrinology laboratory to determine how much hormone was taken up by the tissue. (See Figure 15.)

Results from the endocrinology laboratory revealed that in those women treated with just estradiol the concentration of estradiol in the breast tissue was 200 times greater than those not treated with it (placebo gel). Breast tissue concentrations of progesterone were 100 times greater in women who used progesterone than placebo. These findings clearly demonstrate that both hormones are well absorbed transdermally (through the skin) and accumulate in target tissues in the same manner as endogenous (made in the body) hormones. This is important because it is common for conventional doctors to claim that transdermal progesterone isn't absorbed, and as you'll discover in the chapter on progesterone, transdermal application is preferable.

The effect of these hormones on cell proliferation rates was equally clear. Estradiol increased cell proliferation rate by 230 percent, whereas progesterone *decreased* it by more than 400 percent. The estradiol/progesterone combination cream maintained the normal proliferation rate. Again, this is evidence that unopposed estradiol stimulates hyperproliferation of breast cells and progesterone protects against this.

When progesterone is used transdermally, blood tests don't show a measurable rise, and this is why so many doctors believe it isn't absorbed. It is important to note that progesterone levels rose dramatically in the breast cells of women using transdermal progesterone, and this proves that progesterone is well absorbed when applied to the skin. However, the blood tests showed no measurable increase of progesterone concentration. This is an excellent illustration of the fact that blood testing cannot be reliably used to determine the bioavailable level of progesterone when it is delivered through the skin, because bioavailable pro-

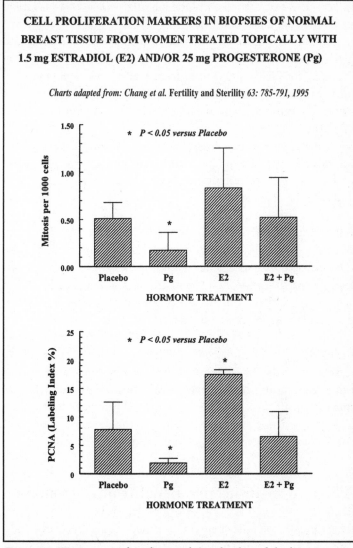

CELL PROLIFERATION MARKERS IN BIOPSIES OF NORMAL
BREAST TISSUE FROM WOMEN TREATED TOPICALLY WITH
1.5 mg ESTRADIOL (E2) AND/OR 25 mg PROGESTERONE (Pg)

Charts adapted from: Chang et al. Fertility and Sterility 63: 785-791, 1995

Figure 15: Women treated with topical (on the skin of the breast) proges-terone alone prior to surgery had much lower proliferation (cell division) rates than women given nothing, (placebo) and women taking estrogen alone (E2) or with progesterone (E2 +Pg).

gesterone is not carried in blood plasma, which is what's measured in a standard blood test.

The above studies demonstrate that estrogen dominance in general stimulates breast tissue: Premenstrual women who are estrogen dominant often suffer from breast swelling and tenderness. Progesterone is the hormone that brings maturation; it brings the cells back into balance, and thus can eliminate breast tenderness.

Be aware that not all estrogens are equivalent in their actions on breast tissue. Among the three major natural estrogens, estradiol is the most stimulating to breast tissue, estrone is second, and estriol by far the least. During pregnancy, estriol is the dominant estrogen, being produced in great quantities by the placenta, while ovarian production of estradiol and estrone are minimal. Since all estrogens compete for the same receptor sites, it is probable that sufficient estriol impedes the carcinogenic effects of estradiol and/or estrone. Lemon et al. reported in a 1996 JAMA article that women with breast cancer excreted 30 to 60 percent *less* estriol than noncancer controls, and remission of cancer in patients receiving endocrine therapy occurred only in those whose estriol quotient *rose*. That is, low levels of estriol relative to estradiol and estrone correlate with increased risk of breast cancer, and higher levels of estriol from endocrine treatment correlate with remission of cancer. Further, rodent studies show that estrone and estradiol are carcinogenic for breast cancer in males or castrated females whereas estriol is not.

The Cancer-Protective Benefits of Progesterone

The cancer-protective benefit of progesterone is clearly indicated by a beautiful prospective study done by Johns Hopkins Medical School and published in the *American Journal of Epidemiology* in 1981. How would you test the cancer protection of progesterone? One good way would be to measure women's estrogen and progesterone levels and then divide them into two groups: one with normal progesterone levels and one with low progesterone levels.

You take 20 years to accumulate enough people, and then you follow them for another 20 years to see what happens. Johns Hopkins Private Obstetrics and Gynecology Clinic did just that, and reported the results in the *American Journal of Epidemiology*. When the low progesterone group was compared with the normal progesterone group, it was found that the occurrence of breast cancer was 5.4 times greater in the women in the low progesterone group; that is, the incidence of breast cancer in the low progesterone group was more than 80 percent greater than that in the normal progesterone group. This difference was not explained by when a woman began menstruating, when she reached menopause, her history of oral contraceptive use, her history of benign breast disease, or her age at first birth of child: No other factor dislodged this ratio of 5.4 times more breast cancer in the low progesterone group. When the study looked at the low progesterone group for *all* types of cancer, they found that women in the *low* progesterone group experienced a tenfold increase from all malignant cancers, compared with the normal progesterone group. This would suggest that having a normal level of progesterone protected women from nine-tenths of all cancers that might otherwise have occurred. And of course this study was published and disappeared without a ripple—there was no money to pursue the obvious implication that progesterone deficiency plays a major role in cancer.

In a 1995 study published in the journal *Fertility and Sterility*, researchers did a double-blind randomized study examining the use of topical natural progesterone (cream) and/or topical estrogen in regard to breast duct cell growth. Forty premenopausal women scheduled to have breast surgery for removal of a presumably benign lump were studied. They were divided into four groups and asked to apply a gel to their breasts daily for 10 to 13 days before surgery. One group received a placebo, one group received progesterone, one group received estrogen (estradiol), and one group received a combination of progesterone and estrogen. Blood tests were taken the day of surgery, and breast tissue taken during surgery was tested for hormone levels and the rate of cell growth. The women using progesterone had dramatically reduced cell multiplication rates compared with the women using either the placebo or the estrogen. The women using only estrogen had significantly higher cell multiplication rates than any of the other groups. The women using a combination of progesterone and estrogen were closer to the placebo group.

This exciting study provides some of the first direct evidence that both estradiol and progesterone are well absorbed through the skin, that 10 to 13 days of transdermal (on the skin) hormone application significantly increases the concentration of hormone levels in breast cells, that estradiol significantly increases breast cell hyperplasia (increased cell growth), and that progesterone impressively decreases cell proliferation rates, even when estrogen is also supplemented.

Since duct cell hyperplasia (an increased rate of cell growth in breast duct cells) is recognized as a major risk indicator for breast cancer, it seems clear that progesterone, contrary to the synthetic progestins, is protective against breast cancer.

Because the blood tests did not reflect the increased levels of progesterone that had reached the breast cells, this study also shows that testing blood plasma levels of progesterone is not useful in measuring transdermal progesterone absorption. A salivary hormone test would be a more accurate reflection.

In the late 1990s, researchers B. Formby and T. S. Wiley published a study in the *Annals of Clinical and Laboratory Science* (1998) showing that estrogen added to breast cancer cell cultures activated the oncogene (cancer-causing gene) Bcl-2, whereas progesterone activated the cancer-protective gene, p53. A study from France and published in the journal *Climacteric* provides the first real clinical evidence that it is the progestins in HRT, not the progesterone, that increases breast cancer risk. B. de Lignieres et al. compared different categories of HRT but this time included progesterone (oral, as it happened). They found that long-term HRT using topical estradiol gel (in much smaller doses than when taken orally) and progesterone had no increased risk of breast cancer compared to nonusers.

They concluded that there is no reason not to use HRT made of estradiol gel and progesterone, and they regard this type of HRT to be "beneficial for quality of life, prevention of bone loss and cardiovascular risk profile, without the activation of coagulation and inflammatory protein synthesis measured in users of oral estrogen." This is a good step, I believe, in showing that progesterone is much better than Provera when used in HRT, and that lower-dose transdermal estrogen can be used safely.

The real point made by this study is that the safety and efficacy of HRT depends on what kind of HRT is being used. It's not a matter of HRT or no HRT, it's a matter of using the right HRT.

Also very interesting is research done by Jose Russo, M.D., a Senior Member of the Fox Chase Cancer Center in Philadelphia, Adjunct Professor of Pathology and Cell Biology at Jefferson Medical School, and Adjunct Professor of Pathology and Laboratory Medicine at the University of Pennsylvania Medical School. We interviewed Dr. Russo for the *John R. Lee, M.D. Medical Letter*, and this is an excerpt of what he had to say about pregnancy hormones and differentiation of breast tissue:

> Humans have areas of breast tissue that are highly proliferative [have a tendency to grow] and are much more vulnerable to damage by any given carcinogenic agent (something that causes breast cancer), such as those found in the environment, estrogen and radiation. During pregnancy, hormones cause changes in the breast, called differentiation. These changes appear to protect breast tissue against carcinogens. The immature breasts of young girls contain structures called lobules type 1 that have a high proliferative activity, and those are the areas that are more susceptible to damage from a given carcinogen. For example, in the atomic bombing of Hiroshima and Nagasaki, in Japan, a lot of radiation was created. Girls who were between 10 and 14 years old at the time, and who were exposed to the radiation, later developed breast cancer at a much higher rate than the general population. The reason is because their breasts contained a lot of these undifferentiated, more vulnerable lobules type 1 at the time of the bombing.
>
> When the breast is stimulated by the sequential cascade

of the hormones released during pregnancy the [breast] gland differentiates and with that process specific genes are activated that make the tissue more resistant to cancer. Cells that are differentiated have a better ability to repair the damage induced in the DNA (genetic material). These have allowed us to postulate a biological law that is "The differentiation of the mammary gland determines its susceptibility to carcinogenesis." We are using this concept to develop strategies for preventing breast cancer.

Even though Mother Nature set it up so that young girls could get pregnant and be protected against breast cancer, that doesn't happen often in Western countries. So how do we protect the breasts in women who may not be getting pregnant until their mid-twenties to their mid-thirties? We started looking for a way to stimulate differentiation in the breast without pregnancy. In experiments with rats, we found the best protection using human chorionic gonadotropin (hCG). When administered to nonpregnant animals, it induces the same level of differentiation as pregnancy. The remarkable effect that this produces is a resistance to the development of cancer when these animals are challenged with a chemical carcinogen.

The hormone hCG has two pathways of action. One is through the ovary by increasing the levels of estrogen and progesterone, which creates differentiation in the mammary glands. We found out that hCG also has a direct effect on the mammary tissue. It binds to a specific receptor and elicits a cascade of events that include the activation of a nonsteroidal glycoprotein called inhibin. Inhibin regulates cell proliferation and induces the activation of genes that control programmed cell death and differentiation.

We also have found that when we use this hormone in patients with primary breast cancer, the proliferative activity of the cancer tissue is significantly reduced after seven doses of this hormone in a two-week period. These data are important because they also indicate that the differentiation of the mammary tissue could be achieved in cells that are already cancerous.

I believe that Dr. Russo's work is highly significant and could represent a major step in how to protect women—especially women who have children late or don't have them at all—from breast cancer, as well as a major step in how to treat breast cancer itself. This is exactly the type of research that can be difficult to find funding for because it is for a natural substance (hCG) and not a drug.

Hormone Receptors in Breast Cancer

Tests have been developed that show whether a breast cancer has receptors for estrogen and progesterone. What if the cancer tests positive for progesterone? Is that a sign that a woman shouldn't be using progesterone? Quite the opposite. One must keep in mind the "message" (effect) of the hormone. In the case of progesterone, the hormone will be beneficial in helping to keep the cancer cells under control. The positive progesterone receptor test is merely a sign that the cancer is receptive to the balancing and anticancer effects of progesterone.

Hormones float through the bloodstream and the fluid around the cells, and they work only if they unite with a receptor in the cell that is already designed to be there. The hormone fits into the receptor like a lock in a key. If the receptor is there, they hook up and make their way to the nuclear chromosomes, and activate the appropriate gene site of a chromosome to produce an effect, a hormone action in that cell. Then, once that message has been sent, so to speak, the hormone is released.

Hormones work only if the receptor site is present in the cell. Thus, when people call and write me to ask about the wisdom of using progesterone in cases of breast cancer that are positive for progesterone receptors, I explain that if the cancer is progesterone receptor positive, that's the only way the progesterone could ever work! If the cancer is estrogen site positive, she should not have estrogen, because estrogen causes the cell to multiply. Progesterone causes the cancer to stop multiplying.

When estrogen and progesterone receptor testing of breast cancer cells is done, it is generally the rule that progesterone receptors are not found unless plenty of estrogen receptors are present. Estrogen stimulates the emergence of progesterone receptors. Since estrogen stimulates cell proliferation (which is not desirable in cancer cells) and progesterone inhibits proliferation in favor of cell maturation, it would seem wise to supply the needed progesterone.

It should be recalled that the breast cancer growth rate is quite variable; the doubling time ranges from one month to over two years, with the average doubling time being about three months. Even at that relatively rapid rate of growth, it is estimated that the time from the emergence of a single cancer cell to its growth to a size sufficient for diagnosis by palpation (touch) is typically about eight to ten years (diagnosis by mammogram may be made, at most, two years earlier). This lag time between onset and diagnosis means that many breast cancers start during the 10 to 15 years before menopause, which is the premenopausal time when estrogen dominance is so common. Thus progesterone supplementation in women with low progesterone levels during these years may help prevent breast cancer.

What About Mammograms?

Mammograms are low-energy X-ray views of breasts obtained for the purpose of detecting breast cancer earlier than by palpation, in the hope that the risk of dying from breast cancer can be reduced. Though this hope may appear sensible to most, appearance and reality are not necessarily the same thing. The lag time between cancer inception and diagnosis even by mammograms may well be over eight years. Diagnosis by palpation can be made about one year later. If the cancer is one that is prone to metastasize, why would it not have metastasized during the years before the mammogram? Where is the evidence that this one-year difference in time of diagnosis will make any difference? And if a given test is found negative, how often should mammograms be repeated? If one accepts the argument that the one-year time interval between mammogram diagnosis and palpation diagnosis is crucial, to be consistent one would have to argue that, to be effective, mammograms should be performed at least every two years. Good evidence for answers for all of these questions is lacking.

Then we have the problem of reliability. Just how good are mammograms at accurately detecting breast cancer? A large Canadian study found that women utilizing mammograms experienced a higher mortality from breast cancer than women who did not have mammograms. This study was discounted by the pro-mammogram spokespeople on the basis of the quality of the mammograms done. If this argument is correct, how does a woman know whether the mammogram she had was a good one or not? It is common knowledge that 30 percent of positive readings turn out to be false and, when cancer is present, a negative reading is reached 10 to 20 percent of the time. For example, Patricia was a trim and youthful 42-year-old woman who came into my office for a routine examination. As I was showing her how to do a breast self-exam, I discovered a small lump in one of her breasts. She told me she had found the lump a year before and, after several months of procrastination, had seen a doctor who ordered a mammogram, which, she was pleased to say, had been negative. She had been advised to wait a year before repeating the test. On my advice she obtained an excision biopsy of this easily palpable lump. The biopsy found breast cancer, and she decided to have a simple mastectomy. Now, 10 years later, she is healthy and active. Reliance on the negative initial mammogram increased her danger by delaying prompt treatment of a suspicious lump.

Recently I received a letter from a woman named Shirley, who, at age 42, detected a firm lumpiness in her left breast. During the next two years she had annual mammograms, all showing a suspicious nonspecific area of density. A surgical biopsy signified the lump was negative. Her doctor, for reasons unknown, placed Shirley on oral contraceptives. The lumps increased in size. A third mammogram a year later showed that the original suspicious area was still there and had become even more suspicious. Shirley then had another biopsy, which found cancer, and she underwent a mastectomy and was given a course of chemotherapy. A year and a half later, her chest X ray showed suspicious nodules at the base of her left lung. Following a surgical biopsy of these nodules, it was found that Shirley's cancer had metastasized, and she died, a tragic consequence of delay wrought by overreliance on nondiagnostic mammograms and a misguided or inept surgical biopsy.

Given this state of inaccuracy in readings of such import, it should not be surprising that the typical mammogram report these days is neither a clear "yes" or "no" but a highly qualified "maybe." A perfect pair of breasts, mammogram-wise, is a rare thing. The mammogram reader often reports a finding of some suspicious nature (a vague sense of localized density or perhaps some minute calcifications here and there) and suggests some concern, along with the advice to check further or obtain a repeat test at some later date. The doctor and her patient are left with uneasy choices. Should they try a needle biopsy or open excision biopsy, or merely follow along with repeat tests, and, if so, how long should she wait? If the biopsy is done and no malignancy found, does it mean that perhaps the malignancy was missed? If she opts for later reevaluation rather than biopsy, what happens to the risk of metastases if malignancy is in fact present? The patient faces unpleasant choices: unnecessary surgery versus possible increased chance of death. Chronic cancer anxiety can become her normal state of mind.

Muriel came into my office at age 50 with multiple scars on both breasts from seven different excision biopsies, all of which found dense fibrocystic breasts. She readily admitted chronic cancer anxiety. In addition, she suffered from reactive hypoglycemia. She performed breast self-exams routinely and the finding of each new lump aroused fear and trepidation because of her cysts. Now, at menopause, she wanted hormone replacement therapy. Instead of traditional HRT, I recommended physiologic dosages of progesterone without estrogen. Her breast fibrocysts disappeared within six months, her sense of energy and libido returned, her hypoglycemic episodes became a thing of the past, and her tennis game improved. Further, serial bone mineral density (BMD) tests over the subsequent 10 years remained good, and her cancer anxiety faded away with the improvement in her breasts.

The efficacy of screening mammography was evaluated by a recent overview study. After analyzing 13 studies, the authors concluded that mammography offers no benefit to women under 50 years of age, but appears to reduce breast cancer mortality in women aged 50 to 74. The authors admit, however, that their study could not determine whether competent breast exam by palpation would have provided the same benefit. Several peculiarities of the study should be noted. The magnitude of the apparent mammogram benefit in women over 50 was similar regardless of the number of mammographic views, screening interval, or duration of follow-up (7 to 9 years versus 10 to 12 years). That is, it did not matter whether single or double views were used, or whether the test was done yearly or every 33 months. The magnitude of the mammogram benefit in this age group is given as about 25 percent. That is, if breast cancer incidence in this age group is one case per 30 women, or 33 cases in 1,000 women, it means that for every 1,000 women having mammograms, 25 percent of the 33 cases of breast cancer found, or about 8 women, would be less likely to die of breast cancer during the next 12 years, according to this report. My hunch is that if those same women or their physicians would perform an adequate breast self-exam for breast cancer, the results would very likely be the same. In the Canadian trial, mammography did not reduce breast cancer mortality beyond the reduction achieved by clinical examination alone.

Another explanation for the presumed benefit of mammography concerns the question of the diagnosis of duct cell "carcinoma in situ." The phrase "carcinoma in situ" implies the finding of suspicious-looking cells scattered here and there in breast tissue, and not growing as a clump or tumor-mass. At one time (prior to 1992), some pathologists used this term to indicate cells they thought might be actual cancer cells at an early stage. Since 1992, most pathologists agree that these cells do not, in fact, progress to actual cancer with any risk of true cancer—in fact the "cure" rate is said to be 99 percent. These are cases found by mammograms (and not by palpation) that resulted in breast surgery, irradiation, or chemotherapy and were counted as "cancer cures" by mammogram proponents. Since they were not true cancers, these apparent "cures" created the illusion that mammograms and early treatment were effective when, in fact, no treatment was necessary.

I believe the jury on mammograms is still out and that women can probably achieve the same benefit by carefully examining their own breasts once a month. Nobody knows your breasts better than you do. You've lived with them for decades and know how they are supposed to feel. If you don't know, I suggest you begin getting better acquainted with them, starting today. I have had women come into my office who were able to detect breast lumps the size of a grain of rice. If you don't know how to do a breast exam, ask your doctor to show you, or ask for a brochure that describes the procedure.

Tamoxifen and Aromatase Inhibitors

Tamoxifen is a drug given to women who have had breast cancer or who are at a high risk for breast cancer. It competes in the breast with estrogen for estrogen receptors, much as phytoestrogens do. Like phytoestrogens, tamoxifen has mild estrogenic properties, but is considered an anti-estrogen since it inhibits the cell proliferation activity of regular estrogens in the breast. When added to chemotherapy for women who have undergone mastectomy but with positive nodes for cancer that demonstrated positive estrogen, tamoxifen, taken orally, improved disease-free survival. Further studies have shown that when used preventively in those at high risk for breast cancer, tamoxifen lowers the risk of getting breast cancer for a few years. However, this doesn't take into account the many and sometimes deadly side effects of tamoxifen, including an increased risk of uterine cancer, strokes, liver damage, and eye damage. Uterine cancer induced by tamoxifen is much more deadly than uterine cancer not due to tamoxifen.

Aromatase inhibitors are another type of anti-estrogen drug used to treat breast cancer, usually after surgery, chemotherapy, and radiation. They block the (aromatase) enzymes that allow the conversion of androgens (male hormones) to estrogen.

Aromatase inhibitors don't appear to have as many or as danger-ous side effects as tamoxifen, but again, they address only part of the breast cancer picture, leaving out the beneficial effects of progesterone. Using aromatase inhibitors in postmenopausal women is an attempt to reduce estrogen levels down to as close to zero as possible. This is not advisable—all adults need some estrogen, just as all adults need some testosterone. Furthermore, without estrogen there are no progesterone receptors, so any ben-efit that might be had from progesterone cannot occur. The point is not in how low you can take someone's estrogen level; the important thing in cancer protection is to create the proper balance between progesterone and estradiol.

Endometrial Cancer

The only known cause of endometrial (uterine) cancer is un-opposed estrogen. Here again, estradiol and estrone are the cul-prits. Estrogen supplements (ERT) given to postmenopausal women for five years increase the risk of endometrial cancer six-fold, and longer-term use increases it fifteen-fold. In pre-menopausal women, endometrial cancer is extremely rare except during the 5 to 10 years before menopause when estrogen dom-inance is common. I believe that the use of natural progesterone in women who are estrogen dominant during these years has the potential to significantly reduce the incidence of endometrial cancer (as well as breast cancer, as noted above), and that in postmenopausal women, endometrial cancer is always a result of excess estrogen relative to progesterone. This is why unopposed estrogen replacement therapy is so strongly contraindicated in women who have a uterus.

In a manner similar to progesterone, the progestin medroxy-progesterone acetate (MPA, Provera) also effectively prevents against estrogen-induced endometrial cancer. However, MPA has many undesirable side effects not found with real proge-sterone. We now know that one of the side effects of this progestin is breast cancer. Thus progesterone is far superior to MPA.

When estrogen is prescribed to postmenopausal women, it is not uncommon that vaginal spotting or bleeding may occur. Given the uncertainties of the significance of vaginal bleeding at this age, the doctor usually recommends an endometrial biopsy or D and C (dilatation and curettage). A common finding is endometrial hyperplasia (areas of excessive endometrial cells) or dysplasia (suspicious-looking endometrial cells). Since many doctors believe hyperplasia and/or dysplasia are a step along the way in cancer development, this finding is hardly reassuring. Quite often, the doctor then recommends hysterectomy, believing that the uterus in postmenopausal women is a useless organ, and it is better to be safe than sorry. With the uterus out, estrogen can be resumed for all its supposed benefits. This line of reasoning is not only condescending to women, but self-serving to her doctor. In pretending to act as protector of his/her patient, he/she manages to convert a side effect of a drug he administered into a lucrative surgical operation.

Nancy, a conscientious, health-minded housewife, had been my patient for many years. At menopause she had developed weight gain and some loss of energy, and was fearful of old age and osteoporosis. A gynecologist she saw at the time prescribed estrogen, which resulted in breast swelling, more weight gain, and no discernible benefit. She refused to take more estrogen. I recommended that she use a progesterone cream, which relieved her breast swelling, helped her lose weight, and brought back her energy. At my retirement, she was 61 years old and doing well on progesterone. She transferred her care to an eminent gynecologist in San Francisco. He convinced her to abandon the over-the-counter progesterone cream and resume estrogen therapy. Again she developed breast swelling, weight gain, and lethargy. Her doctor increased her estrogen dosage. She then developed vaginal spotting. This led to endometrial biopsy and a finding of hyperplasia. He indicated this was precancerous and she should see a gynecologic surgeon for a hysterectomy. In the process, her medical insurance carrier on renewing her policy increased her premiums and included a rider excluding her from any coverage for gynecologic problems. In a panic she called me about this calamitous turn of events.

I asked her to request a copy of her medical records to be sent to me. Despite written requests by herself and me, the records did not arrive. Her doctor deferred to the surgeon who performed the biopsy and was recommending the hysterectomy. After several more letters and phone calls, the information finally arrived. The pathology report indicated nothing more than estrogen-induced endometrial hyperplasia. I told her to discontinue the estrogen, resume the progesterone, and to submit to nothing more than another endometrial biopsy in three months. She accepted my advice, and three months later the biopsy report was entirely normal. I wrote a letter to her insurance carrier pointing out that no pelvic disease existed and that the previous finding was merely the result of a therapeutic misadventure. I added that there was no reason to exclude gynecologic problems from her coverage and indicated I was sending a copy of the letter and the reports to the state insurance board.

Shortly thereafter, Nancy called me to report that a new policy had arrived with full coverage and that she had discovered that the surgeon to whom her doctor had referred her was the wife of her doctor, operating (no pun intended) under her own name. She also said she had found another doctor, one who agreed that natural progesterone would be fine to use. Now, many years later, she is doing well.

This kind of scenario is being repeated with many thousands of women every year. Without casting any stones, it is difficult to resist the observation that the practice of medicine, like any other human endeavor, is not immune to self-interested manipulations and questionable secondary gains at the patient's expense. How many of the annual half million unnecessary hysterectomies are generated by such questionable medical practices? If the doctor or his colleagues are rewarded financially by the logical consequences of women using estrogen, what impetus is there for change?

Endometrial cancer is a relatively "safe" cancer, in that it generally shows itself early by abnormal vaginal bleeding and metastasizes relatively late in its course. It can be cured if a hysterectomy is performed before the cancer metastasizes. Women treated by hysterectomy for endometrial cancer are advised, however, to avoid "hormones" forever. Like patients with a history of breast cancer, they face a future of possible progressive osteoporosis, vaginal atrophy, and recurrent urinary tract infections without recourse to hormonal therapy. These are the women for whom I first began prescribing natural progesterone therapy. Not only did progesterone reverse their osteoporosis and, in many cases, correct their vaginal atrophy, but also none, to my knowledge, have ever developed cancer of any sort. (If vaginal atrophy remains a problem, intravaginal estriol would be the treatment of choice. Estriol is available by prescription at a compounding pharmacy.) Further, among those with intact uteri, none have ever developed any uterine problems of any kind. The evidence is overwhelming that natural progesterone is safe, and only estradiol, estrone, and the various synthetic estrogens and progestins are to be avoided to reduce one's risk of endometrial cancer.

Transcultural Factors in Breast and Uterine Cancer

Although the true incidence of breast and uterine cancer in all geographic areas of the world may not be known with complete accuracy, it is generally acknowledged that these two cancers are relatively rare in nonindustrialized countries. When individuals from these areas emigrate to industrialized cultures, their cancer rates soon rise to match the general rates of their new country. The same is true of heart disease, for example. In the case of heart disease, the change in risk follows the change in diet. Diet is probably a major risk factor in both breast and uterine cancer as well.

The Western, or industrialized, cultural diet is relatively high in meat protein, fat, sugar, and refined carbohydrates—everything but fish, fruits, vegetables, whole grains, nuts, seeds, and fiber, which are exactly the foods we need to eat to maintain optimal health. Diets in industrialized cultures are also high in calories compared to energy needs. In other words, we tend to eat more calories than we can burn off, so we gain weight. The

Third World, or nonindustrialized, cultural diet is relatively high in fiber and largely plant based, and calorie intake is often considerably lower.

It is clear that calories in excess of energy needs increase estrogen levels, which essentially means that obesity increases estrogen levels. When energy needs exceed calorie intake, estrogen declines, reducing fertility. When calorie intake exceeds energy needs, estrogen rises accordingly. Dr. Peter Ellison of Harvard, who has conducted worldwide assays of salivary hormone levels, believes this is the primary reason for the high estrogen levels seen in premenopausal women in industrialized cultures. The estrogen levels he found in Western women are so high in comparison to levels in women of the developing world that they should be considered abnormal. He has stated, "Only at our peril can we assume that ovarian function in the Western world is somehow a model of health."

The primary components of our high calorie intake are sugar and refined carbohydrates. Even though Americans have learned to cut the fat from their diets, they're compensating by increasing their consumption of these other unhealthy foods. Excess intake of sugar and refined carbohydrates causes not just obesity, but also high insulin levels, which when combined increases the risk of almost all types of cancer.

To add insult to injury, literally, our food chain is awash with xenoestrogens, petrochemical by-products from herbicides, pesticides, plastic manufacture, solvents, and emulsifiers that have potent estrogenic effects. In addition to being highly estrogenic, these compounds are nonbiodegradable and fat-soluble, meaning they accumulate in fatty tissues, including in the breasts. The widespread use of petrochemical products in Western cultures makes them difficult to avoid. However, we can greatly lessen our exposure simply by avoiding pesticides and herbicides at home, and by eating organic foods whenever possible.

Other transcultural factors related to breast and uterine cancer include the following:

- The Western diet is woefully deficient in plant-based nutrients that contain cancer fighters such as sulforaphane, phenethyl isothiocyanate, indole-3-carbinol, flavonoids, vitamin C, folic acid, allylic sulfide, capsaicin, genistein, p-coumaric acid, chlorogenic acid, carotenes, vitamin E, and others still unknown, all of which work synergistically to protect us from cancer.

- The Western diet is deficient in fiber, which is found only in plants.
- Western culture is full of laborsaving devices, thus reducing exercise and energy expenditure and creating an abnormal energetic balance.
- Western culture splinters family units and other societal support mechanisms for dealing with stress, loss, and depression, promoting alienation. All of these contribute in one way or another to increased cancer risk.

Breast and endometrial cancer, heart disease, and osteoporosis are some of the greatest fears that women face as they approach menopause. Under present circumstances, these fears are well grounded in reality. However, they need not be. When the cause of any given cancer is known, prevention becomes a reality. Lung cancer, for example, can be almost completely prevented by never smoking. For many cancers, the cause is still unknown. However, for breast and endometrial cancer, a great deal is known about their major hormonal factors. The only mystery is, why hasn't this information permeated the halls of contemporary medicine? The carcinogenic effects of unopposed estradiol and estrone and the anticancer benefits of estriol and progesterone are well established for these two cancers.

Because of its many benefits, its great safety, and particularly its ability to oppose the carcinogenic effects of estrogens, natural progesterone deserves far more attention and application than it is generally given in the prevention and care of women's health problems today.

CHAPTER 16

GETTING OFF CONVENTIONAL HRT AND ON TO NATURAL HORMONES

The Women's Health Initiative (WHI) study was canceled because of a high risk of breast cancer, heart disease, and stroke associated with using HRT (hormone replacement therapy). The study analyzed the health of 16,000 women aged 50 to 79 years. After five years, those using HRT (Premarin and Provera or PremPro) had a 29 percent higher risk of breast cancer, a 26 percent higher risk of heart disease, and a 41 percent higher risk of stroke.

If we extend those numbers out to the general population of women who were taking HRT, nearly 40,000 women were harmed by taking these drugs over the past decade. That number doesn't include women who suffered the typical side effects of conventional HRT, which include weight gain, fatigue, depression, irritability, headaches, insomnia, bloating, low thyroid, low libido, and gallbladder disease and blood clots.

To readers of my books and newsletters, the risks and side effects of conventional HRT are not news—the evidence of harm has been showing up in research for at least a decade. This particular study was finally large and prestigious enough that conventional medicine was forced to pay attention.

Questions and Answers About Natural Hormone Replacement Therapy

Q: Do the results of the WHI apply to your recommendations of using natural estrogen and progesterone?

A: Not at all. What I recommend is first measuring saliva hormone levels to find if there is a hormonal imbalance. Then, if necessary, correcting the imbalance using natural hormones in physiologic doses, which means ordinary doses that the body would naturally produce itself. Another way to look at this is, from puberty until menopause, a healthy woman's body is making its own natural hormones in synchrony and balance, without giving her cancer, heart disease, or strokes. What I recommend is attempting to regain this natural balance as closely as possible.

Conventional HRT not only fails to measure hormones and use physiologic doses, it uses synthetic "hormones" that are foreign to the human body and may cause a long list of unwanted side effects, rather than natural (bioidentical) hormones.

Q: How Do I Get Off of PremPro?

A: Most women simply need to lower their dose of estrogen and replace the progestin (the "pro" part of the PremPro) with progesterone cream.

Estrogen is a prescription-only medication in the United States, so you'll need to ask your doctor about a separate prescription for estrogen, preferably either estradiol, or a combination of estradiol and estriol, or estriol alone. Even Premarin, although ethically objectionable to many people because of the way it is obtained from pregnant mares, will work if it is used in the lowest dose needed, and in combination with natural progesterone. If you discontinue estrogen suddenly, you're likely to suffer from hot flashes and night sweats. Hot flashes and night sweats are less likely if the estrogen dose is decreased in gradual steps.

Unless a low dose of estrogen is already prescribed, many

women begin with half the dose when adding progesterone cream in place of the progestin. Many menopausal women don't need any estrogen at all, and can gradually taper (over three to four months) their dose down to nothing. Although transdermal progesterone alone will alleviate menopausal symptoms for many women, some women may need a little bit of estrogen to control their symptoms. Symptoms of estrogen deficiency can include hot flashes, night sweats, and vaginal dryness.

Q: My doctor says that I can't use estrogen and progesterone cream, because progesterone cream won't protect my uterus the way the progestins do.

A: Progesterone cream protects the uterus just fine. Not only did I not have any problems in my hundreds of menopausal patients before I retired from practice, I am in touch with dozens of physicians who have tens of thousands of patients between them, who have not reported problems (some of them have been doing this for nearly twenty years). Furthermore, a double-blind, placebo-controlled study by Helene Leonetti, M.D., showed that progesterone cream protects the uterus adequately. Her study compared the uterine protection of PremPro with an estrogen/progesterone cream combination. In short, the women on the progesterone cream were well protected against estrogen-induced endometrial cancer.

You might also ask your doctor how he thinks that your pre-menopausal body protected itself against estrogen effects! It was the progesterone that your ovaries made every month!

Q: My doctor says that because blood tests don't show a rise in progesterone when progesterone cream is used, it doesn't work, and I should use oral progesterone.

A: Blood tests measure only the serum, which is the watery part of the blood, and progesterone that comes from cream use is carried in fatty components of blood, such as the red blood cells, not in the watery serum. Sex hormones are not soluble in serum. The most accurate way to measure hormone levels is with a saliva hormone level test, which measures your active or bioavailable hormones. When you use progesterone cream, a saliva hormone test will show a rather rapid rise in hormone over a three-hour period, and then it reaches a plateau for several hours and then gradually drops such that 90 percent is gone after 15 hours. This amount of time is an average, and can vary a bit from woman to woman.

Q: I read an article in a major magazine where a doctor is quoted as saying that natural progesterone stimulates tissue growth in the breast and therefore could contribute to breast cancer. Is this true?

A: We have tracked down the source of this information, and once again, it was a progestin, not progesterone, that stimulated the cell growth in the study being referred to. As you'll read in our books, progesterone stimulates cells to grow toward differentiation, which is an anticancer property. Cancer cells are undifferentiated, and thus grow without control. Progesterone also encourages cells to die when they're supposed to (which cancer cells don't do). This topic is covered in detail in *What Your Doctor May* Not *Tell You About Breast Cancer*.

CHAPTER 17

NATURAL HORMONE BALANCE AND PELVIC DISORDERS

The human female pelvis is an engineering marvel. Its tissues are sufficiently elastic and its bony arches sufficiently large for the passage of babies with heads already over 50 percent the size of an adult's. Vaginal tissue during a woman's fertile years, and especially at childbirth, is the best-healing tissue of the body. Vaginal mucus secretions facilitate sexual activity, protect against infection, and promote self-cleansing. The ovaries are placed in the most protected spot of the body. The uterus, normally smaller than a fist, can accommodate a pregnancy by becoming larger than a basketball, retain muscle strength sufficient for successful delivery contractions, and return to normal within six weeks after delivery. Despite its proximity to the rectum and the possibility of coliform contamination (the dreaded *E. coli*), a healthy pelvis is remarkably resistant to infection, despite a monthly discharge of bloody flow that might otherwise be a culture medium par excellence.

Pelvic disorders do of course occur. Conditions such as vaginitis, urinary tract infections, endometriosis, PID (pelvic inflammatory disease), ovarian cysts, *mittelschmerz*, uterine fibroids, and menstrual cramps (dysmenorrhea) are among the most common. Are these disorders to be expected because of some error in Nature's plan, or do they occur because of some preventable cause? Let's take a closer look.

Vaginitis

Vaginitis occurs more often among women taking contraceptive pills. One might argue that taking contraceptive pills implies more frequent sexual activity and therefore such women are more exposed to infectious organisms. Perhaps so, but one could also argue that contraceptive pills prevent the normal hormone-generated mucus from being produced to protect them. After all, birth control pills work by suppressing normal hormones.

After menopause, vaginal dryness and reduced mucus production predispose women to vaginal, urethral, and urinary bladder infections. To treat whatever is causing the infection with antibiotics is only temporarily successful (and sometimes not at all successful) because the underlying and real cause of the problem is the inability of these parts of the body to resist infection, which is caused by a hormonal imbalance. For this reason, using a vaginal application of an estrogen cream often works very well to restore hormone balance, with estriol being the most effective. A recent controlled trial of intravaginal estriol in postmenopausal women with recurrent urinary tract infections found that estriol significantly reduced the incidence of urinary infections compared to placebo (0.5 versus 5.9 episodes per year). In addition, estriol treatment resulted in the reemergence of friendly *Lactobacilli* bacteria and the near-elimination of colon bacteria, as well as the restoration of normal vaginal mucosa and a resumption of normal low pH (which inhibits the growth of many bacteria).

In my care of postmenopausal patients, there are those for whom estrogens are contraindicated by reason of a history of breast or uterine cancer and who are at risk of recurrent urinary tract and vaginal infections. I have been surprised to observe that those who opted for natural progesterone therapy have been remarkably free of these problems. Further, in many, their previous vaginal dryness and reduced mucus production returns to normal after three to four months of progesterone use. This suggests that natural progesterone also provides a direct benefit to vaginal and urethral tissues or may sensitize tissue receptors to the lowered levels of estrogens still present in postmenopausal women.

Pelvic Inflammatory Disease (PID)

PID is a serious inflammation of the uterus and fallopian tubes that can result in pelvic abscesses, chronic pain, and infertility. Its treatment includes antibiotics for both sexual partners and, rarely, surgery. Some of the infections that can cause PID include gonorrhea, chlamydia, and coliform bacteria that come from the colon. The infection begins in the vagina and cervical tissues, then spreads up into the endometrium and out along the fallopian tubes, at which point the inflammation is called *salpingitis* or pelvic inflammatory disease (PID).

Preventing PID is dependent upon reducing the opportunity of vaginal contamination by wiping from front to back after a bowel movement, making sure sexual partners are uninfected, keeping the vaginal mucus healthy, and increasing your resistance to infections. In all of these strategies, vaginal mucus is an important factor. Normal vaginal mucus results from a normal balance of natural hormones and nutritional factors, such as beta-carotene, vitamins E, C, and B6, as well as the minerals zinc and magnesium. It is unlikely that synthetic hormones (contraceptive pills and menopausal hormones) provide the hormone balance or action necessary for the most balanced vaginal mucus.

Estriol is the estrogen most beneficial to vaginal and cervical tissue, the sites that act as the first line of defense against infection. Estriol is a product of estrone metabolism. Contraceptive synthetic estrogens, which inhibit the production of natural hormones, do not contain estriol and are not metabolized to form estriol. Progestins similarly inhibit the function of natural progesterone.

After menopause, progesterone levels fall to near zero and estrone levels are also very low. Thus the protection against infection offered by estriol and progesterone is lost unless natural hormones are used in supplementation.

Ovarian Cysts and *Mittelschmerz*

Ovarian cysts in young women are almost always caused by excess sugar and refined carbohydrates in the diet. These foods create chronically raised insulin levels, which stimulate the production of androgens (male hormones) from the ovary, which stimulates the production of the cysts. This is why conventional medicine uses diabetes drugs that lower blood sugar to treat polycystic ovary disease (PCOS). This is a typically misguided conventional medical approach, as these drugs can be very hard on kidney and liver function, and a change is diet is a very quick and effective approach. My experience is that ovarian cysts clear up within two to four months of cutting sugar and refined carbohydrates from the diet.

Mid-cycle pain is a product of failed or disordered ovulation. As I have described earlier, one or more ovarian follicles is developed monthly by the effects of follicle-stimulating hormone (FSH). Luteinizing hormone (LH) promotes actual ovulation and the transformation of the follicle (after ovulation) into the corpus luteum, which produces progesterone. During a young woman's early years of menstruating, ovulation may coincide with a small amount of bleeding where the follicle has ruptured to release the egg. This can cause abdominal pain, often with a slight fever, at the time of ovulation (in the middle days between periods) and is commonly called *mittelschmerz* (German for "middle" and "pain"). Treatment might consist only of some ibuprofen, reassurance, rest, and perhaps a warm pack. It is unlikely to recur and portends no future problems.

Later in life, usually after their mid-30s, women sometimes develop an ovarian cyst that may not cause any symptoms, or it may cause pelvic pain ranging from mild to severe. The cyst may simply collapse and disappear after a month or two, or it may persist and increase in size and discomfort during succeeding months. Such cysts are caused by a failed ovulation in which, for reasons presently unknown, the ovulation did not proceed to completion. With each succeeding month's surge of LH, the cyst swells and stretches the surface membrane, causing pain and possible bleeding at the site. Some cysts may become as large as a golf ball or lemon before discovery. Treatment may require surgery. (Removing the ovary along with the cyst used to be the standard procedure, but I recommend asking your surgeon to leave the ovary intact if at all possible.)

An alternative treatment for ovarian cysts is natural progesterone. The signaling mechanism that shuts off ovulation in one ovary each cycle is the production of progesterone in the other. If sufficient natural progesterone is supplemented prior to ovulation, LH levels are inhibited and both ovaries think the other one has ovulated, so regular ovulation does not occur. (This is the same effect as contraceptive pills.) Similarly, the high estriol and progesterone levels throughout pregnancy successfully inhibit ovarian activity for nine months. Therefore, adding natural progesterone from day 10 to day 26 of the cycle suppresses LH and its luteinizing effects. Thus the ovarian cyst will not be stimulated and, in the passage of one or two such monthly cycles, will very likely shrink and disappear without further treatment.

Endometriosis

Endometriosis is a serious condition in which tiny islets of endometrium (inner lining cells of the uterus) become scattered in areas where they don't belong: the fallopian tubes, within the uterine musculature (adenomyosis), and on the outer surface of the uterus and other pelvic organs, the colon, the bladder, and the sides of the pelvic cavity. With each monthly cycle, these islets of endometrium respond to ovarian hormones exactly as endometrial cells do within the uterus—they increase in size, swell with blood, and bleed into the surrounding tissue at menstruation. The bleeding (no matter how small) into the surrounding tissue causes inflammation and is very painful, often disabling. Symptoms begin 7 to 12 days before menstruation and then become excruciatingly painful during menstruation. The pain may be diffuse and may cause painful intercourse or painful bowel movements, depending on the sites involved. Diagnosis is not easily established, as there is no lab test to identify endometrial islets, nor are they usually large enough to show on an X ray or sonogram. Laparoscopy (a minimally invasive surgery enabling a doctor to look into the abdomen with a small scope) can be very useful in this regard.

The cause of endometriosis is unclear. Some authorities argue that these endometrial cells wander out through the fallopian tubes. Others suggest they are displaced through some sort of embryologic mix-up when an embryo is just forming its tissues. The fact is, however, that endometriosis seems to be a disease of the 20th century. Given the severity of the pains and the association with monthly periods, it seems unlikely that earlier doctors would not have described the condition. Now that we know about xenoestrogens and the fact that the tissues of the developing embryo are especially sensitive to the toxic effects of xenoestrogens, it is tempting to speculate that our petrochemical age has spawned diseases we've never known before—and that endometriosis is one of them.

Mainstream treatment of endometriosis is difficult and not very successful. Surgical attempts at removing each and every endometrial implant throughout the pelvis are only temporarily successful. Many of the tiny islets are simply too small to see, and eventually they enlarge and the condition recurs. Another surgical venture is even more radical: the removal of both ovaries, the uterus and the fallopian tubes, the aim being to remove or reduce hormone levels as much as possible—not a pleasant prospect.

When women with endometriosis delay childbearing until their 30s, they are often unable to conceive. Pregnancy often retards the progress of the disease and occasionally cures it. With this in mind, other medical treatments attempt to create a state of pseudopregnancy, with long periods of supplemented progestins to simulate the high progesterone levels of pregnancy. Unfortunately, the high doses needed are often accompanied by side effects of the progestin and breakthrough bleeding.

As an alternative, I have treated a number of endometriosis patients, some after failed surgery, with natural progesterone and have observed considerable success. Since we know that estrogen initiates endometrial cell proliferation and the formation of blood vessel accumulation in the endometrium, the aim of treatment is to block this monthly estrogen stimulus to the aberrant endometrial islets. Progesterone stops further proliferation of endometrial cells. I advised such women to use natural progesterone cream from day 6 of the cycle to day 26 each month, using one ounce of the cream per week for three weeks, stopping just before their expected period. This treatment requires patience. Over time (four to six months), however, the monthly pains gradually subside as monthly bleeding in these islets becomes less and healing of the inflammatory sites occurs. The monthly discomfort may not disappear entirely but becomes more tolerable. Endometriosis is cured by menopause. This technique is surely worth giving a trial, since the alternatives are not all that successful and laden with undesirable consequences and side effects.

Fibroids

Otherwise known as *myoma* of the uterus, fibroids are the most common growth of the female genital tract and the most frequent reason that women over age 40 visit a gynecologist. Fibroids are roundish, firm, benign (i.e., noncancerous) lumps of the muscular wall of the uterus, composed of smooth muscle and connective tissue, and are rarely solitary. Usually as small as a hen's egg, they commonly grow gradually to the size of an orange or grapefruit. They often cause or are coincidental with heavier periods, irregular bleeding, and/or painful periods. After menopause, they usually wither away.

Fibroids are also one of the most common reasons that women in their 30s and 40s have a hysterectomy. Some particularly skillful surgeons are capable of removing only the fibroid, leaving the uterus intact, but they are the exception. Most would rather remove the uterus because it's a much simpler surgery—simpler for the surgeon, that is.

Fibroids tend to grow during the years before menopause and then atrophy after menopause. This suggests that estrogen stimulates fibroid growth, but we also know that once they get larger progesterone, too, can contribute to their growth. Many doctors prescribe Lupron injections to block all sex hormone production. This causes the fibroids to shrink but they regrow when the injections are stopped, and Lupron is certainly not an appropriate long-term therapy. The anti-progesterone drug RU-486 is also used to reduce the size of larger fibroids.

Women with fibroids are often estrogen dominant and have low progesterone levels. In women with smaller fibroids (the size of a tangerine or smaller), when progesterone is restored to normal levels, the fibroids often shrink a bit and stop growing, which is likely due to progesterone's ability to help speed up the clearance of estrogens from tissue. If this treatment can be continued through menopause, hysterectomy can be avoided.

However, some fibroids, when they reach a certain "critical mass," are accompanied by degeneration or cell death in the interior part of the fibroid and will have an interaction with white blood cells that ends up with the creation of more estrogen within the fibroid itself. It also contains growth factors that are stimulated by progesterone. Under these circumstances, surgical removal of the fibroid (myomectomy) or the uterus (hysterectomy) may become necessary. When you think of treating smaller fibroids you should be thinking in terms of keeping your estrogen milieu as low as possible, and when treating large fibroids, all hormones should be kept as low as possible.

The last thing you want to do if you have fibroids is to take estrogen, which will stimulate them to grow. If you're estrogen dominant, it's important to use a supplemental progesterone, usually in doses of 20 mg per day during the luteal phase of the cycle. Sometimes this approach works to slow or stop fibroid growth, and sometimes it doesn't. It is worth a try. Reducing stress, increasing exercise, and reducing calories are also good strategies for slowing fibroid growth.

Ultrasound tests can be obtained initially and after three

months to check results. A good result would show the fibroid size had not increased or had decreased by 10 to 15 percent. With postmenopausal hormone levels, fibroids usually atrophy.

There are a number of techniques for removing fibroids without removing the uterus. If your doctor doesn't know about these, find another one who does! The difference in recovery time alone between laparoscopic removal of fibroids (for example) and hysterectomy is three weeks versus three months.

Endometrial Cancer

This pelvic disorder is another example of estrogen dominance. Unopposed estrogen is the only known etiology of endometrial carcinoma. Both natural progesterone and some of the synthetic progestins give a protective effect from this disease. This important topic is discussed more thoroughly in Chapter 15, "Hormone Balance and Cancer."

Hysterectomy

I have included hysterectomy here because it almost always falls under the category of an iatrogenic (i.e., physician-induced) pelvic disorder. Total hysterectomy has come to mean the removal of a woman's uterus and ovaries. Technically, a hysterectomy is only the removal of the uterus, and an *oophorectomy* or *ovariectomy* is the removal of the ovaries. Since women who have had hysterectomies go into instant, surgically induced menopause, they are immediately put on hormone replacement therapy.

Dr. Stanley West, chief of reproductive endocrinology and infertility at St. Vincent's Hospital in New York and the author of *The Hysterectomy Hoax*, believes that, in general, a hysterectomy is never necessary unless a woman has cancer. How did it come to be that every year 600,000 women are getting hysterectomies and more than 500,000 of them are unnecessary? As West points out, it has more to do with outdated views of women than any physical problem women are having. West quotes an M.D. who gave a speech to the American College of Obstetrics and Gynecology as saying, "After the last planned pregnancy, the uterus becomes a useless, symptom-producing, potentially cancer-bearing organ and therefore should be removed." I'm sure these physicians have good intentions, or at least do not intend to harm their patients, but they are sadly misguided in using hysterectomy as a routine treatment.

Removal of the ovaries is also known in medical terminology as female castration. Think of how men would respond if their doctors wanted to remove their testicles and prostate gland once they had all the children they wanted, and then put them on synthetic testosterone drugs. It's almost inconceivable. And yet removing a woman's ovaries is no less a violation and has equally devastating consequences, not the least of which are the side effects of the synthetic hormones she is put on to replace her own. Removing the ovaries as a matter of course has gone somewhat out of fashion lately. Doctors now tell their patients that sparing the ovaries will allow them to keep producing hormones, but this is not accurate. The blood supply of the ovaries is a branch of the uterine artery that is ligated (cut and tied off) in the usual hysterectomy. The loss of this blood supply by the ovaries routinely results in loss of ovarian function. Even in cases in which the ovaries appear to be saved, they often quit functioning in one to three years. It is as if somehow the ovaries know there is no longer a uterus there and within a few years they atrophy and stop producing hormones. Hysterectomy means castration, whether or not the ovaries are involved.

Hysterectomy is lucrative for the physician doing the surgery, lucrative for the pharmaceutical companies supplying the replacement hormones (600,000 new lifelong customers each year!), and physically, mentally, and emotionally expensive for women who undergo them. The aftereffects of hysterectomy tend to be played down by the physicians who do them, but they are frequent and include fatigue, depression, headaches, heart palpitations, mood swings, hair loss, loss of sex drive, vaginal dryness, and urinary tract problems. Women who are put on estrogen after a hysterectomy have to cope with all the side effects of unopposed estrogen and, if a progestin is added, all those side effects as well. Women who have had a hysterectomy are at a higher risk for heart disease, arthritis, and osteoporosis.

Before you submit to a hysterectomy, I strongly recommend you reconsider, unless you clearly have a malignant cancer. The leading reasons given for hysterectomies are fibroids, uterine prolapse (the uterus falls from its normal position), and endometriosis. As you have read here, fibroids and endometriosis can usually be effectively helped with some natural progesterone cream, and there are many other ways to deal with uterine prolapse.

If you've already had a hysterectomy and are struggling with the side effects of synthetic hormone replacement therapy, ask your doctor to use natural hormones. I have my patients wean themselves off HRT by gradually (over a period of three to four months) reducing their dosage, while at the same time using progesterone cream. In those very few women who still have hot flashes or vaginal dryness, I give them some estrogen cream, usually estriol, to use intravaginally for a few months, and they are then able to taper that off.

Staying Naturally Healthy

The monthly rise and fall of natural estrogen(s) and progesterone not only prepares your body for procreation, in the sense of ova production, but also predisposes you to be healthy. Many of women's pelvic complaints arise from an imbalance of their hormones. This imbalance is most often a deficiency of progesterone. There are many factors that bring this about: nutritional deficiencies, stress, environmental xenoestrogens, toxins, depletion of follicles, and the hormonal imbalance induced by contraceptive pills composed of synthetic hormones. Progesterone deficiency and estrogen dominance can be recognized and handily treated by supplementation of natural progesterone, especially when combined with diet and supplements.

CHAPTER 18

HORMONE BALANCE AND OTHER COMMON HEALTH PROBLEMS

Until rather recently, women's ailments were regarded simply as evidence of some design flaw or inherent weakness of women's constitution. Women who had ailments with causes unknown to their male doctors were often treated with a condescending pat on the hand and a prescription for a tranquilizer to calm fragile nerves. During my own time in medicine, a great change has occurred. In my medical school class (of 1955), there were 112 men and 3 women. Now women constitute 30 to 60 percent of medical school classes. The era of condescension and not-so-benign neglect is passing. Surely medical progress will soon catch up to the real causes of women's ailments.

We now know that hormone balance is an important factor in a woman's overall health. Estrogen, testosterone, and progesterone are potent substances. They affect every organ and tissue of the body. Their effects are both complementary and opposing to each other. The sum total of all their effects is dependent not only on the quantity of a given hormone, but also on the relative quantity or balance of the hormones in relation to each other. Understanding this will help us understand (and correct) conditions that we call women's ailments.

Premenstrual Syndrome (PMS)

When I was in medical school more than 40 years ago, there was no such thing as premenstrual syndrome (PMS). Now it's a household word in Western industrialized countries. There's no doubt that PMS exists and can make a week or so out of every month miserable for everyone involved. The symptoms tend to occur consistently a week or 10 days before menstruation begins and go away shortly after. Women often report a "tidal wave" of symptoms at their onset and dread the approach of each premenstrual time of the month. A good diet and exercise help, but the root of the problem is—you guessed it—hormone imbalance. Progesterone has been wrongly accused of being the hormone responsible for PMS because it's the one that's high just before menstruation. The truth is, however, that women with PMS tend to have *lower* progesterone than normal at that time in their cycle, when progesterone is supposed to be dominant, so that estrogen is dominant instead.

My book *What Your Doctor May* Not *Tell You About Premenopause* (coauthored with Dr. Jesse Hanley and Virginia Hopkins) goes into great detail about PMS, as well as other hormonal and health factors that can affect women between the ages of 30 and 50. However, in this chapter let's take a broad look at PMS and some of the other common health problems that can afflict women of all ages.

What Is PMS?

I've seen lists of PMS symptoms that include dozens of complaints, but the most common symptoms include several or all of the following: bloating, weight gain, headache, backaches, irritability, depression, breast swelling or tenderness, loss of libido, and fatigue. Do these symptoms sound familiar? They are also the symptoms of estrogen dominance.

But the full range of symptoms includes confusion and disorientation, intemperate judgments and decision making, mood swings, body aches, anger and verbal abuse, lethargy alternating with increased energy, alienation, guilt (at having abused friends), lack of self-esteem, and cravings for sweets, especially for chocolate. Further, every system in the body can be affected: immune, digestive, circulatory, nervous, endocrine, and dermatologic (skin). Victims of PMS may experience any combination of the above and with all degrees of severity, from mild to overwhelming.

There are two important realities to understand about PMS. They are:

1. Yes, it is real.
2. No, you are not crazy.

Diagnosis of PMS rests on the range and monthly timing of symptoms. Since the exact mechanisms to explain the symptoms are unknown, the malady is correctly called a syndrome— a collection of recognizable signs and symptoms. To my mind, the hormone connection is most intriguing. It is obviously linked with the monthly hormone cycle; it never occurs prior to a year or so before menarche, and never after menopause (unless you're on HRT).

Treatment of PMS has in the past included diuretics, tranquilizers, dietary changes, aerobic exercise, psychiatric counseling, thyroid supplements, herbs, acupuncture, and vitamin and mineral supplements. While each may provide some relief, none has proved to be a panacea.

The Role of Progesterone

More than a decade ago, after reading of the work of Dr. Katherina Dalton in London, who defined PMS and found success using high-dose progesterone administered as rectal suppositories, I decided to add natural progesterone cream to my treatment of patients with PMS. The results were most impressive. The majority (but not all) of these patients reported remarkable improvement in their symptoms, including the elimination of their premenstrual water retention and weight gain. I have received hundreds of phone calls and letters from women and their doctors over the past few years who report that PMS has been alleviated with the use of natural progesterone. Dr. Joel T. Hargrove of Vanderbilt University Medical Center has published results indicating a 90 percent success rate in treating PMS with oral doses of natural progesterone.

As described in previous chapters, estrogen is the dominant sex hormone during the first week after menstruation. With ovulation, progesterone levels rise to assume dominance during the two weeks preceding menstruation. Progesterone blocks many of estrogen's potential side effects. A surplus of estrogen or a deficiency of progesterone during these two weeks allows an abnormal monthlong exposure to estrogen dominance, setting the stage for the symptoms of estrogen side effects. If you want to test this for yourself, have your doctor measure your serum or saliva progesterone levels during days 18 to 25 of your cycle. Low progesterone levels undoubtedly affect hormone regulatory centers in the brain, resulting in increased production of hormones such as LH and FSH. These may also play a role in the complex symptomatology of PMS. However, for most women, simple correction of the progesterone deficiency will restore normal biofeedback and pituitary function.

PMS, Thyroid, Adrenal Function, and Blood Sugar

It's important to note here that not all of the symptoms of PMS may be caused directly by a progesterone deficiency. Hypothyroidism, or low thyroid function, for example, may cause fatigue, headaches, and loss of libido, and thus simulate PMS. Estrogen dominance impairs thyroid hormone activity and will simulate hypothyroidism. How do you know whether you have a progesterone deficiency or hypothyroidism? Ask your doctor to test serum thyroid levels (T3 and T4) and thyroid stimulating hormone (TSH). Normal T3 and T4 levels with elevated TSH suggest impaired thyroid hormone activity rather than a true deficiency of thyroid hormone production. In this case, estrogen dominance is probably interfering with your thyroid function.

Adrenal exhaustion or low adrenal reserve, which I believe is epidemic among working mothers in their mid-30s, can cause fatigue, unstable blood sugar, mood swings, foggy thinking, and impairment of steroid hormone synthesis; these reactions can throw sex hormones out of balance and cause PMS. Long-term high cortisol levels caused by chronic stress (which usually precedes adrenal exhaustion) can create an overall hormone resistance. In this case all hormones are affected, including thyroid, insulin, and melatonin. When hormone resistance occurs, it takes more of the hormone to have the same effect on the body.

Similarly, women with idiopathic (i.e., without a known cause) unstable blood sugar or hypoglycemia often experience symptoms similar to PMS and will benefit from dietary adjustments. However, it should be known that estrogen predisposes one to blood sugar imbalance, whereas progesterone enhances blood sugar control.

Other Factors in PMS

It is likely that a hormone imbalance directly or indirectly caused by progesterone deficiency is the major factor in the majority of PMS cases, but other factors may also deserve attention, especially for those who do not find complete relief with progesterone treatment.

Nutrition plays a role. For example, when your body has finished using estrogen, it is dumped, via the liver and bile, into the intestines to be excreted. Here, fiber plays an important role in binding the estrogen and holding it for elimination. A lack of fiber in the diet can cause estrogen to be reabsorbed and recycled. Because beef cattle are often fed estrogens to fatten them up for market, eating too much red meat can unnaturally increase estrogen levels. Exposure to xenoestrogens may also play a role in hormone imbalance.

Many women experience PMS for the first time after going off contraceptive pills, suggesting that synthetic hormone use and the prevention of normal ovulation may leave one's ovaries less able to function normally. All factors must be considered in understanding and treating PMS, and yet the problem of normalizing hormone balance remains a key factor in proper treatment.

It is entirely likely that PMS, like many other diseases, is multifactorial, and that adrenal exhaustion (or lack of adrenal reserve) is another factor in this syndrome.

Hypothyroidism (Low Thyroid)

Thyroid hormone is now the most common of all drug prescriptions. The premise of thyroid is simple—the thyroid gland makes thyroid hormones that set the metabolic rate (the rate at which energy is used) for all the cells of the body. Thyroid hormone is said to be the throttle, or gas pedal, or governor for all metabolic activity. There is a computer in the hypothalamus gland in the brain that monitors and modulates thyroid hormone levels to control metabolic activity. This computer makes a hormone called *thyrotropin releasing hormone* (TRH), that signals the pituitary gland in the brain to make another hormone, *thyroid stimulating hormone* (TSH) (also called thyrotropin) that instructs the thyroid gland to make more or less thyroid hormone for circulation throughout the body. This sets the body's metabolic rate. If the hypothalamic computer detects a lagging metabolic rate, it signals the pituitary to make more TSH, which activates the thyroid gland to make more thyroid hormone. If the metabolic rate is too high, it reduces TSH to slow the production of thyroid hormone. What a beautiful system! A low TSH reading may indicate high thyroid levels, whereas a high reading may indicate low thyroid levels.

But then things get a bit more complicated. One would think that by measuring the thyroid level in the bloodstream, or the level of TSH, or TRH (a more difficult test), one could easily determine whether thyroid hormone supplementation was necessary. As it turns out, many factors affect how much thyroid hormone is produced and how efficiently it is being used by the cells in your body. Just because your thyroid level is in the lab's "normal" range, that does not mean that all is well with your thyroid or metabolic regulation. If someone is lacking energy, or is cold all the time, or not feeling up to par (all symptoms of hypothyroidism—low levels of thyroid hormone), the underlying cause may be lack of sleep, the need for a vacation, bad diet (high insulin levels), stress (high cortisol levels), a nutrient deficiency (low iodine levels), or hormonal imbalance (estrogen dominace). If we succumb to the erroneous belief that "normal" thyroid tests rule out thyroid problems, there are plenty of other suspects to consider, and the potential thyroid problem is ignored.

The Basics on T3 and T4

Here's a closer look at how thyroid hormone really works. Thyroid hormone is a remarkably simple compound, made of a single amino acid (protein building blocks) called tyrosine plus the addition of some iodine atoms. Actually, the thyroid gland makes two thyroid hormones, thyroxine (with 4 iodines) and triiodothyronine (with 3 iodines). In medical parlance, thyroxine is called T4, and thyronine is called T3, indicating the number of iodines in each molecule.

T4 blood levels are higher than that of T3, but T3 is four times more potent. Normally the body converts T4 to T3 as needed. The total thyroid effect is a combination of both T4 and T3. Though not common in conventional medicine, ideal thyroid replacement therapy should consider the use of both T4 and T3. The most commonly prescribed thyroid medication is Synthroid, which is only T4.

What Thyroid Hormone Does

Thyroid hormone increases the number and activity of mitochondria, those little intracellular inclusions (they exist separately from the cell but are found inside the cell) that convert food we eat (particularly carbohydrates) into energy for the body. Mitochondria can also be thought of as small organelles within each cell of the body that act as furnaces that burn the food we eat to release heat and energy that is stored for later use. Thyroid increases the efficiency of these intracellular furnaces, allowing them to burn the nutrients we consume more efficiently, thus creating heat and energy. When thyroid isn't operating properly, the mitochondrial furnaces will not burn fuel properly and we suffer from lower body temperature and lack of energy. Low body temperature and fatigue are two of the most common symptoms doctors use to diagnose low thyroid.

Thyroid increases protein synthesis (for growth and repair), excites the nervous system (for alertness and quicker reflexes), and stimulates the endocrine (hormone) system in general. Thyroid deficiency can cause an amazing variety of symptoms. A brief list of symptoms includes general fatigue, feeling more chilly than most people, difficulty in losing weight, muscle aches and pains, mental sluggishness, dry skin, dry hair and hair loss, waking up tired, anxieties and/or depression, increased menopausal symptoms, slow pulse, and digestive problems. Each of these symptoms might well be caused by something else but when enough of the whole set is present, it is wise to think of hypothyroidism. People with underactive thyroids also show an increased tendency for autoimmune disorders.

Low thyroid can intensify the ill effects of other diseases because all metabolic actions require energy, and thyroid hormone sets the energy level. If thyroid is low, your energy is low and your body is less able to deal with other conditions. Examples are chronic stress, poor sleep, colds and other viral or bacterial infections, malnutrition, anemia, injuries, or surgery. Without good thyroid levels, recovery is delayed.

Potential Causes of Hypothyroidism

Why should thyroid deficiency be so common now? Historically, iodine deficiency was the most common cause of hypothyroidism and goiter (enlarged thyroid gland). Without sufficient iodine, thyroid hormone production results in thyroxine being stored in the gland rather than being released into the circulation. This leads to engorgement of the gland, causing goiters. The condition was most prevalent in populations that did not live near the sea, because all ocean fish, crustaceans, and seaweed contain iodine. Now that iodine is added to salt, and seafood is widely available, iodine deficiency is not as common. Our present epidemic of thyroid problems is not due to iodine deficiency. We must look elsewhere.

The Estrogen Dominance Factor.   No hormone works in isolation from other hormones; they all function within a complex, subtle web of interconnectedness. If thyroid is low, cortisol and sex hormone production lags. Estrogen inhibits thyroid hormone activity, and thus exacerbates thyroid deficiency. In contrast, progesterone, cortisol, and testosterone are thyroid allies. Hypothyroidism occurs predominantly in women, especially during the perimenopausal period (around the time of menopause) when estrogens dominate and progesterone is low. Persistent estrogen dominance, which is most likely to occur during the perimenopausal period, creates a cycle of lowered thyroid function, decreased SHBG, and further increases in the bioavailable levels of estrogens. Breast cancer incidence begins to rise sharply during this period. Progesterone therapy often restores normal thyroid activity, perhaps by its antiestrogenic actions. Here again, estrogen dominance, unopposed by progesterone, underlies the link between thyroid dysfunction and breast cancer.

Dr. David Zava often sees what he describes as thyroid resistance, where thyroid parameters measured in blood are normal (i.e., normal TSH, T4, and T3), but symptoms characteristic of low thyroid are present. These individuals nearly always suffer from severe imbalances in their steroid hormones. In monitoring salivary hormones and symptoms, Dr. Zava finds that estrogen dominance (usually associated with normal or high estrogen, but always low progesterone), and adrenal dysfunction (low or high cortisol) correlate closely with symptoms common to low thyroid. If your doctor is telling you that your thyroid hormones are normal, but you have most of the classic thyroid symptoms, you may want to test your steroid hormones in saliva.

The Autoimmune Factor.   The immune system is also a major factor in hypothyroidism. In particular, antithyroid antibody disease (Hashimoto's thyroiditis), once considered rare, is now a common finding, especially among women. The antibody attack on the thyroid causes chaos in the hormone cycle. It may provoke hyperthyroidism (elevated T4 levels or excess thyroid) or classic hypothyroidism (low T4 levels). Since the cause is usually unknown, conventional treatment consists of thyroid supplementation sufficient to drive TSH to very low levels, thus effectively stopping endogenous (made in the body) thyroid hormone synthesis.

The Fluoride Factor.   The thyroid molecule is simply a thyronine molecule with some iodines attached. Thyroid only works if iodine is attached there. Iodine is a halogen, one of a group of nonmetallic elements that also includes fluorine, chlorine, and bromine. If you look at the periodic table of elements, you note that they all are short by one electron of having a complete outer ring of electrons. They all seek to acquire an extra electron. In chemical reactions, a more reactive halogen will replace a less reactive halogen. Iodine is the largest of the four common halogens and its chemical activity is the least among them, whereas fluorine is the smallest of the halogens and is the most chemically active.

In the past two generations, fluoride exposure has increased greatly due to fluoridated water and toothpaste. Prior to fluoridation, the common daily intake of fluoride was about 0.1 mg per day. Now, fluoride intake even in unfluoridated communities is 30 to 40 times greater. If fluorine replaces iodine in the structure of thyroxine, it would make it unsuitable for thyroid hormone effect. Years ago, fluoride was used to treat hyperthyroidism. Why is this fluoride poisoning now ignored? Not only is fluoridated tyrosine unsuitable for thyroxine construction, but it may stimulate antibody formation, leading to thyroiditis.

The Xenohormone Factor.   Many petrochemical toxins are also known as endocrine disrupters or xenohormones (see Chapter 5 for details), and thyroid is among the endocrine systems disrupted by these pollutants. In the case of thyroid, a plausible mechanism for damage is known. The thyroxine molecule has a remarkably similar structure to that of polychlorinated biphenyls (PCBs), widespread industrial pollutants that are not only estrogenic but also toxic to the thyroid gland itself. The development of the inner ear in human embryos requires thyroid hormone. If exposed to PCBs, the cochlear development is inhibited, causing low tone hearing loss. Animals exposed to PCBs develop thyroid tumors, now common in cats, for instance. It is entirely possible that the chlorinated biphenyls are perceived by the immune system as abnormal thyroxine. In the process, one's antibodies attack the thyroid gland. Thus, industrial pollutants known as PCBs or other similar petrochemical endocrine (hormone) blockers may be a major cause of hypothyroidism caused by thyroiditis.

Supporting Your Thyroid Gland with Nutrition

The thyroid gland is a resilient gland; many people with terrible nutrition have normal functioning thyroid glands. However, several nutrients are important to proper thyroid gland function, and iodine, of course, is crucial. The synthesis and secretion of thyroid hormone requires sufficient amino acids (proteins) for normal albumin levels and, in particular, for tyrosine or the amino acids from which we can make tyrosine. The essential nutrient for thyroid hormone synthesis is iodine. Before this was discovered, people living well away from the sea were prone to develop enlarged thyroid glands (goiter) and, in more advanced cases, cretinism (arrested physical and mental development with lowered metabolic rate) or myxedema (dry, waxy swelling of the skin and mucus membranes). Eventually it became clear that eating fish or seaweed products prevented these disorders and in time, it was found that the missing nutrient was iodine. Now iodides (salts of iodine) are added to table salt and iodine deficiency is rare. A diet that includes occasional ocean fish or the taking of kelp concentrate easily meets one's iodine requirements. If one were to avoid iodized salt, I would recommend daily kelp concentrate for its iodine content. Paradoxically, excessive iodine intake can also lead to goiter.

Fibrocystic Breasts

In the late 1970s, Dr. Regine Sitruk-Ware of France found that women with fibrocystic breasts were estrogen dominant (i.e., their ratio of estrogen to progesterone was high compared with control women). He referred to the fibrocystic breast condition as "benign breast disease" (BBD). The BBD women were treated with transdermal progesterone and Dr. Sitruk-Ware observed that the majority of them cleared and their breasts returned to normal within 3 to 4 months. This was published in *Obstetrics and Gynecology* in 1979. As the story goes, Dr. Sitruk-Ware was challenged to prove that the hormone ratio had been changed by the progesterone treatment, but blood (serum) tests did not reflect much change. The work of Chang, done in 1995 and described in the chapter on estrogen, proved through biopsy that not only was progesterone absorbed, it caused remarkable changes in breast cell replication, all without significant changes in serum progesterone levels. Because of the blood test results, Sitruk-Ware's critics discounted his good work and his discovery of an effective treatment of fibrocystic breasts was lost for 16 years. Dr. Sitruk-Ware did not know that progesterone absorbed transdermally circulated in blood by red blood cells, not in the serum. However, Dr. Sitruk-Ware was correct: Estrogen dominance is the cause of fibrocystic breasts and topical progesterone supplementation is the preferable treatment. Most physicians today are still unaware of that.

Many women present themselves to their doctors with breast swelling or tender, painful breasts occurring each month before their menstrual periods. Exam by palpation may find exquisitely tender lumps in the breast. Even though he knows with almost 100 percent certainty that the problem is due to fibrocystic breasts, the doctor is aware of the liability of overlooking any breast lump and therefore often orders a mammogram (especially painful in this condition). Mammogram readings are often couched in terms of caution and the advice to rule out potential underlying cancer. (Cancer lumps in breasts are rarely if ever painful.) A trial of vitamin E and avoiding caffeine and other methyl xanthines (coffee, tea, colas, chocolate) may have little or no result.

From my women patients I learned that fibrocystic breasts were most often merely a sign of estrogen dominance—relatively high estrogen and low progesterone. In my experience, using natural progesterone routinely resolves the problem. I also recommend adding vitamin E in dosages of 600 IU at bedtime, supplemental magnesium (300 milligrams a day), and vitamin B6 (50 milligrams a day). I cannot recall a case in which the result was not positive. Once the cysts have cleared up, you can reduce the progesterone dose to find the smallest dose that is still effective each month and continue the treatment as needed through menopause. This treatment is simple, safe, inexpensive, successful, and natural. Do keep in mind that because progesterone keeps estrogen receptors active, an estrogen-dominant woman who starts on progesterone cream may experience anywhere from a few weeks to a few months of increased estrogen dominance symptoms caused by an up-regulation of estrogen receptors. This will balance out within a few menstrual cycles.

Migraine Headaches

Migraines are serious headaches, most often occurring only on one side of the head, and often preceded by a vague sense (aura) that the sufferer learns to recognize as an impending headache. Migraines are thought to be related to overdilation of blood vessels in the brain. They very likely have an allergic or chemically mediated trigger and are related to stress. They vary in severity, sometimes becoming almost unendurable without medication, and can be accompanied by nausea and vomiting. Routine conventional medical treatment involves serotonin receptor agonists such as sumatriptan and naratriptan which can cause heart attacks, or ergotamine medication (often combined with caffeine), which, to achieve success, may result in side effects of muscle pains, numbness and tingling in the fingers and toes, rapid (or slowed) heart rate, and nausea and vomiting. Not medications to take lightly. Migraine victims live in fear of their next headache.

When migraine headaches occur with regularity in women only at premenstrual times, they are most likely due to estrogen dominance. These are the lucky patients. By now I have hundreds of letters in my files from women whose premenstrual migraines have been dramatically improved or cured with the use of progesterone cream. This is because estrogen causes dilation of blood vessels, and thus contributes to the cause(s) of migraines. One of the many virtues of natural progesterone is that it helps restore normal vascular tone, counteracting the blood vessel dilation that causes the headache. Here again, progesterone is safe and treats the cause in a normal, physiologic way. The more dangerous pharmaceutical drugs can be reserved for the rare case that does not respond completely to progesterone.

Skin Problems (Acne, Seborrhea, Rosacea, Psoriasis, and Keratoses)

Acne is more common in males than in females. It is especially common in males around and just after puberty. It may last for decades, but does not occur in eunuchs (castrated men). Androgens (testosterone and others) are involved in acne. Scattered throughout the skin, but more common around the hairline, nose, and ears, are little skin (sebaceous) follicles that make an oily wax known as *sebum*. Sebum keeps skin smooth and supple. Extra androgens stimulate excess sebum production; drying sebum blocks the gland outlet at the skin surface, causing retention of sebum. A common benign bacterium (*Corynebacterium acnes*) multiplies in the incarcerated sebum, causing low-grade inflammation. Vitamin A deficiency can aggravate acne and make it more difficult to heal. Vitamin A or beta-carotene and zinc aid the resolution of acne. Many dermatologists prescribe tetracycline antibiotic because it inhibits bacterial growth and thus reduces inflammation. Tetracycline does not cure acne; it merely reduces the inflammation. It also kills friendly intestinal bacteria, leading to "leaky gut" syndrome and yeast overgrowth known as *candida*.

When a woman in her late 30s or early 40s develops acne, I suspect increased androgen production. In almost all adult female patients with this condition, supplemental progesterone clears the skin. My hypothesis is that ovarian follicle depletion leading to progesterone deficiency results in increased adrenal production of androgens. When progesterone is resupplied, androgen production goes down and the skin clears. (The same hypothesis does not apply to men.) But in women, topical progesterone cream does wonders for acne.

Seborrhea is a related condition of the sebum-producing follicles. It causes flaking and itching skin without specific inflammation of the skin follicles. It, too, clears rapidly with topical progesterone cream.

Rosacea is a rose-colored, flaking inflammation of skin, usually on the face symmetrically adjacent to the nose or forehead, sometimes with itching. It tends to be chronic and recurring. Its cause is unknown, but I have seen it well controlled with vitamin B12 injections. Cortisone creams suppress the inflammation but do not cure rosacea. Continued use of fluoridated cortisone preparations results in atrophy of skin cells with permanent detrimental results. My patients using topical progesterone who happened to have rosacea have applied the cream directly to affected skin areas and report excellent results, though I don't know what the mechanism of action could be.

Similarly, patients with psoriasis (a normally intractable skin disorder characterized by red, scaly patches) have reported impressive remissions of the condition when progesterone cream was applied. In some cases, psoriatic skin lesions that had been present for many years cleared completely. Since progesterone skin creams providing physiologic dosages have no side effects, I see no reason not to try it.

Keratoses are generally small skin lesions composed of dry, hardened skin cells (keratinized epithelial cells) in discrete patches or protuberances considered "hornlike" to early doctors. They are thought by some to be precursors of later squamous cell skin cancers. People spend considerable time and money having dermatologists remove them. My patients using proges-terone cream report that keratoses soften and disappear when the cream is applied directly to them. (See Chapter 15, "Hormone Balance and Cancer," for details.)

Candida

Candida, short for *Candida albicans*, refers to yeast that usually lives companionably on our skin and (sometimes) our mucous membranes. On mucous membranes (mucosa), candida form whitish patches visible to the eye. The patches do not scrape off easily and cause itching and irritation. In the mouths of babies and young children, candida infection is called *thrush*. Under normal conditions the immune system protects us very well from unwarranted yeast overgrowth. However, if our immune system is dysfunctional, candida overgrowth becomes rampant, infecting the mucous membranes of the intestinal tract, mouth, and lungs. Another factor in candida control is the many help-ful bacteria that live with us. Bacteria and yeast compete for sus-tenance. Bacteria suppress candida growth. When these helpful bacteria are killed by prolonged, potent antibiotics, candida overgrowth can result.

Candida like to live in the vagina. They grow well wherever it is warm, moist, and well supplied with their favorite nutri-ent—glucose. Skin and vaginal mucus contain glucose. Estro-gen dominance increases mucus glucose, thereby facilitating candida growth. In males, candida can survive (but not flourish) under the penis foreskin, sometimes causing an irritation and other times causing no discernible symptoms. In sexual inter-course, candida are easily passed from one partner to the other.

Numerous medications are very effective at suppressing can-dida growth, but the conditions within the vagina are such that reinfection is probable. Candida are often found in the skin folds of the anus, from which they reinfect the vagina. Success-ful treatment of candida includes a diet low in sugar and simple carbohydrates, good hygiene and protection from reinfection by one's sexual partner by using condoms or douching after sex, appropriate treatment of one's self and sexual partners with an over-the-counter yeast infection remedy (ask your pharmacist), and correction of estrogen dominance in the woman. This correction is accomplished by supplemental natural progesterone. When hormone imbalance is restored to normal balance using progesterone, candida growth is less likely to persist. The normal benign bacteria are restored and the body heals itself of its candida population.

Some writers have claimed that progesterone supplementation increases the risk of candida. This may be true of excessively high dosing of progesterone, which creates hormonal havoc. Sadly, many health care professionals don't understand that more is not better when it comes to hormones, and they grossly overdose their patients with progesterone cream or more often, with oral progesterone. When the patients inevitably develop side effects from the overdose, the health care professional concludes that it's the progesterone.

Allergies

Potential allergy-causing substances are abundant in everyone's environment. They do not provoke an allergic response unless the allergen load exceeds our body's ability to deal with it. Adequate cortisone blocks the histamine response to allergens. Progesterone is the precursor not only to estrogen and testosterone, but also to all the corticosteroids made by the adrenal gland. Adrenal exhaustion is the result of stress, vitamin C deficiency, and progesterone deficiency. Many of my patients using progesterone tell me that their allergy problems are much reduced. One woman called me from her supermarket to tell me that when she walked by the aisle with all the decongestants and antihistamines, she suddenly realized that since she began using progesterone she had not been plagued by her chronic sinus congestion. This is not an isolated incident; it is a common experience that I hear often.

Arthritis

Athritis is a generic Greek word that usually means only that one's joints, or the tissue around one's joints, hurt or are inflamed. It does not refer to any specific cause or any specific mechanism of action. It is more a Greek translation of a symptom than a diagnosis.

If your joints ache, or the connective tissue around your joints aches, your doctor is inclined to call it arthritis and prescribe nonsteroidal anti-inflammatory drugs (NSAIDs) such as aspirin, ibuprofen, or any of a dozen similar medications. You must realize that your joint aching is not due to NSAID deficiency, and your doctor's prescription is merely treating symptoms, not causes.

Connective tissue aches and pains have a variety of causes. Some of them include:

- nutritional deficiencies;
- repeated trauma to cartilage and the connective tissue that holds joints together (as in pianist's hands and fingers);
- repeated strain causing microscopic tears in connective tissue around joints and tendon sheaths (like carpal tunnel syndrome);
- inflammatory reactions to these connective tissue strains due to prostaglandin imbalance secondary to dietary choices (like too much milk and meat and not enough foods with omega-3 and omega-6 fatty acids); and
- lack of physiological cortisone responses to check the inflammatory reactions.

This is where progesterone comes in. Natural progesterone has anti-inflammatory properties that the synthetic analogs do not have. Many of my patients using natural progesterone cream report relief of chronic aches and pains, and other doctors have also reported this to me. You can rub progesterone cream or oil directly on the joint or tissue that hurts. I do not have a good explanation for why it works, but the consistency of the reports makes me believe it does. Here is another excellent opportunity for research.

Autoimmune Disorders

Autoimmune disorders are those disease states in which your own antibodies attack some gland or tissue in your body. Normally your antibodies protect you from harmful invaders, but in this case they go after normal tissue. The actual cause is generally never found. Autoimmune disorders, in general, are more common in women. Why should this be? It is natural to suspect estrogen, the one hormone that is more plentiful in women than men over the course of a lifetime. After follicle depletion or menopause, some women make less progesterone than men of the same age. The onset of autoimmune disorders is often in middle age, when estrogen dominance becomes common. Hashimoto's thyroiditis, Sjögren's disease, Graves' disease (toxic goiter), and lupus erythematosus are all not only more common in women, but appear to be related to estrogen supplementation or estrogen dominance. Recent studies have shown that women who use hormone replacement therapy containing estrogen are more likely to get lupus.

Many of my patients with autoimmune disease who began using natural progesterone to relieve menopausal symptoms reported that their disease symptoms also gradually abated. This is a clinical question that haunts my mind: Is this an unrecognized symptom of estrogen toxicity, or the fact that progesterone itself may "tune down" the antibody-modulated disorder? Further research is needed.

Urinary Tract Problems

Urinary urgency and incontinence are big business these days, as we know from media advertising. The present hype calls these conditions "overactive bladder," a phrase I intensely dislike because it lumps together many different problems—which have different causes and treatments—as if there were just one problem causing urinary urgency or incontinence in women. And it incorrectly suggests that the problem is with the bladder and implies that a single pill will correct it.

The truth is that there can be many sources of urinary tract problems. Here are the most common causes, as well as solutions.

Sagging Ligaments and Muscles

Some women with urinary urgency or incontinence have stretched-out pelvic ligaments and muscles. This condition allows the bladder to sag down (prolapse) in a manner that distorts the urethra (the tube through which urine passes) and allows urine leakage, especially when coughing, laughing, or lifting something heavy, such as a grocery bag.

The most frequent causes of the stretched or weakened tissues are difficult births or multiple births of large babies, followed by hormone imbalance, particularly low testosterone. The stretched or weakened tissues may be healed by supplemental testosterone (physiologic doses in a cream), the major anabolic (tissue-building) hormone for ligaments and muscles, and Kegel exercises, which can strengthen the muscles that hold urine in the bladder, prevent prolapse of the pelvic organs, and correct the urinary problem.

Inflammation, Infection, and Low Estrogen Levels

Some women with urinary urgency and incontinence have chronic, low-grade inflammation or infection of the urethra. This is particularly true in postmenopausal women, many of whom have chronic recurring urinary tract infections. It should be remembered that infections have two underlying factors: pathogens (bacteria or viruses) and host resistance.

All external surfaces of our body are exposed to pathogens of many sorts, which nevertheless cause no disease because our bodies resist them (host resistance). This is especially true of the vagina, which is continually exposed to coliform pathogens, such as the varieties of *E. coli* found in stool. In most premenopausal women, the vaginal cells are healthy and well keratinized (with strong cell membranes) as a result of good estrogen levels. In some women, estrogen levels after menopause decline so far that vaginal dryness develops and vaginal cells become weaker, or even atrophy. As a result, host resistance is lost.

Raz and Stamm reported in the *New England Journal of Medicine* in 1993 that intravaginal (applied as a vaginal cream) low-dose estriol is remarkably effective in preventing urinary tract infections in postmenopausal women. Their study showed that estriol treatment resulted in the reemergence of friendly *Lactobacilli* bacteria, and the near elimination of colon bacteria, as well as restoration of normal vaginal mucosa and normal low pH, which inhibits the growth of many germs.

Without the estrogen treatment, antibiotic treatment alone is doomed to fail since it is almost always followed by recurring infections. Antibiotics, as we know, not only lead to resistant bacteria but also kill the friendly bacteria we need to protect us.

Good pelvic hygiene—including the hygiene of one's sexual partner—is also important in preventing urinary tract infections. It can be helpful for both men and women to urinate within a half hour or so after intercourse to flush out the urinary tract.

Low Progesterone and Estrogen

Progesterone also plays several roles in preventing vaginal and urinary tract infections. It is often forgotten that estrogen and progesterone help each other. Estrogen is necessary for cells to make progesterone receptors, and progesterone helps make estrogen receptors more sensitive. When progesterone is deficient, estrogen receptors become less sensitive to estrogen. Thus, many women with sufficient estrogen will nevertheless have signs of estrogen deficiency, such as vaginal dryness and hot flashes, as well as estrogen dominance symptoms. When progesterone is restored to normal physiological levels, estrogen receptors become more sensitive and signs of estrogen deficiency disappear:

Hot flashes diminish in intensity and frequency, vaginal lubrication returns, and urinary tract problems go away.

Also, it should be remembered that progesterone is part of our immune defense system that prevents infections: Progesterone aids in the formation of secretory IgA, an immune globulin that traps germs before they enter mucosal tissues such as those found in the vagina. This is why many women who begin using progesterone cream find that their allergies and sinusitis clear up. Therefore, whenever estrogen is given, or progesterone is deficient, it is wise to supplement with normal physiological doses of progesterone to optimize one's immune defenses.

Imbalances, Food Sensitivities, Stress, and Drugs

Urinary urgency and incontinence does not necessarily imply infection from germs. The vagina is host to many bacteria including the so-called friendly bacteria that keep the "unfriendly" bacteria in check.

I recall one patient with vaginal and urinary tract irritation that her doctor thought was due to candida (yeast) or trichomonal infections. In my exam I could find no such pathogens. Mystified, I referred this patient to an OB/Gyn specialist who finally learned that she used high doses of B vitamins, especially B1 (thiamine), and that her blood level of vitamin B1 was very high. After stopping the vitamin pills, the vaginal irritation cleared up. Apparently the vitamin stimulated an overgrowth of "friendly" bacteria sufficient to have caused the irritation.

Some women (and men, too) develop urinary urgency and incontinence from food sensitivities. In particular, coffee and other high-caffeine products can become irritants to the bladder. I have had some patients who, strangely, I thought, developed bladder urgency from coffee but not from tea, which also contains caffeine. When they switched to decaffeinated coffee, the problem persisted. For these people, it is not only the caffeine but also other components in coffee that can cause bladder irritability.

In addition, stress can cause urinary tract problems. The

muscles involved with normal urination are essentially autonomic in function; their performance is not directed by conscious effort. When we are under stress, the combination of
bladder contraction and sphincter relaxation are not in perfect
synchrony. The result can be that urination is not complete, and
the bladder retains significant amounts of urine. Since the flow
of urine from the kidneys down to the bladder is continuous, it
does not take long for the bladder to fill up again and signal the
need for urination. This is more common in men than in
women. In both sexes, however, stress can lead to frequent and
urgent urination.

Many drugs can affect the autonomic processes necessary for
proper urination. These drugs include antihypertensives (drugs
for high blood pressure), diuretics, certain tranquilizers, and selective serotonin reuptake inhibitors such as Prozac. It is wise not
to start another drug to treat a urination problem until you review the known side effects of any present drug you are taking.

Recurrent urinary tract infections also seem to be related to
birth control pills. Because of this link, it is often assumed that
urinary tract infections are due to sexual promiscuity. However,
they may be due instead to the suppression of progesterone production by the synthetic progestin in the birth control pills.

The most important thing to remember is this: The key to
treating urinary tract problems is to look for the source of the
problem, not just treat the symptom. Taking the time to play detective could spare you much needless waste of time, energy, and
money and could spare you from unnecessary drug side effects.

Gallbladder Disease and Bile Flow

Most people don't even know where their gallbladder is located,
never mind what it does; yet, gallbladder disease is the most
common digestive disease in the United States. It affects over 20
million Americans, with a million new cases diagnosed each
year. Half of those go on to have surgery to remove gallstones or
the gallbladder. Women are twice as likely as men to develop
gallstones, probably largely due to unidentified estrogen domi-

nance and the excessive estrogen used in hormone replacement therapy (HRT).

So-called gallbladder attacks are extremely painful. These pains are often felt in the upper right quadrant of the abdomen, the right collarbone area, or under the right scapula of the back (the wing-shaped bone below the shoulder and overlying the upper ribs in back). Not being at the location of the gallbladder itself, these pains are called "referred" pain. Other symptoms include bloating, gas, nausea, and stomach pain, especially after meals.

If the bile duct is blocked, jaundice (yellowing) may develop in the skin and the sclera (the whites of the eyes). The good news is that most women can avoid gallstones and gallbladder disease altogether by knowing a few simple guidelines for preventing them.

Other risk factors besides conventional HRT include diet in general, especially diets involving rapid weight loss, and obesity. By common wisdom, fried foods are thought to bring on gallbladder attacks, but, when studied objectively, this connection is inconsistent. Similarly, attempts to identify "trigger" foods that prompt gallbladder attacks are inconsistent. Most patients find it difficult to associate any specific food with their gallbladder attacks.

The Inner Workings of the Gallbladder

Bile production by the liver is controlled by a several factors including the food we eat and a variety of gastrointestinal polypeptide hormones. One of these hormones, somastatin, is a major regulator within the central nervous system (produced by the pituitary), but is also made by the adrenal medulla, the pancreas, and the gastrointestinal tract, a fact that confirms the essential unity of the brain and body. These hormones are autonomic and cannot be altered by voluntary control. However, sex hormones and fiber also play a role in bile flow and bile constituents, and these *are* under our control. To understand their roles, one must understand how bile is carried to the intestines and the factors that influence the fluidity of bile.

The Common Bile Duct

The liver is a large organ functionally divided into two lobes. Within an inch or so of exiting the liver, the two hepatic (liver) ducts merge to form the *common hepatic duct*. In another inch or so, a small convoluted duct branches off to the gallbladder, a pear-shaped hollow bag about the size of a man's thumb. As a result some bile is drained into the gallbladder to form a reservoir for extra bile, should circumstances require it. The main bile duct beyond the branch leading to the gallbladder is called the *common bile duct*.

The common bile duct passes under the pylorus (the sphincter through which food exits from the stomach) to the duodenum (the first 10 inches or so of the small intestine) to reach the Sphincter of Oddi, which, by constricting or dilating, controls the flow of bile into the duodenum. The duodenum follows a C-shaped path, and is plastered, so to speak, against the back of the abdomen, holding it securely in place, unlike the rest of the 20 feet of intestine that freely moves around in the abdomen. Thus, the duodenum is a fixed site for the entrance of the common bile duct.

Interestingly, the pancreas is also secured against the back of the abdomen, sitting like a beached flounder with its head in the concavity of the C-shaped path of the duodenum. The pancreas secretes insulin into the bloodstream but also secretes digestive enzymes through a duct from its "head" into the same Sphincter of Oddi. The passage of secretions from two different organs through a single sphincter is truly quite remarkable.

Keep the Bile Flowing

The flow of bile is very important to health. Its two major functions are excretory and digestive. In its excretory function, bile acts as a carrier for toxins and waste products being excreted from the body. For example, red blood cells become "senescent" (old, unable to function) in 120 to 140 days. The spleen and liver select out these older cells, save the iron, and excrete the rest as bilirubin via the liver. It is the bilirubin that gives bile its characteristic color. Undesirable solids such as sand, soot, and metal particles are also captured in the liver and disposed of through bile.

The digestive action of bile is twofold: First, its high bicarbonate content creates a pH of about 8, which is very alkaline. This is necessary to counteract the high acidity of gastric juice arriving from the stomach and allows intestinal and pancreatic enzymes to work effectively to digest food. Second, bile is a wonderful emulsifier, which means that it breaks up the fats that you've eaten into tiny droplets so that they are readily digested by the pancreatic enzyme lipase.

Pancreatic enzymes are very potent—amylase digests starches; protease digests proteins; and lipase digests fats. It is a wonder to me how the pancreatic duct can carry these potent enzymes and not be digested itself.

The flow of bile and pancreatic secretions through the Sphincter of Oddi is primarily a matter of (1) the size of the sphincter opening and (2) the fluidity of the secretions. If the sphincter is constricted, flow is decreased. Progesterone (and not estrogen, testosterone, thyroid, or insulin) causes a relaxation of the sphincter, thus increasing bile flow. Thus, people with estrogen dominance (relative progesterone deficiency) are more likely to have a constricted Sphincter of Oddi. Perhaps that's why so many women tell me their digestion is so much better after they correct their estrogen dominance with progesterone supplementation.

Another Reason to Get Plenty of Fiber

Fiber helps prevent viscous (thick) bile by reducing cholesterol absorption in the intestines, and also reducing cholesterol synthesis. A primary ingredient of bile is cholesterol, much of it in the form of cholesterol monohydrate crystals. This, along with calcium bilirubinate granules, creates biliary sludge. Biliary sludge can obstruct the Sphincter of Oddi. In addition, these crystals and granules can coalesce to make gallstones, which totally obstruct the Sphincter of Oddi, or they can accumulate in the gallbladder, leading eventually to surgical removal of the gallbladder.

When the sphincter is obstructed, bile backs up into the pancreatic duct. This is particularly disastrous since the addition of the emulsifying effect of bile combined with the potent digestive pancreatic enzymes causes damage to pancreatic tissue and leads to pancreatitis. Biliary sludge is the probable cause of 30 to 50 percent of the incidence of recurrent pancreatitis, which is not only extremely painful and difficult to treat, but is also quite often fatal.

Other factors contributing to sluggish bile flow are sugar and highly refined starches, overeating, and a couch-potato lifestyle. Once a person has pancreatitis, all alcohol must be discontinued.

GUIDELINES FOR PREVENTING GALLBLADDER DISEASE

- Avoid fried food, especially if you've had attacks after eating fried food.
- Avoid sugar and highly refined starches.
- Drink plenty of good water.
- Recognize estrogen dominance and correct it.
- Make sure you have adequate progesterone (saliva test best for this).
- Aim for 20 to 24 grams of fiber a day. Fiber supplements can help.
- Do not be afraid to consume olive oil and good omega-3 fatty acids such as fish.
- Keep your liver healthy.
- If you've had any attack of pancreatitis, avoid all alcohol.
- Do not overeat.
- Avoid rapid weight-loss diets.
- Chew your food well. Take time to eat in a leisurely fashion, setting aside anger and stress.

SOME HIGH-FIBER FOODS

fruits	seeds
prunes	popcorn
vegetables	brown rice
beans	whole grain breads
wheat and oat bran	whole grain cereals
nuts	

PART III

CREATING AND
MAINTAINING
HORMONE BALANCE

CHAPTER 19

HOW TO USE PROGESTERONE SUPPLEMENTATION

The purpose of this chapter is to review the types of progesterone available and to give you details about using progesterone. For the most part, how you use natural progesterone will depend first on whether you are premenopausal or menopausal rather than on your list of individual symptoms. If you're currently taking HRT or have migraines, you'll need special instructions, and information about this is covered later in the chapter. The dosage you use and the exact days of your cycle (if you still have one) you use it will vary according to your individual biochemistry. I will review those criteria shortly.

Types of Progesterone Supplementation

If progesterone supplementation is decided upon, a woman can choose between skin creams and oils, sublingual (i.e., under the tongue) drops, and capsules.

Creams and Oils

My preference among the various available forms of progesterone supplements remains the transdermal route, meaning "through the skin." My reasons have to do with the appropriateness of hormone supplementation. Remember that the goal is *physiologic* hormone *balance*. By physiologic, I mean that the dosages approximate (and not exceed) normal hormone needs and responses. When intervening in a system of biofeedback controls, it is unwise to exceed the normal responses of the healthy gland. In the case of hypothyroidism or adrenal deficiency, supplemental dosages greater than normal will suppress normal function of the target gland. Dr. William Jefferies, in his book *The Safe Uses of Cortisol*, makes this same point in a convincing manner. I try to follow the same principle in regard to sex hormone supplementation, and I strongly recommend dosages that approximate the ovaries' normal expected production of progesterone. What we are treating is progesterone deficiency secondary to follicle depletion. We do not wish to suppress whatever function of the ovary still remains.

The fact that transdermal progesterone is well absorbed, as shown by the good concentration of it in target tissues such as breasts, without a demonstrable rise in plasma (blood) levels, is perplexing to some. In fact, some doctors argue that because they give their patients progesterone cream, take a blood test a month later, and no rise in progesterone is shown, this is proof that progesterone is not well absorbed when applied on the skin. The explanation, however, is quite simple.

Progesterone is fat-soluble and, as such, is not soluble in the watery blood plasma, which is the part of the blood tested for hormone levels. When passing through the liver, progesterone becomes protein-bound, making it soluble in the plasma. However, protein-bound progesterone is not biologically available. The protein-binding interferes with progesterone bonding to its receptor in target tissue cells. When serum or plasma is used in "blood" tests, more than 90 percent of the progesterone found is already protein-bound and no longer bioavailable, and only 1 to 9 percent of it is "free" (not protein-bound). In contrast, when progesterone is absorbed across skin or mucous membranes (such as the mouth), it is not protein-bound and only a small fraction of it is found in plasma. The majority of it rides through the bloodstream on red blood cells, much as pollen is carried by bees, or seeds are carried by birds. There it is nicely compatible with cholesterol, vitamin A, vitamin E, and other components of the fatty structure of the cell membrane. For these reasons, progesterone carried in this manner is close to 100 percent biologically available, as shown by salivary hormone assays.

Transdermal progesterone is absorbed through the skin into the underlying fat layer, from which it diffuses into the capillaries permeating the fat, where it can be taken up in the blood as needed. It begins circulating in the blood within seconds of application, and reaches its peak in about 3 to 4 hours. After about 8 hours levels begin dropping, and most of the progesterone is cleared from the body within 12 hours of application. When I first wrote this book, there was much debate in the medical community about whether or not it was really absorbed. Since then, a number of good studies have come out showing irrefutably that the progesterone is very well absorbed. Furthermore, conventional medicine now uses estrogen and progestin patches for HRT and contraception, so as far as I'm concerned the debate is over.

Transdermal progesterone comes in creams and oils. The oils can be thick and sticky used transdermally; you can dilute them with olive or coconut oil at the time you are using them, or simply rub the oil briskly into your palms, where it is quickly absorbed.

Transdermal progesterone cream is very easily and quickly absorbed into the body, so you can apply it almost anywhere with success. However, I do recommend rotating the areas you apply it to avoid saturating any one area. It is best absorbed where the skin is relatively thin and well supplied with capillary blood flow, such as the face, neck, upper chest, breasts, inner arms, and the palms of the hands and soles of the feet.

Some people claim that transdermal progesterone accumulates in the fat cells and creates extremely high levels of progesterone in the body. Being fat-soluble (as endogenous progesterone and all endogenous sex hormones are) it will naturally be soluble in fat cells, just as endogenous progesterone is. The only problem these critics have is with excessive dosing. To the best of my knowledge, all of these people were using very high doses of cream, some up to 100 mg per day. As I explained before, this is medical mismanagement and is almost guaranteed to cause side effects. I have never seen an overdose occur when the physiologic doses that I recommend were used.

Sublingual or Buccal Drops or Oil

Progesterone now comes in a variety of forms that can be put in the mouth and held there (without swallowing) for a few minutes. It is important not to swallow for at least a minute after applying the drops this way so the drops are absorbed rather than swallowed. If not swallowed, they are absorbed through the mucous membranes of the mouth within minutes, leading to prompt elevation of progesterone levels. However, the levels fall in three to four hours due to rapid metabolizing and excretion, or absorption by body fat. Thus, to maintain stable blood levels, the drops should be administered three to four times a day, increasing the chance of overdosing. The number of drops to be applied varies with the product, so you'll need to check saliva levels and experiment to find out what works best for you.

These types of liquid formulations can also be applied to the skin.

Capsules

Progesterone dissolved in peanut oil is commercially sold as capsules under the trade name, Prometrium. It is often used by fertility specialists to treat women with luteal phase defect, meaning that they don't produce enough progesterone after ovulation to maintain a pregnancy. Prometrium is only available by prescription.

The disadvantage of taking oral (by mouth) capsules is that they need to be given in very large doses, 100 to 200 milligrams per day, to compensate for the 85 to 90 percent that will be metabolized or excreted before having a chance to enter the bloodstream. This is 10 to 20 times greater than transdermal doses just to get the 10 to 15 milligrams of progesterone circulating in blood. I see no reason to put the liver to all this work when transdermal application is much more efficient.

Physicians tend to believe that the use of progesterone capsules gives them a more precise dose than the transdermal creams, but this is a mistaken notion. In fact, the capsules give a much more unpredictable dose. This is because when progesterone is taken orally, it (like other fat-soluble nutrients) is taken up by the portal vein, which transports it directly to the liver, where much of it is metabolized and conjugated (combined with glucuronide) for excretion in bile. This is termed the "first pass loss" through the liver. Some undoubtedly is absorbed by chylomicrons, tiny bits of fat that float in the bloodstream, and will circulate through the body, but the rate at which this happens varies greatly according to the health of the digestive tract and liver, stress levels, diet, and many other factors, including basic individual biochemistry, and thus it is unpredictable. In general, oral doses of progesterone (even in the micronized versions) must be greater than transdermal doses to create the equivalent biologic effects. For example, the success of Dr. Joel Hargrove from Vanderbilt University in using progesterone for PMS requires 300 to 400 milligrams or more per day to accomplish what I have observed in patients using only 30 to 40 milligrams per day by the transdermal route.

Because of the great safety of progesterone and the freedom from side effects, I am not aware of any danger in using the larger oral dosages over the short term. However, I see no reason to subject the liver to this extra work, and long term both estrogen and progesterone receptors will be shut down, resulting in hormone imbalances and a return of symptoms. In addition, some women taking oral progesterone complain that it makes them sleepy, indicating that they are getting a larger dose than needed. I have a further concern that liver-generated metabolites of oral progesterone may have diminished or different effects from the natural progesterone molecule.

Testing Hormone Levels

Saliva Testing

The usual way to test hormone levels has been with a blood test that measures the blood serum or blood plasma content of the hormones. These tests are inherently irrelevant since bioavailable "free" hormone is not soluble in serum. Bioavailable sex hormones are fat soluble and circulate in blood via fatty substances not found in serum, such as red blood cell membranes. What is important is how much progesterone circulates through the target tissues for progesterone action. We now know that the non-protein-bound hormone molecule, when circulating through the saliva tissue, will filter directly into the saliva, whereas protein-bound (nonbioavailable) hormone does not. Thus, saliva levels reflect tissue levels of sex hormones, and serum tests do not.

Hormones made in the ovaries, testes, or adrenals are wrapped in protein envelopes called either sex hormone–binding globulin (SHBG) or cortisol-binding globulin (CBG) so they can be carried in the blood. These protein-bound hormones are not fully biologically active. The more important and relevant hormone levels are the 1 to 10 percent that are unbound and thus biologically active. Saliva contains only the unbound, biologically active hormone molecules. When progesterone is absorbed through the skin, it is not coated with protein and is carried in the blood's fatty components, such as chylomicrons or red blood cell membranes. Only when absorbed progesterone exceeds the carrying capacity of the fatty material in blood will it "slop over," so to speak, into the serum. Thus, when serum levels of progesterone are seen to rise, it is probably a sign of overdosing. Conversely, transdermal progesterone absorption is quick and efficient, showing up in saliva within just a few hours, indicating that it is well absorbed and available to cells in biologically active form.

Saliva testing is quicker, less expensive, and less painful than blood tests, and is a reliable way for your doctor to measure hormone levels and test for hormone deficiencies. It will confirm that the hormones you are taking are being absorbed and utilized; it doesn't involve a trip to a lab or drawing blood; and it's inexpensive enough that you can do a number of tests, such as over the course of a day or a month. For those women who wish to monitor their own hormone levels to find out if they are ovulating, for example, the tests can be ordered and easily done at home without a doctor's prescription.

Salivary testing done by Dr. David Zava at ZRT Lab in

Beaverton, Oregon, to test the absorption of transdermal progesterone creams confirms that this form works better than other methods or routes because the hormone is absorbed more efficiently, the effect is longer lasting, and it doesn't create the highs and lows created with the oral (swallowed) or sublingual (held in the mouth) drops. Though these latter two forms reach peak levels even faster than the creams, they are also excreted faster. My guess is that the interrupted highs and lows of a hormone like progesterone is confusing to the hypothalamus, leading to physiologic levels that may actually "tune down" or down regulate the receptor response. My goal is to mimic normal physiologic levels of progesterone, to simulate what the ovaries would be doing if their follicles were in working order.

Blood Serum or Plasma Testing

Serum levels of progesterone will rise in about three months of using progesterone cream. This may be a sign of overdosing, and it is wise to check a saliva test. If your doctor wants to measure your serum progesterone levels, here are some guidelines: Normal, untreated (not on HRT) postmenopausal women will show an initial serum progesterone level of 0.03 to 0.3 ng/ml, and after three months of transdermal progesterone, this level rises to 3 to 4 ng/ml, or about 10 times higher. In normal premenopausal women, luteal (midcycle) phase serum progesterone levels are 7 to 28 ng/ml. Note that this is a fourfold range. Since some women have more sex hormone protein-binding than others, the serum level cannot indicate how much of that 7 to 28 ng/ml concentration is composed of "free" hormone or protein-bound (nonbioavailable) hormone.

Not All "Wild Yam Extract" Is Progesterone

A word of caution: Not all products with labels claiming "wild yam extract" actually contain any progesterone. Some do; others don't. By historical practice, many nutritional products have merely listed their ingredients by such nonspecific labeling.

Thus "wild yam extract" may be ground-up wild yam, it may be diosgenin (an extract of wild yam), or it may be progesterone. If progesterone is not specifically listed on the label, the only way to find out if there is any in there is to call the company. Furthermore, some of these "wild yam creams" contain very small amounts of progesterone, so if the amount of progesterone is not listed on the label or in a brochure, make sure to find out how much it contains. Because there are many excellent progesterone creams available at reasonable prices, the best approach may be to stick with creams that are clearly labeled.

Progesterone is obtained by extracting specific components from plants (e.g., diosgenin from wild yams or soybeans) and then converting them to actual (in other words, *bioidentical*) progesterone in the laboratory. As I mentioned in earlier chapters, the synthetic progestins are also made from the diosgenin found in wild yams and soybeans. The key difference is that the molecular structure of the progestins is not found in nature, and certainly not in the female body! Even though progesterone is synthesized in a laboratory, it is still "natural" progesterone. Since there is only one molecule called *progesterone*, if it's not progesterone it can't be called progesterone. Products with some progesterone-like actions are progestins.

Progesterone (U.S. Pharmacopeia) is available on the wholesale pharmaceutical market. It is used by the major pharmaceutical companies as the base from which they synthesize their estrogen, testosterone, cortisone, and, of course, their progestin products. Unfortunately, the early alternative nutritional companies who incorporated this same progesterone in their products saw fit to list it as "extract of wild yam." Now, with the success of progesterone supplementation, many companies are producing products listed as containing wild yam extract, but they actually contain no progesterone. What many of these "wild yam extract" products contain is diosgenin, which is indeed the *laboratory* precursor to progesterone and other hormones, but there is *no* evidence that the human body converts diosgenin to hormones. In fact, rodent and human studies of diosgenin supplementation show only that it sometimes creates a drop in cholesterol levels.

Another word of caution: Even when a cream contains progesterone, it will not be effective if it isn't suspended in the proper medium. Products containing mineral oil or wax may prevent the progesterone from being absorbed into the skin. Other products haven't properly stabilized the progesterone, so it deteriorates over time with exposure to oxygen and may be dissipated by the time you get to the bottom of the jar.

How and When to Use Natural Progesterone

Women differ in almost every aspect of their physiology. Although genetically all humans are 99 percent the same, that 1 percent difference can account for an astounding variation in how the details work. It's not rational for a doctor to order the same dose of any given medicine for every patient, and the same is true of natural progesterone.

Though medical professionals can give you guidelines to work within, it's up to you to find the best dose for your body. Ideally, you should be able to find the minimum amount you can use to gain and sustain relief from your symptoms. Because natural progesterone is so safe, it won't hurt you to use a little more than your optimal dose. That leaves plenty of room for experimentation.

On the other hand, as with most substances, too much progesterone can cause problems. As the use of progesterone has increased in popularity, health care professionals have developed many different schools of thought about how to use it, and many of them prescribe very high doses of progesterone. This practice is counterproductive and leads to further hormone imbalance, not to mention a handful of interesting theories about why the progesterone isn't working the way Dr. Lee says it does. Here's the answer folks: *It's the overdose!*

Chronically high doses of progesterone over many months eventually cause progesterone receptors to turn off, reducing its effectiveness. Using excessive doses of progesterone can also cause the side effects listed next. But keep in mind, not all women suffer from these side effects when they use excessive doses of progesterone.

Possible Side Effects of Progesterone

I used to say that there are no known side effects of progesterone when it is taken in small physiologic doses, that is, 20 or so milligrams per day. However, after nearly a decade of having millions of people read my books and newsletters, I've learned that to make such a blanket statement is to invite mail that informs me to the contrary. However, 99 percent of the time I find that these so-called side effects have good reasons to exist. The most common reason for progesterone cream side effects is gross overdose. I have heard tales of health care professionals and pharmacists recommending 100 mg daily of progesterone cream. This type of medical mismanagement is guaranteed to cause not just side effects, but serious hormonal imbalances including a shutting down of hormone receptors. Another common cause of side effects are the creams that include a mix of other hormones such as estrogen and testosterone. Transdermal hormones should be taken individually so that you can regulate dosage if you get symptoms of overdose or deficiency.

Extremely large doses of progesterone can cause sleepiness, although most women report they simply feel calm. Enormous doses can cause an anesthetic or drunken effect. Some women report estrogen dominance symptoms for a week or two after starting progesterone, but this is caused by a sensitization of estrogen receptors and generally disappears within a few weeks. In some women it may take a few months for hormones to balance out. If you're still having periods and you take progesterone out of phase with your cycle, it may change the timing of your period or cause some spotting.

Overall, the percentage of women who genuinely suffer from side effects is extremely small and may be due to rare individual variations in biochemistry, or some type of autoimmune reaction.

Lethargy/sleepiness   This is probably an effect of allopreg-nanolone, a by-product of progesterone, on the brain.

Edema (water retention)   Probably caused by excess conversion to deoxycortisone, a mineralcorticoid made in the adrenal glands that causes water retention.

Candida   The bacteria present in a yeast infection; excess progesterone can inhibit anti-candida neutrophils (white blood cells).

Bloating   Excess progesterone slows gastrointestinal (GI) transport, and with the wrong kind of gastrointestinal flora such as candida this can lead to bloating and gas. (During pregnancy the high levels of progesterone slow food transport through the GI tract to enhance absorption of nutrients.)

Lowered libido   Excess progesterone blocks an enzyme called *5 alpha reductase*, which normally causes conversion of testosterone to DHT. Testosterone is good for libido in both women and men. Excessive progesterone may also lower one's libido because it saturates and down-regulates progesterone receptors, just as too much light in your eyes reduces your light sensitivity.

Mild depression   Excess progesterone down-regulates estrogen receptors and brain response to estrogens is needed for serotonin production.

Symptoms of estrogen deficiency   Excess progesterone down-regulates estrogen receptors and desensitizes tissue to estrogen. Because progesterone receptors are dependent on estrogen priming through the estrogen receptor, excess progesterone in the absence of estrogen can cause a lot of problems. This can be especially true in women who have very low estradiol and are taking large doses of progesterone.

Then there's the question of progesterone metabolites (some mentioned in the list above), the by-products created by excessive progesterone. In addition to the above-listed side effects, they certainly put an extra and unnecessary burden on the liver as it works overtime to excrete them. This happens most frequently when women use oral progesterone (pill form). As much as 90 percent of an oral dose is destroyed in the gastrointestinal tract within 15 minutes or so of taking it. The progesterone that is destroyed becomes by-products or metabolites that enter the liver where they and the real progesterone are transported into the bloodstream. Several research groups, including one in France (Nahoul) and another in the United States (Levin), using highly sophisticated methods of analysis, came to the conclusion that about 80 percent of what is measured as progesterone by conventional blood tests is really inactive metabolites of progesterone. Therefore, if you are taking 100 mg of oral progesterone and your blood test comes back as 10 ng/ml, the real progesterone level is more likely only to be about 2 ng/ml and the rest of it inactive metabolites, or metabolites that are causing side effects rather than benefits. These metabolites are not as likely to get into saliva, and therefore a measurement of bioavailable progesterone (through a saliva test) will give far more accurate levels than serum (or plasma) levels.

Although some women take too much progesterone, there are also creams out there with virtually no progesterone in them (5 to 10 mg per jar of cream), and women who use those creams are underdosed. Ten mg of progesterone per jar of cream is not enough to oppose the effects of estrogen or to build bone. These creams are *not* recommended.

I always prefer that women work in partnership with a skilled and competent health care professional when balancing their hormones. It is notoriously difficult to be objective in diagnosing and treating oneself and tracking whatever changes might be taking place. With or without a health care professional to work with, it's a great idea, at least for the first few months of beginning a hormone balance regimen, to keep a daily journal that records what you ate, what you took in the way of supplements, and how you feel.

Dosage Recommendations for Progesterone

All the dosage recommendations in this chapter are based on using a 2-ounce container of progesterone cream that contains 900 to 1,000 mg of progesterone per 2-ounce container (a 1.6

to 2.0 percent progesterone cream). This amounts to about 40 mg per ½ teaspoon, 20 mg per ¼ teaspoon, and 10 mg per ⅛ teaspoon. Most premenopausal women need only 15 to 20 mg of progesterone daily during the luteal phase of the cycle—about what the body would make if it was making its own progesterone. Some women do better with closer to 30 mg; others do fine with closer to 10 mg. People and their metabolic needs differ.

Another way of looking at it is, if a premenopausal woman uses 20 mg of progesterone per day for 14 days each month, the monthly dose is 280 mg, approximately one-third of the 2-ounce container. When using the creams with the concentration I recommend, this 20-mg dose is found in ¼ of a teaspoonful of cream. This is commonly a very acceptable dose. I don't recommend the super-high dosage creams that contain 3,000 mg, which are typically listed as 10 percent creams and which contain about 100 mg of progesterone per ¼ teaspoon. It's way too easy to get too much cream with these doses, and we are striving for balance.

If you are taking a physiologic dose (an amount approximating what your body would make itself under normal circumstances) and your symptoms don't go away after four to six months, or if they return, it's best to continue to work in partnership with a competent health care professional to find out why. In many cases other hormone imbalances need to be corrected, most commonly estrogen deficiency, androgen deficiency (particularly problematic in women who have had a complete hysterectomy), poor adrenal function causing low or high cortisol levels, or thyroid deficiency. There is never a reason to add an estrogen supplement to a woman still having monthly periods; the very fact that she is menstruating is evidence that she is making plenty of estrogen.

After menopause, the ovaries continue to make small amounts of estrogen and testosterone. In addition, estrogen continues to be made by body fat. In two-thirds of women after menopause, estradiol levels are sufficient.

A progesterone-deficient woman who starts using natural progesterone cream in the recommended doses will find that in three to four months, the progesterone in her body fat will reach physiologic equilibrium. Most women will be able to judge for themselves, based on symptoms, that the previous hormone imbalance is now corrected.

In a menopausal woman (who is not preparing her uterus for pregnancy), I have found that 10 to 12 mg of progesterone per day for 24 to 25 days of the calendar month works well. That is one-half of a quarter teaspoonful. A 2-ounce container will easily last for at least three months.

Ultimately, how you achieve your monthly dosing goal will probably come down to personal preference under the guidance of your health care professional. How you're feeling will be a good indicator of whether it's working for you. In a very few women, the first few weeks of starting a hormone balance regimen can involve some worsening of symptoms and even new ones, but that phase generally passes quickly. If a woman felt fine for four to six months on a given dose, and then finds it not working as well, this is usually a sign that she should reduce her dose. A saliva test will come in helpful here.

The cream can be applied once or twice a day. The optimal approach is a divided dose, with a larger dose at bedtime and a smaller dose in the morning. Getting each dab of cream to be exactly the right size isn't that important here, because there's a buffering effect as the progesterone is absorbed into subcutaneous (under the skin) fat. The release of the hormone from body fat serves to make the progesterone effect relatively steady even if daily doses vary a little.

How to Get the Most Out of Progesterone Cream

Here are some general guidelines on how to get the most out of your progesterone cream dose:

- The larger the area of skin the dose is spread on, the greater the absorption.

- You should apply the cream to thinner skin with high capillary density—such as places where you blush. Through testing at his lab, Dr. David Zava has found that the best spots are the palms (if they aren't callused), chest, inner arms, neck, and face. The soles of the feet are also good if they're not thickened from walking barefoot.
- Progesterone cream should be applied after, not before, a warm bath or shower.
- If you use the cream at bedtime it can be calming and help you sleep. If you apply it twice a day, use a larger dab at night and a smaller one in the morning.
- Because other ingredients of the cream are generally not absorbed, continual use of any single skin area will eventually saturate that area, and this might reduce progesterone absorption. Rotate among three or four different skin sites on different days.

When During the Month to Use Progesterone Cream

In this section, we're going to first give you general information on when to use progesterone cream, and then we'll go into different ways of using it for specific problems. Again, please keep in mind that it is not helpful to use too much progesterone cream.

Menopausal women (not having menstrual cycles) can use progesterone cream for 24 to 26 days of the calendar month. Women who experience a recurrence of hot flashes or other symptoms during the break can try reducing the dose gradually over a 2- to 3-day period before taking the break, or if that doesn't work, reduce the break time to just 3 days completely off. The monthly break is important since postmenopausal women still make estrogen and the addition of progesterone may cause the recurrence of menstrual periods. It is wise to allow complete shedding, which usually occurs when you allow the progesterone to fall for several days. If regular periods resume, then return to the premenopausal schedule of using progesterone two weeks each menstrual month, stopping a day or two before the expected period. When the periods stop for three to four months, then you can resume the 24- to 26-day schedule again. If spotting continues, it is wise to consult with your doctor. The use of progesterone cream will not prevent menopause from occurring.

Premenopausal women with signs of estrogen dominance and progesterone deficiency can use progesterone during the two weeks prior to their period, stopping a day or two before the expected period. When a woman is progesterone-deficient, estrogen receptors become less sensitive. When progesterone deficiency is corrected, these estrogen receptors regain normal sensitivity. This can cause breast swelling and tenderness in some women for a few weeks to two to three months. This breast swelling is due to the estrogen effect in breasts that causes fluid retention in breast cells and usually resolves in two to three months. Women with this problem should try smaller doses of the progesterone cream.

If you have an average 26- to 30-day menstrual cycle, you can begin your first month of progesterone cream use between day 10 to 12 of your menstrual cycle *counting the first day of your period as day 1*. Continue until a day or two before your expected period, which for most women is between 26 and 30 days. (If you don't know how long your cycle is because you have had irregular bleeding, or if your cycles have been very short or very long, use your intuition and pick a day.) If your period starts before your chosen last day, stop using the cream and begin counting again to day 10, 11, or 12. It may take 2 to 3 cycles to find the synchrony your body desires.

It can be perfectly normal to have a menstrual cycle as short as 18 days and as long as 32 days. If your cycle is shorter or longer than average, use the following method to determine when to take the cream: Use the calendar to figure out when the first day of your next period is expected, then count backward two weeks. This is when you should start taking the cream. The reason for this is that the number of days from day 1 of your period to the day you ovulate can vary greatly, but for nearly all women, the number of days between ovulation and the start of the next period is 14 days. The closer you can get to taking the progesterone when you ovulate or just after, the more in tune with your own cycle you will be.

Even if you can tell that you have ovulated, it does not mean that you do not need progesterone supplementation. Ovulation does not guarantee continued progesterone production throughout the luteal phase. In many women, progesterone production may fall shortly after ovulation and they become estrogen dominant again in the week before their period. This is called *luteal phase failure* and it is common in U.S. women after age 35. Luteal phase failure is a common cause of irregular cycles and infertility.

It may take up to three months of progesterone use to restore normal menstrual cycles. As women approach menopause, estrogen production often becomes more variable. Under such circumstances, it may be unrealistic to expect to have regular cycles, even with progesterone cream.

It's best to synchronize your natural progesterone supplementation with your body's own hormonal cycles as much as possible. Menstrual dysfunction is usually the result of more than just progesterone deficiency. Factors such as stress, diet, and cortisol or thyroid hormone play important roles in this matter. The cooperation between the *hypothalamus* (the part of the brain that controls the endocrine system), the *pituitary gland* (the "master gland" that sends out instructions to other glands throughout the body), and ovaries may be out of sync because the body is out of balance. Adding progesterone at the right times in the right amounts helps this complex system regain its equilibrium.

Ovulation often begins to be irregular 8 to 10 years before actual menopause. Each anovulatory cycle sends a woman deeper into estrogen dominance as body fat progesterone stores are depleted. Very thin women with little body fat go into estrogen dominance much more quickly. In women with long-standing progesterone deficiency, their body fat is devoid of progesterone. In such women, the first one or two months of transdermal progesterone are used to replenish body fat stores, so it makes sense to use higher doses during that time. After two to three months of progesterone use, the dose can usually be reduced with good effect. Women who start out using ¼ of a teaspoon of cream twice a day (40 mg/day) for the two weeks prior to their period usually find that they can reduce the dose in half (20 mg/day) for these same two weeks each month and continue to have good results.

We can't emphasize enough that the bottom line in progesterone dosing is always observed physiologic effects. Are your PMS symptoms improved? Are you gaining less weight before your periods? Are your breast or uterine fibrocysts getting smaller? Are your moods steadier? Are you less anxious? It's all about working to find the dose that corrects the problem, then reducing that dose to the minimum needed to maintain the desired effect.

Guidelines for Menopausal Women

The majority of menopausal women can simply use 10 to 15 mg of progesterone daily for 24 to 26 days in a row of the calendar month. Many women find it easiest to start using the cream on the first of the month and stop from day 24 to 26 until the next month. Other women prefer to take their hormone break the first 5 to 6 days of the calendar month and then use the cream until the end of the month. It's best to use the cream in divided doses: half before bed and half in the morning. However, if that doesn't work well for you, don't be concerned, just pick one time of the day when it's most convenient to use it and use the whole dose.

Guidelines for Premenopausal Women Who Are Menstruating but Not Ovulating

Salivary assays done during the luteal or midcycle, when progesterone levels would normally be at their highest, can determine whether you're having anovulatory cycles. If your progesterone levels are low, that indicates either that you haven't ovulated or the follicle is unable to produce the proper amount of progesterone. Dr. David Zava finds with saliva testing that anovulation is usually associated with both low estradiol and low progesterone, and occurs frequently in women who have been on birth control, particularly Depo Provera. These women often suffer with symptoms characteristic of both estrogen and progesterone deficiency.

In contrast, ovulation with luteal insufficiency is associated with normal to high estrogen and low progesterone, along with a host of estrogen dominance symptoms. If you have estrogen dominance symptoms, that's a pretty good indicator that your progesterone production is inadequate. Your health care professional can help you determine where you are.

In one study on a group of 18 regularly cycling women, with an average age of 29, 7 (39 percent) were found to be anovulatory and were not producing progesterone during the luteal phase. Many women who appear normal for their age group are actually not ovulating and have very low progesterone levels.

If this is you, try using one-third of a 2-ounce container of cream that contains approximately 900 to 1,000 mg per container during the time from presumed ovulation to a day or so before your expected period (⅛ teaspoon twice daily). That will provide you with about 300 mg of progesterone per month. Since the daily progesterone produced by women with good functioning ovaries ranges from 12 to 24 mg/day, your goal is to restore progesterone to those normal levels.

Women's sensitivity to hormones differs tremendously, so your dose will depend on your individual sensitivity. Because progesterone is such a safe hormone, do not be afraid to experiment a bit to find the dose that serves you best. What is normal for one woman is not necessarily normal for another. As mentioned previously, in premenopausal women who have been progesterone deficient for years, it's common that the initial application of progesterone will cause water retention, headaches, and swollen breasts—symptoms of estrogen dominance. This happens because the estrogen receptors shut down by progesterone deficiency are "waking up." It's important to remember that these symptoms will usually disappear in two weeks to two or three months.

Guidelines for Women with Endometriosis

Endometriosis involves small islets of endometrial tissue scattered here and there about the uterus, other pelvic organs, the wall of the colon, and even in the lungs. Though the cause is not clear, these islets of endometrial tissue respond to estrogen just as the endometrial cells in the uterus do—they fill with blood each month, causing severe pain. During pregnancy, endometriosis recedes, only to recur after the pregnancy when normal periods return. This suggests that the higher levels of progesterone during pregnancy inhibit estrogen-stimulated endometriosis.

During regular menstrual cycles, estrogen production rises around day 7 to 8 of the cycle and falls a day or so before your period begins. Progesterone production, on the other hand, starts after ovulation (around day 12), reaching levels several hundred time greater than estrogen, and falls abruptly a day or so before the period. Using this concept as a model, transdermal progesterone can be given in doses similar to that of early pregnancy, starting at day 8 and continuing until day 26 of a usual 28-day cycle. Experience shows that this treatment is often effective in relieving the symptoms of endometriosis. Your goal is to find the lowest dose of progesterone necessary to control endometrial stimulation.

During the early weeks of pregnancy, progesterone production doubles or triples, from the normal 12 to 24 mg/day to 40 to 60 mg/day. These levels are easily reached using ¼ teaspoon of progesterone cream twice or three times a day during these 18 days of the cycle. Many women find success using a 2-ounce jar or tube of the recommended cream each monthly cycle. Improvement is usually noted after several months of progesterone cream used in this manner. If improvement is not found in two months, the dose can be raised to 1 ounce per week. It can take up to six months for symptoms to be controlled, and even then they may not dissipate entirely. If the symptoms eventually disappear, the progesterone dose can be decreased gradually to find the lowest effective dose. (Otherwise use the dose that's most effective to control symptoms.) This must usually be continued until menopause is passed since recurrences are common if the progesterone protection is lowered too much. If a flare-up occurs, increase the dose to the previous effective level. If high doses of progesterone cream make you sleepy, that's an indication that you're taking too much. Reduce the dose until the sleepiness goes away.

Guidelines for Women with Uterine Fibroids

Women with fibroids are often estrogen dominant and have low progesterone levels. In women with smaller fibroids (the size of a tangerine or smaller), when progesterone is restored to normal levels, the fibroids often shrink a bit and stop growing, which is likely due to progesterone's ability to help speed up the clearance of estrogens from tissue. If this treatment can be continued through menopause, hysterectomy can sometimes be avoided.

However, some fibroids, when they reach a certain "critical mass," are accompanied by degeneration or cell death in the interior part of the fibroid and will have an interaction with white blood cells that ends up with the creation of more estrogen within the fibroid itself. It also contains growth factors that are stimulated by progesterone. Under these circumstances, surgical removal of the fibroid (myomectomy) or the uterus (hysterectomy) may become necessary. When you think of treating smaller fibroids you should be thinking in terms of keeping your estrogen milieu as low as possible, and when treating large fibroids, all hormones should be kept as low as possible.

Taking estrogen if you have fibroids will stimulate the fibroids to grow. If you're estrogen dominant, it's important to use a supplemental progesterone, usually in doses of 20 mg per day during the luteal phase of the cycle. Sometimes this approach works to slow or stop fibroid growth, and other times it doesn't. It may be worth a try. Reducing stress, increasing exercise, and reducing calories are also good strategies for slowing fibroid growth.

Guidelines for Women with Breast Fibrocysts

Breast fibrocysts are fluid-filled fibrous cysts, usually tender and painful, more so during the last 7 to 8 days of the menstrual cycle, primarily due to estrogen dominance over a prolonged period of time. This is a sign that your ovaries are not producing enough progesterone. Breast fibrocysts respond remarkably well to topical progesterone, a fact which the French first recognized some 30 years ago.

Progesterone cream, at 15 to 20 mg per day from ovulation until the day or two before your period starts, will usually result in a return to normal breast tissue in three to four months. Some of my patients found it helpful to apply the progesterone cream to the breasts every few days. You can also take 400 IU of vitamin E at bedtime every night, as well as 300 mg of magnesium and 50 mg of vitamin B6 a day. For many women it helps to cut out caffeine (coffee and certain soft drinks), and reduce sugar and refined starches in the diet. Once the fibrocysts are under control, the natural progesterone is usually tapered down to the minimum dose needed to help prevent recurrence.

Guidelines for Women Using Estrogen Supplements

Some women who have irregular bleeding are prescribed estrogen by their doctors. This is a misguided approach. Irregular periods are due most often to progesterone deficiency. Without the normal rise and fall of progesterone each cycle, the uterus just doesn't know when to shed its lining. There's really no good reason to give estrogen to women who are still menstruating. Unless you're close to actual menopause and experiencing blatant estrogen deficiency symptoms such as hot flashes, night sweats, and vaginal dryness, the very fact that you're menstruating indicates that you are not deficient in estrogen.

Some reduce the estrogen dose by half when adding progesterone, and gradually taper off the estrogen to find the right dose, which might well be no supplement at all. Approximately two-thirds of women up to age 80 continue to make sufficient estrogen after menopause, and therefore need no estrogen supplement.

Saliva testing usually shows 1 to 2 pg/ml of estradiol. The healthy ratio of progesterone to estradiol is 200 to 300 to 1. Therefore you would want the saliva progesterone level to be around 400 to 500 pg/ml. Without progesterone supplementation, the saliva progesterone level is often less than 50 pg/ml. In addition to progesterone deficiency, many women are deficient in testosterone. Saliva testing is invaluable for proper hormone balancing. If you are using estrogen tablets and need a half dosage, the tablets can be cut in half.

Estrogen patches deliver a low, steady state of estrogen and in this sense more closely mimic production by the ovaries. Most available patches are overdosed, however, leading to weight gain, extra body fat, water retention, and other signs of estrogen dominance. The producers of these patches do not use saliva tests but instead increase the estrogen dose until it appears in the serum tests. Some of the more recent patches are made like a honeycomb and can be cut into pieces and used as smaller doses. In addition, many women discontinue the patch because of skin irritation caused by the adhesive in the patch.

There are also estrogen creams available, which work well, but like the patches are given in excessive doses. Here, again, saliva testing helps restore proper dosages.

Guidelines for Specific Premenopause Problems

For women with PMS. PMS usually involves stress and higher levels of the hormone *cortisol*. Excessive cortisol not only reduces progesterone production but also competes with progesterone for common receptors, so you may need a higher progesterone dose than usual. For the first month or two, it is common to use up a full 2 ounces from day 10 to 12 to day 26 to 30. Women treating PMS can try using the cream in a crescendo pattern, with small dabs at night starting on day 10 to 12 and gradually increasing to two dabs per day morning and night. Finish off the last three or four days with bigger dabs, or by applying the cream three times a day. When symptoms subside, the dose may be reduced to find the lowest effective dose. Since PMS is a syndrome with multiple causative factors, it is wise to seek guidance in matters of stress management, diet, and other nutritional advice.

For women with menstrual migraine.   Use natural progesterone during the 10 days before your period (day 16 to 26). My
patients who feel the characteristic "aura" that usually precedes
migraines apply ¼ teaspoon of cream every three to four hours,
until their symptoms cease (usually this happens in only one or
two applications). You can also apply the cream directly to your
neck or your temples.

Guidelines for Women Who Have Had a Hysterectomy or Ovariectomy

Complete hysterectomy, a term some doctors use inappropriately to mean removal of both the uterus and the ovaries, is also
known as "surgical menopause," and its abruptness is hard on
the body. If you have had your ovaries surgically removed, all the
ovarian hormones are lost. Hormone replacement in these circumstances should include low-dose estrogen and natural progesterone cream in normal physiological doses for 24 to 26 days
of the calendar month. Many women, after removal of their
ovaries, also have testosterone deficiency, causing low energy
levels, depression, and lack of libido. The best way to confirm
the diagnosis is by measuring "free" testosterone levels (as in
saliva hormone assay), and not by regular blood tests. If present,
testosterone deficiency can be effectively treated by transdermal
testosterone in doses as low as 0.15 mg/day. (See Chapter 20 for
details on supplemental testosterone.)

Restoring hormone balance in castrated (ovaries removed)
women requires attention to all three of the sex hormones. If
only the uterus was removed (hysterectomy), progesterone levels fall in one to two months, and estrogen levels fall in one or
two years, as in normal menopause. Because hysterectomy seriously reduces the blood supply to the ovaries, hormone balancing is a bit more complex than with ordinary menopause.
Attention must be paid to estrogen, progesterone, and testosterone as in the hormone loss from ovary removal (oophorectomy). As stated before, under no circumstances should
estrogen be given without progesterone.

Will Progesterone Cream Raise the Levels of My Other Hormones?

This has been extensively tested by Dr. David Zava of ZRT Lab using saliva hormone level tests and the answer is no, progesterone cream does not raise the levels of other hormones. The body does use endogenous (made in the body) progesterone to create other hormones, but this does not occur with supplemental progesterone. The use of supplemental progesterone in someone who is deficient will keep estrogen receptors working efficiently, and it will improve thyroid function.

Can I Use Natural Progesterone if I'm Taking Birth Control Pills?

The honest answer to the above question is that I just don't know for sure. I suspect that the more potent progestins in the birth control pills will block progesterone from its receptors, but progesterone has many effects in different parts of the body, so it could have some benefit anyway. On the other hand, it isn't clear whether or not progesterone will interfere with the action of oral contraceptives. I suspect it won't, but don't know for sure. More research is needed to study this question.

If I'm Menopausal and Take Progesterone, Will My Periods Start Again?

Not usually. The buildup of blood in the uterus is strictly a function of estrogen. At menopause, production of estrogen does not fall to zero; it falls to a level just below that needed for monthly periods. It is likely, however, that progesterone production is very close to zero. Without progesterone, estrogen receptors are less sensitive. When progesterone is resumed, estrogen receptors become more sensitive, that is, more likely to respond to estrogen. Thus some women may notice that after a week or two of progesterone some vaginal bleeding may occur due to their own estrogen. At that point, a woman may stop the progesterone for a week and then start up again for three weeks, as she would if she were still menstruating. The cycle should be three weeks on progesterone and one week off. During the week off progesterone, there may be some bleeding. This is due to the persistence of estrogen production, which will diminish over time. This is the advantage of stopping progesterone for one week each month: It allows the estrogen-induced blood buildup to be shed if it's there.

Later, when no monthly bleeding occurs, the progesterone can be continued on a calendar basis: 24 days of progesterone, then stopping for the remainder of the month. In cases of persistent spotting or vaginal bleeding, consult your physician.

Where to Find Natural Progesterone

At this time, natural progesterone cream is available over the counter and by prescription at compounding pharmacies. You can usually find it in health food stores, and it's easy to find on the Internet. Be sure that you're getting the real thing. If the label says "wild yam extract," don't buy the product without calling or e-mailing the company and confirming that it contains the necessary amount of progesterone and not diosgenin or dioscorea, which are precursors of progesterone in the laboratory, but do *not* "convert" to progesterone in the body.

Your doctor can order a progesterone cream from a compounding pharmacist, but be careful of the 10 percent creams that contain very high amounts of progesterone. Taking a higher-than-recommended dose does not contribute to hormone balance. I recommend a 1.6 percent cream by weight, with about 450 to 500 mg of progesterone per ounce. In ¼ teaspoon of cream this amounts to about 15 to 20 mg of progesterone.

Many natural progesterone creams contain ingredients other than progesterone that may be active, including "wild yam extract," which is usually diosgenin, as well as a variety of herbs and aromatic oils. We do not know which are active and which aren't, or what biochemical effects these ingredients may or may not have, nor do we know what effect they may have when used by women who are pregnant or nursing. In an extensive screening of hundreds of herbs traditionally used for hormonal imbalances, Dr. David Zava has yet to identify one that has activity similar to natural progesterone. For this reason, we feel that progesterone creams containing herbs should be avoided by women who are trying to get pregnant, who are pregnant, or who are nursing. Women who make this choice are advised to use one of the creams that contain only progesterone as the active ingredient. (This is not to say that the other ingredients aren't helpful for women with hormone imbalances—we suspect they probably *are*.)

Some herbs have traditionally been used to stop pregnancy (abortifacients), to induce menstrual periods (emmenagogue), or to induce labor. In his research, Dr. Zava has found that these herbs interact with progesterone receptors but do not activate the receptor in the same manner as natural progesterone. In fact, many behave more like an anti-progesterone, which is consistent with their use.

If a progesterone cream feels grainy or sandy, that probably means the progesterone has precipitated out, and you should return or exchange it. Do not use creams that contain DHEA or any other hormone besides progesterone.

In the Resources section at the back of this book you'll find a list of progesterone creams that contain my recommended dose of progesterone. The manufacturers have not paid to be on this list; it is offered as a service to my readers. There are plenty of perfectly good progesterone creams that aren't on this list, many of them private-label versions of these creams. Because of space limitations it was impossible to list them all. Neither author of this book sells progesterone cream or makes any money from the sale of any progesterone cream.

A Final Reminder

This chapter has covered a lot of ground concerning the use of natural progesterone. I have explained why transdermal progesterone is the preferred delivery system. Oral dosing is inefficient and results in excessive progesterone waste products. The advantages of transdermal application are a more gradual absorbtion and the avoidance of first-pass loss through the liver. Sublingual drops are absorbed very quickly and also excreted more quickly than transdermal cream application. I have also explained why saliva hormone testing is superior to the usual blood tests. It is important to think in terms of physiological dosing, rather than pharmacological dosing, and the knowledge of "free" hormone status is the key. Keep in mind that individuals differ; we are not all stamped out of the same cookie cutter. Individualization in hormone balancing is a necessity. Knowing how things work is a great advantage in getting them right.

CHAPTER 20

HOW TO USE ESTROGEN, DHEA, PREGNENOLONE, THE CORTICOSTEROIDS, TESTOSTERONE, AND ANDROSTENEDIONE

If you are truly deficient in a steroid hormone it's probably a good idea to supplement it, but never to the point where you then create an excess. Always remember when supplementing steroid hormones: Optimal balance means minimal risk and side effects. This means having a saliva hormone level test when you begin supplementing. If your symptoms resolve, your hormone levels are probably fine; if not, you may want to have another test six months after supplementing to see what's still out of balance. If you are at risk for breast cancer or a recurrence of the disease, I recommend that you not use supplemental hormones, except for progesterone, unless your hormone levels are well below normal. Even then, if you know you're not going to carefully track your hormone levels for as long as you're taking supplemental hormones, then *don't* do it.

If you have had a "complete" hysterectomy, are plagued by hot flashes and night sweats, or have no libido at all, or are losing bone mass, even when using progesterone cream, supplemental estrogen and/or testosterone is a consideration. It's important to have a saliva hormone level test first, to make sure that the symptoms you're experiencing are truly a hormone deficiency and/or imbalance. For example, if you've had breast cancer, your low libido might have as much to do with emotional trauma as with low testosterone, and you do not want to add testosterone to your body unless you truly need it.

Estrogen

About a third, or 35 percent, of postmenopausal women (usually those with less body fat) may benefit from low-dose estrogen supplementation. HRT doses of estrogen are typically greater than a postmenopausal woman needs. Overdoses of estrogen prescribed to postmenopausal women are a large factor in causing many of the illnesses they experience.

As Dr. Cummings et al. found in 1998 in an article published in the *New England Journal of Medicine*, when measuring estradiol levels in postmenopausal women aged 65 to 80, only one-third of them were actually deficient in estrogen. It was also found that conventional ERT or HRT estrogen doses were 8 to 10 times higher than needed. In a recent report from *Lancet*, for example, the dose of estradiol for optimal bone effect in women with osteoporosis was 0.25 mg per day rather than the 1 to 2 mg usually given. Keep in the mind the fact that progesterone won't work without at least a little bit of estrogen to prime its receptors.

After a "total" hysterectomy (ovaries also removed), the problem is a bit different. With the ovaries removed, all the ovarian hormones are removed. Commonly, physicians prescribe only estrogen. This is an error; these women certainly need progesterone, not only for its own benefits, but also to balance supplemental estrogen. *No one should be taking unopposed estrogen without progesterone.*

If you are so inclined, you can try using some of the more gentle phytoestrogens first, such as eating some soy (see page 344 on soy for details), or red clover extract, and see if those help relieve your symptoms. If you aren't at risk for breast cancer, then it's fine to use appropriate amounts of estrogen *if you need it.*

Natural estrogens (for humans) are estrone, estradiol, and estriol. All of the available evidence we have so far indicates that estriol is safe to use to control menopausal symptoms and that it may even be protective against breast cancer. The research is divided on whether estriol builds bone, but indications are that it does have at least some bone-building properties. If you are experiencing vaginal dryness, night sweats, or hot flashes, you may want to try some supplemental estriol, which is available by prescription from a compounding pharmacist.

We can't emphasize strongly enough that no woman, with or without a uterus or ovaries, should ever take estrogen of any kind alone. It should *always* be combined with natural progesterone.

The dosage of estrogen to use can vary a great deal from woman to woman, and its effect is variable depending on whether you're using oral doses or creams. Since estrogen is a prescription-only hormone, I recommend that you work with your doctor to find the lowest dose that will alleviate your symptoms and that you use regular saliva hormone level tests to track your estradiol and estrone levels.

DHEA

When people with low levels are given DHEA they tend to experience a boost in energy, immune function, ability to adapt to stress, feelings of well-being, and sex drive. DHEA can have masculinizing effects on women, and in excess it can have the opposite effect of the low dosages, increasing your risk of diabetes and heart disease. This is more true of women than men. If you start to see changes like acne, hair loss, or the growth of facial hair, stop taking it or reduce your dose. These side effects are reversible with discontinuation of DHEA.

Supplemental DHEA can convert to estrogen and theoretically could increase estrogen levels more than you would want. Recent research even shows that DHEA itself has a stimulatory effect on breast cells, particularly when estrogen is low. However, other studies have shown an association between low DHEA-S levels and metastatic breast cancer, but epidemiological studies haven't found an association between DHEA levels and breast cancer.

Thus, if your DHEA levels are *low* (the normal range for middle-aged women is quite broad), taking enough to restore mid-normal levels may be beneficial, but keep in mind that an excess of DHEA could be harmful. If you decide to use it, keep a close watch on your overall hormone balance levels, testing every six months or so.

The recommended dose of DHEA for women is 5 to 10 mg a day. If you have your DHEA levels checked with a blood test, remember that DHEA-S is the relatively inactive form. Saliva DHEA testing is a more accurate measurement of the active DHEA in the blood.

Pregnenolone

Pregnenolone is made from cholesterol by mitochondria and is the compound within cells from which DHEA, progesterone, estrogens, cortisol, and testosterone are created. It would seem that taking large doses of pregnenolone would be a good way to reach hormone balance, giving the body what it needs to make its other steroid hormones. Unfortunately, it doesn't necessarily work that way. Pregnenolone is an intermediary in the biosynthesis of other steroid hormones. If the ovaries or testes have lost the ability to create these other steroid hormones, the presence of pregnenolone will not change that situation. In other words, if your ovaries are functioning properly, supplemental pregnenolone may be turned into other steroid hormones. If your ovaries are malfunctioning, they may not be able to use pregnenolone to make other hormones—pregnenolone is not a reliable way to supplement hormones.

Pregnenolone does appear to have some benefit on rheumatoid arthritis symptoms. Those who have this autoimmune disease may want to try 10 to 50 mg three times daily. Give it at least a month to work. Some clinicians use doses of 100 to 200 mg daily, but please use these amounts only under the supervision of a health care professional who will monitor your health.

Researchers have recently discovered that pregnenolone blocks receptors for the neurotransmitter GABA (gamma-aminobutyric acid). High GABA levels can have the effect of blocking memory and pregnenolone seems to offset that effect. It also increases brain cell activity. Those who have problems learning or remembering may benefit from 50 to 100 mg of pregnenolone between meals, but again, at these doses please work in partnership with a health care professional and monitor your hormone levels.

The Corticosteroids

Corticosteroids are made by the adrenal cortex in response to long-term stress. They include cortisol, which is a gluco-corticoid that regulates immune response, opposes insulin, and stimulates conversion of proteins to glucose in the liver (gluco-neogenesis). Other corticosteroids such as corticosterone help regulate mineral balance. Aldosterone is the most potent of these, acting on the renal tubule (kidney) to promote retention of sodium and the increased excretion of potassium. You might also see these hormones referred to as *cortisones*, which has become a generic term for adrenal cortex hormones. These hormones respond to any stressors that increase energy require-ments. Fasting, infection, intense exercise, pain, or emotional stress stimulate the secretion of a releasing hormone from the hypothalamus in the brain, which tells the adrenals to secrete extra cortisol. There's also a regular daily cycle of cortisol release into the bloodstream, with peaks in the morning and late after-noon and lows in midafternoon and during deep sleep.

Cortisol is extremely important to survival when stress of any sort is present. If an animal can be made stress-free, the lack of cortisol is not life-threatening. But without the corticosteroids, we couldn't survive even the slightest stress. People who have had their adrenal glands removed or whose adrenals don't make enough cortisol are in danger of death from even mild illness. These people must use cortisol replacement for the rest of their lives, increasing their dose at any sign of extra stress or infection.

Excessive cortisol, on the other hand, creates a broad range of undesirable side effects including truncal obesity, elevated blood glucose, hypertension, "moon" face, fatty accumulation called a "buffalo hump" behind the neck and upper thorax, osteoporosis, easy bruising, a susceptibility to fungal infections, and disorders of the immune system. If produced by excessive stimulation by pituitary hormones, the resulting disease is called Cushing's disease. If resulting from excessive adrenal production independent of pituitary control, the disease is called Cushing's syndrome.

Chronic stress leads to chronic high levels of cortisol in the bloodstream, which leads to a greater need for both DHEA and progesterone to maintain balance. In addition to the symptoms of Cushing's disease and syndrome, chronic excessive cortisol is toxic to brain cells in high concentrations and can cause short-term memory loss. A lifetime of high cortisol levels may be a primary cause of Alzheimer's disease and senile dementia. High cortisol is also a primary cause of osteoporosis because it blocks the bone-building effects of progesterone. High cortisol also blocks the action of the steroid hormones and thryoid.

The way this hormone is used in conventional medicine is another good example of the dramatic difference between physiologic and pharmacologic dosing with hormones. People who take powerful synthetic cortisone drugs like prednisone, prednisolone, and dexamethasone for their anti-inflammatory effects suffer side effects like swelling of the face, acne, unwanted hair growth on the face and body, lowered resistance to infection, weight gain around the midriff, menstrual irregularities, and psychological problems ranging from depression to anxiety to outright psychosis. With long-term use, these medications cause adrenal cortisol production to shut down completely, so that stopping the drug can cause fatal complications.

In contrast, natural hydrocortisone or cortisone acetate, used in small doses several times a day, has very little incidence of side effects, and it has been used successfully to treat symptoms of adrenal insufficiency. Supplementing natural hydrocortisone or cortisone acetate in doses of 2.5 to 5 mg two to four times daily can be a safe and effective way to replenish depleted adrenals.

(Too much taken later in the day can cause insomnia, so adjust your dosage accordingly, or don't take it later in the day.) Proper use of natural cortisols can correct problems as diverse as asthma, rheumatoid arthritis, and chronic fatigue. However, it's very important to combine the cortisone supplementation with lots of rest, good nutrition, and hormone balance, with the goal of healing the adrenal glands and not having to use it every day long-term. Once you have brought your body back into balance you can use it occasionally as needed, which you'll know by your symptoms.

I suggest that you use natural cortisone supplementation with the guidance of a health professional, because even natural cortisone isn't safe if you take too much, and it's a delicate balance to maintain. If you take it when you don't really need it, it can cause problems. If your doctor doesn't know about William McK. Jefferies' groundbreaking book, *Safe Uses of Cortisol* (Charles C Thomas, Springfield, Illinois, 1998), inform him or her that it contains all the necessary information on how and when to prescribe physiologic amounts of natural cortisone.

If you don't have the symptoms of cortisol deficiency but are living an extremely hectic life, working and playing too hard and not taking time to get enough sleep and to relax, you're probably making too much cortisol. Even if your adrenals can sustain that kind of energy without ever running down, you're still at risk from chronically high cortisol levels. Optimal health is achieved with a balance of activity and rest.

Testosterone

If you have used progesterone cream for at least six months and still have a low libido, check your testosterone and DHEA levels to see whether the problem could be due to low androgens. You should first check your androgen levels to make sure the low libido is caused by low androgens, because this problem is often caused by other hormonal imbalances such as low thyroid or high stress hormones like cortisol. In testing saliva, Dr. David Zava has seen many cases where women had perfectly normal and sometimes high androgen levels and low libido. These women usually had other problems such as high stress and symptoms of low thyroid caused by estrogen dominance. Excessive estrogen or excessive natural progesterone replacement therapy can also suppress libido, so if you are taking these hormones check the levels of estradiol and progesterone to make sure you are not using too much.

Testosterone deficiency can cause loss of energy, depression, memory lapses, vaginal dryness, incontinence, and loss of libido. Similar symptoms to those listed above for testosterone deficiency can also be caused by adrenal exhaustion or thyroid deficiency. These, too, should be sorted out by a physician.

Dr. David Zava has found with saliva testing that the majority of women who have had a total hysterectomy suffer from low androgens (testosterone, DHEA-S, and androstenedione). A recent study found that women after "complete" hysterectomy (i.e., ovaries removed) often suffer low energy, depression, and lack of libido. Testing "free" testosterone (not the usual serum testing) showed that these women were testosterone deficient. Transdermal testosterone, in doses of 0.15 mg/day, raised their "free" testosterone levels fivefold and effectively relieved their symptoms. Clinicians report that they successfully use doses of 0.15 to 1 mg per day, with the average dose for a menopausal woman being 0.5 mg daily.

Testosterone is available in the form of cream, sublingual drops, oral tablets, and transdermal patch. A compounding pharmacist can make up testosterone creams and sublingual drops. In questioning practicing clinicians who use supplemental testosterone, I have found that combining testosterone and progesterone into one cream is not recommended. It's so easy for women to get too much testosterone that they need to be able to adjust their dosage if they notice symptoms of excess.

Testosterone is available only by prescription. If you're interested, talk with your physician. Be sure to use only a natural form, as synthetics like methyltestosterone are powerful and can have unpleasant side effects.

Androstenedione

This steroid hormone is a precursor to testosterone and estrogens, and it can theoretically act as a DHEA precursor. Secreted from the adrenals and the ovaries into the circulation, it has its own jobs to do before being converted into other hormones in the liver. In older women it travels from the ovaries to the fat cells, where it is converted to estrogen.

Androstenedione is a popular supplement for bodybuilders, who use it to boost their testosterone levels, increase muscle mass, and decrease the length of time needed to recover from hard workouts. Many of the positive effects of supplemental testosterone—including enhanced energy, libido, and sense of well-being—have also been attributed to androstenedione.

Androstenedione may also be involved in maintaining the strength of bones. It's converted to estradiol in the bones themselves, and estradiol helps slow bone loss.

There should be no reason for a menopausal woman to use androstenedione.

CHAPTER 21

NUTRITION FOR
HEALTHY HORMONES

This chapter includes a synopsis of how to bring your hormones back into balance with the help of lifestyle changes, particularly good nutrition. As I mentioned in the Introduction, I don't want you to think of progesterone as a magic bullet or a magic pill. Just taking the simple steps in this chapter to change your diet and lifestyle may very well be enough to bring your hormones back into balance. When we provide an optimum environment, our bodies are remarkably resilient and capable of healing themselves and restoring balance.

Menopause and premenopause are not diseases. They are natural transitions that need no treatment. If undesirable symptoms accompany these normal biological processes it means that something has gone awry in some women. These symptoms are usually caused by a less-than-optimum environment leading to stresses that alter normal metabolic processes, as in situational stress, nutrition, and so forth. My goal in this chapter is to show you how to create the healthiest possible nutritional environment for yourself. And I want you to know that, regardless of what your lifestyle has been in the past, it is *never* too late to get healthier. Every small step you take toward improving your health will make a big difference.

If you've spent decades eating refined and processed foods, avoiding exercise, and being exposed to xenoestrogens, taking these steps toward hormone balance may seem challenging at first. Changing habits is not always easy, and many of the processed foods are comfort foods we eat when we're upset or need to nurture ourselves. This holds especially true for chips, candy, cookies, ice cream, and baked goods. If you know what your comfort foods are, please don't try to eliminate them suddenly and completely from your diet. That's too harsh a step for most of us. If we are eating certain foods to nurture ourselves, then suddenly yank them away, all those parts inside we're trying to nurture are going to rebel. And you know what that means—obsessing about the food, bingeing, and guilt. That's as unhealthy as just continuing to eat the food.

Instead, gradually cut down on the amount you eat. Eat two cookies instead of ten. Eat ¼ of a bag of chips instead of the whole bag. Eat a Hershey's kiss instead of a Hershey's bar. Begin to think of these foods as occasional treats rather than daily sustenance while you find healthier ways to nurture yourself. As your hormones begin to come back into balance and your blood sugar begins to stabilize, you'll find you have much less craving for sweet and salty junk food.

Do I need to tell anyone that they should quit smoking? Just in case, if you're smoking, quit. Now.

I have nothing against alcohol consumption, but I recommend you limit it to no more than two drinks a day. More than that will take a toll on your liver, deplete you of nutrients, and put you at a higher risk for cancer.

Refined Carbohydrates

An inseparable connection between fat and estrogen exists because fat cells are estrogen factories. Women become caught in a cycle where increased body fat raises estrogen levels, and estrogen increases the tendency to accumulate body fat. It was once thought that the Western diet caused weight gain because of its high fat content, but today we know better. The evidence is everywhere: How many people do you know who jumped on the low-fat-diet bandwagon, increased their consumption of low-fat carbohydrate-rich foods, and ended up heavier than they were to begin with? And how many people do you know who *lost* weight on a high-protein and -fat diet such as the one developed by the late Robert Atkins, M.D.?

Dietary fat doesn't necessarily make you fat. In fact, the huge quantities of sugars and refined carbohydrates (breads, pastries, cookies, pastas, bagels) eaten by the typical Westerner have made a far more significant contribution to the expansion of American girths. The elimination of fats from the diet in the attempt to lose weight and improve health made way not for more vegetables and fruits, but for packaged, processed low-fat/high carbohydrate products with lots of calories and little to no nutritive value.

An intracellular insulin-like growth factor called IGF-1, if excessive, can interact with estrogen and increase the risk of greater human breast cancer cell replication rates. The levels of IGF-1 in a woman's body increase with insulin resistance, which is correlated with increased refined carbohydrate intake and body fat. A high-refined-carbohydrate diet sets the body up for weight gain and an increased estrogen burden more than does a diet with balanced amounts of fats from olive oil and whole foods.

Excess Calories, Not Just Excess Fat

The Western diet is relatively high in calories compared to energy needs. Almost every person in the Western world consumes more calories than he or she needs for fuel on a daily basis. The Third World diet is relatively high in fiber and is largely plant-based, calorie intake is considerably lower, and exercise levels are considerably higher.

It is now clear that calories in excess of energy needs are stored as fat, which increases estrogen levels. When energy needs exceed calorie intake, total body fat and estrogen decline. When calorie intake exceeds energy needs, estrogen rises accordingly. This is one of nature's way of reducing fertility during times when food is scarce and increasing fertility when food is abundant. Dr. Peter Ellison of Harvard, who has conducted worldwide assays of salivary hormone levels, believes that excessive caloric intake is the primary reason for the higher estrogen levels seen in premenopausal women in industrialized cultures.

One major source of excess calories in Western diets is refined carbohydrates from such foods as breads, cakes, muffins, bagels, pancakes, and waffles, as well as most cereals and most American pasta—also candy, cookies, pretzels, and sodas and other sweetened drinks. These foods are bad news—not only because they supply plentiful calories without any real nutritive value, but also because they keep blood sugars and insulin levels soaring and then dropping like a roller coaster, and predispose people to adult-onset diabetes. Recent research has shown that insulin resistance, a prediabetic condition caused primarily by excessive consumption of calories and a sedentary lifestyle, increases breast cancer risk and that obesity is a major risk factor for nearly all cancers.

Good Fats and Bad Fats

You need fat in your diet to build and maintain many parts of your body, including cell membranes, cholesterol, steroid hormones, and *prostaglandins*. Prostaglandins are a class of hormones produced within cells throughout the body. They affect a variety of bodily processes, including blood pressure, inflammation, and immune function. Some prostaglandins promote inflammation whereas others inhibit it. However, the prostaglandins that promote inflammation are not necessarily "bad"; your body needs all types of these hormones to function properly. What will cause problems is too much of any one type of prostaglandin. A healthy balance is a key to a healthy body.

The manufacture of prostaglandins is largely driven by the fats and oils we eat. Therefore, it is important to eat the fats that keep our prostaglandins in proper balance. Eating too much red meat, for instance, tends to increase the prostaglandins that are pro-inflammatory, which means that they increase vasoconstriction (blood vessels narrow), platelet aggregation (sticky blood), and cellular proliferation, and suppresses the immune system, thus increasing blood clotting and the risk of stroke. Vegetable and fish oils in the right amounts (e.g., not in excess) tend to be anti-inflammatory, meaning that they create vasodilation (open

the blood vessels), inhibit platelet aggregation, control cell proliferation, and enhance the immune system.

Prostaglandins are yet another example of how the body's systems work to maintain a dynamic balance for good health. Although the entire subject of fats and prostaglandin balance is
quite complex, a major lesson to learn is that fresh, unprocessed
natural fats common to human consumption for the past thousands of years are, in general, much more wholesome and
healthy than are synthetic trans-fatty acids, such as those found
in processed seed oils and deep fat–fried foods so common these
days. I recommend Dr. Mary Enig's book, *Know Your Fats*
(Bethesda Press, 2000), and Andrew Stoll M.D.'s *The Omega-3
Connection* (Simon & Schuster, 2001) if you're looking for scientifically sound and detailed information on this topic. Suffice
it to say that the categories of saturated, mono- or polyunsaturated fats are less important to your health than the distinction
between natural fats and synthetic trans-fatty acids. Learn to
avoid trans-fatty acids, which most often show up on food labels
as hydrogenated or partially hydrogenated oils.

Women who eat more of their fat as olive oil (which is extracted from the olive without high pressure or high temperature) appear to enjoy decreased breast cancer risk compared with
women who eat more of the trans-fats. Test tube and animal
studies show that this could be explained by the effects of these
fats on breast prostaglandin levels. Prostaglandin E2, for example, which is increased by eating excessive quantities of red meat,
increases the activity of aromatase, an enzyme that converts
other steroids into estrogen in breast cells. Studies on rats show
that the omega-6 fats found in unsaturated oils such as corn and
safflower can accelerate the promotion phase of breast cancer by
enhancing the formation of pro-inflammatory prostaglandins,
which may increase free-radical–mediated DNA damage and
stimulate cell proliferation and higher free estrogen levels. In
contrast, the omega-3s seem to promote anti-inflammatory
prostaglandins that inhibit cell proliferation.

This doesn't mean you should entirely give up red meat or
corn oil, it means that you should eat these types of foods in bal-

ance with a wide variety of other wholesome foods. Let's examine what this means more closely.

Here's a general rule of thumb: The good fats are part of whole foods. That means fish, vegetables, nuts and seeds, free-range eggs, whole grains, and legumes. It does not mean that highly processed seed oils are good for you. The processing converts their natural fats into trans-fats for longer shelf life.

Olive oil and modest amounts of butter for cooking and baking are part of a health-supporting diet. Wherever you can, substitute olive oil for other oils that require heavy processing. Look for dark green extra virgin olive oils. They're expensive, but there's nothing better for you to spend your money on than a health-promoting diet. And it tastes so good you'll only need to use a small amount. Avocado oil is another monounsaturated fat that's rich in healthy essential fatty acids (EFAs).

Canola oil is also monounsaturated, but it's highly processed for commercial uses and therefore less desirable because of its content of trans-fats. It's best to use canola oil only very occasionally. If you love potato chips and corn chips and insist on having them, chips fried in canola oil are probably safer that chips fried in highly processed polyunsaturated oils like safflower, corn, sunflower, nut, or seed oils. Polyunsaturated oils are most likely rancid by the time you open the bottle to use them, so you can imagine how far gone they are when they've been sitting on the store shelf for a while, or when they've been heated to high temperatures and used for frying. It's best to completely avoid polyunsaturated or hydrogenated oils made from soy, corn, nuts, and seeds.

Saturated fats such as butter, coconut oil, and lard are solid at room temperature and are very stable. You can leave them sitting out and not worry that they'll spoil, and you can heat them up without creating free radicals. Unrefined coconut oil and butter are best for baking. Again, remember that these fats have gotten a bad name, but only because they've been eaten in excess; in moderate amounts they are beneficial to your health.

Hydrogenated oils are the trans-fatty acids used to make everything from margarines to baked goods to potato chips to frozen desserts, and are now being linked to increased risk of artery disease. It seems that hydrogenated fats directly damage the delicate linings of blood vessels. They also throw off your hormone balance by blocking the actions of "good" fats.

Omega-3 fats are found most abundantly in deep-water fish such as mackerel, herring, sardines, and cod. However, the FDA has recently warned pregnant women away from eating mackerel due to high mercury content, so you can leave that one off the list. Albacore tuna is also a good source, but it, too, can accumulate mercury, although less than mackerel; just be moderate about how often you eat it. Wild pacific salmon is also a good source of omega-3 fats, and if it's fresh it has a very mild flavor that even kids usually don't mind. Try to have omega-3 rich fish two or three times a week.

Green leafy vegetables and walnuts also contain omega-3s.

Flaxseeds are especially rich in omega-3 fats. Flaxseed oil, however, spoils (becomes oxidized or rancid) easily; in fact it is one of the most unstable oils known. It is better to buy whole flaxseeds and grind them at home (with a small coffee grinder) to sprinkle on cereal or salads. Although the omega-3s are beneficial oils, you don't need them in large amounts. For example, I use three heaping teaspoons of flax seeds every few days, added to some whole grain cereal (like old-fashioned oatmeal), or taken with orange juice. That is a very modest amount of omega-3 oils.

Vegetable oils contain omega-6 fatty acids, which are beneficial for you in small amounts. They go rancid easily and thus are best added to the diet by eating plenty of fresh vegetables.

Whole Foods Are Best

Of course, there's more to eating well than the types of fat you eat. Some popular diet books emphasize protein and carbohydrate intake; some focus on specific "superfoods" purported to have miraculous effects on health; some focus on nutritional supplements or vitamins, minerals, and other nutrients from healthy foods. With all of the dietary advice that's available today, making the right choices can seem downright confusing.

If I had to choose one single piece of advice to give you that would most improve your health, it would be to learn to eat modest amounts of fresh, whole, organic, unprocessed foods. They contain vitamins, minerals, and other nutrients you need, in abundance. They contain fiber, which is very important for proper digestion of food and intestinal transit, and for hormone balance.

What does eating whole foods mean? It means eating whole grains such as brown rice, bulghur, millet and quinoa, and amaranth (really a seed), which are tasty and can be used by themselves or in casseroles. Look at the labels on store bread. It may be advertised as whole wheat or whole rye, but the contents listed usually refer to flour made from these grains. Flour means the outer fibrous, mineral-rich coat has been removed and the "germ" of the grain with its fat-soluble vitamins has also been removed. Become a smart shopper. What you're looking for is "whole grain" flour. If your store does not sell good bread, ask the store manager to order some.

Eating whole foods means eating beans, including traditionally prepared soybean products such as tofu, tempeh, and miso. Beans won't cause gas in most people if they are introduced gradually into the diet. It is also helpful if they are soaked overnight and the soaking water discarded. You can also use a product called Beano, which contains the enzyme necessary to digest beans, until your own body learns to make the enzymes. You just put a few drops of it onto the beans before you eat them. Most health food stores and pharmacies carry Beano.

Eating whole, unprocessed foods means emphasizing fresh vegetables. Vegetables contain dozens of natural cancer-fighting compounds (*phytochemicals*) that inhibit cancer initiation and promotion. The awful habit of boiling vegetables until they're mushy and tasteless has given them a bad name. Canning is equally hard on taste. Freezing is somewhat better, but you still lose important enzymes and vitamins when you freeze foods. Fresh vegetables are delicious raw or lightly steamed. Fresh root vegetables such as beets, carrots, turnips, onions, garlic, and potatoes are wonderful baked with some olive oil and fresh herbs. Experiment with some of the more exotic green leafy vegetables such as kale and bok choy. Broccoli, cauliflower, cabbage, and brussels sprouts—vegetables from the *brassica* (cruciferous) family—are especially potent cancer fighters, as are garlic, onions, and leeks (from the *allium* family). Once you become acquainted with these foods, you will find they are quick and simple to prepare and very tasty.

As I mentioned in the section on fats, fish is a highly nutritious addition to a whole foods diet. An excellent source of protein, fish also contains the omega-3 fatty acids EPA (eicosapentaenoic) and DHA (docosahexaenoic acid), which appear to offer some protection against breast cancer as well as heart disease.

And last but not least, eating whole, unprocessed foods means eating fresh fruit instead of desserts loaded with white sugar, fructose, or corn syrup. Before you balk at the idea of spending money on some expensive grapes or a papaya, stop and think how much you would pay for a pie, cake, or ice cream. If you really have a sweet tooth, try sprinkling apples, pears, or peaches with cinnamon and baking them. Even then, your consumption of fruits shouldn't be overdone. They are primarily sugar, which will adversely affect your blood sugar balance if you eat too much. Remember that dried fruit contains all the sugar of the whole fruit, so be moderate about dried fruit too. If you like fruit juice, invest in a juicer and drink only freshly squeezed vegetable and fruit juices. Pasteurization and storage of packaged juices robs them of nutrients and enzymes.

The obvious opposite of eating whole foods is eating processed foods. I don't advocate becoming extreme, but it's best in general to avoid highly refined carbohydrates such as those containing white flour or sugar, as well as foods that contain additives, preservatives, and colorings. You'll find it's easier to maintain overall balance if you have that ice cream cone or chocolate chip cookie now and then, but eating sugary foods daily will set you up for a long list of health problems. If having an ice cream cone is going to send you off on a binge of eating sugar, don't do it; use your common sense here.

Eat Organic Foods Whenever Possible

Nonorganic farming leaves soil fallow, depleted of the minerals it needs to produce healthy, pest-resistant crops. Whatever plants can be eked out of this used-up soil need plenty of harsh fertilizers, herbicides, and pesticides to survive to market. The hybridization of crops—which is what makes those uniformly large, flawless-looking and tasteless veggies you see in the super-market produce section—means further exhaustion of nutrient content. Fruits and vegetables that are conventionally grown are low in nutrients and are hybridized, sprayed, and fertilized with all manner of poisonous compounds, many of them with estro-genic properties, and they don't taste as good as organically grown produce. The pesticide residues left on that nice red apple may be small, but if you add that to all the other pesticides you're exposed to, the toxic load can be too much.

Organic produce is usually locally grown and fresher than conventional varieties. If you have a farmer's market in your area, take full advantage of it. You can usually find plenty of or-ganic foods at reasonable prices because you're buying them di-rectly from the grower. If you don't have a farmer's market, start one in your area! Or, you can tell the produce manager at your local supermarket that you would like organic produce. Super-markets are springing up all around the country that feature hormone-free meat, whole foods, and organic produce in re-sponse to increased consumer demand for these items. If there's one in your area it will be worth the extra few dollars a week to shop there. Think of it as a long-term investment in your health.

Is Vegetarianism Protective?

Although I can't argue with those who are vegetarian for philo-sophical reasons, being a vegetarian isn't necessarily healthier—for most people. Some vegetarians may be healthier because they eat a lot of vegetables, but many have nutritional deficien-cies caused by a lack of the nutrients supplied by meat and dairy products. In other words, you have to know what you're doing, and eat very carefully, if you're going to be a vegetarian. Eating only carrot sticks and bagels won't contribute to nutritional well-being! None of the large, long-term studies looking at meat consumption and breast cancer have shown an increased risk. Although there are good reasons not to overdo it with meat eating, there's no evidence that eating small portions of meat increases your risk of breast cancer. Poultry and beef are nutritious and satisfying accompaniments to vegetables and whole grains. If you don't go overboard with fast-food burgers or huge steaks, there's no reason you can't enjoy these foods as part of a balanced cancer-preventive diet. Rather than seeing meats as the main course, make vegetables the main course and use meat as a condiment.

Opt for Free-Range Meats, Eggs, and Poultry

Range-raised cattle are naturally lean. The fats found in the meat of a cow that's grazed at open pasture are stable, saturated fats, whereas the meat of cattle raised in factory farms contains a conglomeration of polyunsaturated and saturated fats, chemicals, and hormones. Factory-farmed meat may come from cattle that are fed a mishmash of oils, grains, wastes from chemically fertilized crops, old newspapers urinated on by other cattle, and even unsaleable parts of their slaughtered brethren. If you are what you eat, you're also what whatever you eat eats.

Many beef cattle are routinely injected with estrogen pellets to fatten them up for market. This estrogen is still in the meat when it gets to your table. Meat and eggs from conventionally raised chickens contain the antibiotics and petrochemical xenobiotics (e.g., pesticides) they are fed. Many of these toxins are concentrated in the fatty tissues of animal products, which means you're getting a far more potent dose with these foods than with vegetables.

The bottom line here is that you and your family are much better off eating organic meats and eggs. If you're on a tight budget and can afford to buy only some of your foods as organics, these are the ones you should choose. Look for free-range, hormone-free eggs, meats, and chicken.

Cooking methods also make a difference when it comes to meats. Broiling meats in high heat yields substances that are known to initiate cancerous changes in cells. Baking and stir-frying are better alternatives than grilling or broiling over open flames.

Are Dairy Foods Right for You?

Most cultures in the world are allergic to cow's milk and, after puberty, lack the enzymes to digest its lactose. Some northern European cultures can tolerate milk to some degree, but for the most part, there is no good reason I can find for milk to be a staple of anybody's diet. Centuries ago, Eastern Mediterranean people learned to add a bacterial culture to milk to digest the lactose and convert it into lactic acid, the process that produces a rather sour flavor in the product we call yogurt. The bacterial culture may include *lactobacillus acidophilus* or *bulgaricus*, or others with lactose-fermenting powers. This makes the milk less likely to cause gas and indigestion from one's lactose deficiency, but it does not make the product any healthier. Cheese, another milk fermentation product, is largely protein and not containing lactose. Cheese, perhaps as a result of fermentation that changes milk proteins, is not correlated with the problems brought on by liquid milk such as heart disease, for example. With the strong coronary heart disease record of my family, I gave up drinking milk in 1951, during my first year in medical school, but continued eating cheese. Here I am 52 years later, advising my readers to avoid liquid milk but enjoy the good cheeses made from milk.

Magnesium is necessary to utilize calcium for bone building and milk has a poor calcium-to-magnesium ratio. Without adequate magnesium, the milk-derived calcium tends to form calcium deposits in joints, ligaments, and tendons, rather than in bones. Furthermore, dairy cows are forced to exist in intolerably unhealthy conditions and are loaded up with antibiotics and other drugs to compensate. When you drink milk or eat other dairy products, you are getting dosed with these drugs. The amount in any given glass of milk may be minuscule, but added to other sources the effect can be cumulative.

If you want the complete story on why milk doesn't do a body good, read my book *Optimal Health Guidelines Revised and Updated* (BLL Publishing, 2000).

Eat Your Phytochemicals

Natural Defenses Against Cancer

Phytochemicals are plant compounds, many of which have health-supporting effects on the body. It's estimated that there are more than 10,000 different compounds in the plants we eat. Phytoestrogens are a family of plant phytochemicals that have weak estrogen-like activity. Their chemical structures are very similar to the estrogens produced in the body and because of this chemical mimicry they are able to bind to activate estrogen receptors throughout the body. However, their binding is much weaker than estrogens like estradiol and their effects more subtle. At high levels they actually can displace estradiol from its receptors and in doing so act as weak anti-estrogens. They compete for estrogen receptors throughout the body, helping to block the effects of excess or stronger estrogens. If you eat a variety of fresh vegetables and have fermented soy products a few times a week, you'll reap the benefits of these natural estrogen blockers. Some herbs, like red clover, licorice root, anise, and fennel, contain phytoestrogens, but it's wise to consult with an herbalist or naturopathic doctor before using these plants medicinally over a long period of time.

Be wary of the hype around soy. While it does contain phytoestrogens than can help balance your hormones, it also contains other phytochemicals called *phytates* that block the absorption of needed nutrients such as zinc and iodine, and that disable enzymes your body needs to access other nutrients. Fermentation denatures these substances and thus reduces the nutrient-blocking effect of soy. Asian diets utilize mostly fermented soy products such as miso and tempeh in small amounts, and also adds seaweed, which is rich in minerals.

Eat More Fiber

Fiber is indigestible plant matter that passes all the way through the digestive tract. On its way through it has important "roto rooter" effects and also absorbs waste products in the large intestine. People who eat plenty of fiber-rich food have lower rates of all types of cancer, especially colon cancer. Adding supplemental fiber to an otherwise poor diet does not seem to be effective in preventing or slowing colon cancer—the lesson being: Eat whole foods!

Plant cell walls are our only dietary sources of fiber. Fiber is not just a rough broom that makes bowel movements easier; it also serves as a source of important nutrients for our bodies and for the friendly bacteria that live in our digestive tracts. Cellulose, found in most plant foods, binds water in the digestive tract, which makes for easier and more frequent elimination. Other varieties of fiber form gels within which excess dietary cholesterol is trapped and not absorbed. Mucilages are a type of fiber found in beans and around the moist inner layer of seeds, and they have potent cholesterol-lowering effects. Lignins (very small, indigestible fibers) are broken down into compounds that are protective against cancer.

The best possible way to get fiber into your diet is to eat whole, unprocessed foods. Whole grains, fresh fruits, vegetables, legumes, and nuts have plenty of fiber. If your diet presently consists mostly of processed foods, please introduce the fiber gradually so your digestive system has time to adjust.

Dietary fiber carries excess estrogens out of the body. After estrogens have finished their work in the cells, activating growth and development in tissues such as the breast and uterus, they return to the bloodstream. They are carried in the blood to the liver, where they are metabolized to *inactive estrogen conjugates*. These conjugates are then incorporated into bile that carries them into the gastrointestinal tract. There, microbes convert the inactive estrogen conjugates back into "active" estrogens, which can be reabsorbed into the bloodstream. Fiber absorbs both active and inactive estrogen conjugates in the digestive tract, preventing them from being reabsorbed. Elimination of estrogens in feces helps to decrease the body's estrogen load. Estrogens cause more body fat; body fat is aromatized to more estrogen. When estrogen is dominant, your body cannot burn fat for energy. It is a vicious cycle. By maintaining good fiber intake, you excrete more estrogen, and thereby make less fat. In this manner, women who have a good fiber intake are less likely to become fat or have breast cancer, strokes, or heart attacks.

Most plant-eating animals our size living in the wild would take in 30 to 90 grams of fiber a day. The average human gets only about 10 grams a day. Most omnivorous animals move their bowels more than once a day, after meals. As you follow our other dietary recommendations, you'll take in more fiber. An added bonus: On a high-fiber diet you'll feel satiated with less food than on a low-fiber diet. You'll eat less and probably lose a few pounds.

If you need to add even more fiber to your diet (due to constipation, for example) you can take 1 teaspoon of psyllium seed husk in 8 ounces of water or juice every morning. (You need to stir it vigorously and drink it right away.) The pure psyllium you find at your health food store is the same ingredient found in Metamucil and other similar products, without the sweeteners, preservatives, and food colorings.

Drink Plenty of Clean Water

Water is nature's inner cleanser. All metabolic actions require a water milieu in which to function. Most people in industrialized countries don't drink enough water and are chronically dehydrated. They drink coffee, tea, juice, and soda, but rarely water. Coffee, tea, and soda tend to act as diuretics, causing the body to lose more water, and juice contains a fair amount of sugar, so it's not recommended that you drink it in large quantities. Alcohol dehydrates tissues. Drinking clean water will help your body clear away wastes and toxins that can contribute to the development of cancer. Dehydration can create an imbalance of minerals, which can contribute to hormone imbalance.

In my opinion, most water that comes out of your tap is now polluted beyond the point that it is truly safe to drink, and it generally tastes terrible because of the addition of chlorine. Since you can't always trust commercial bottled water to be clean, the best way to get clean water is to put a filter on your kitchen tap. A simple charcoal filter will *not* do the job. Be sure to get a type that filters out chlorine, heavy metals, benzene, and bacteria. You do not have to go to the expense of getting a reverse osmosis system—a ceramic or copper/zinc filter will do the job and just takes a few minutes to install. Check your Yellow Pages under "water."

Take Your Multivitamins

Our food crops today have half the nutrients of crops grown a century ago, and, even though our consumption of food is greater than our need, we consume less of the nutrients than our ancestors (who spent much of the day at hard physical labor). Factor in the fact that we tend to cook a lot of the nutrients out of our vegetables, add the large amounts of processed food that have replaced whole foods in most diets and generally poor digestion, and you see the dismal picture of the nutritional intake of the average modern American.

Because of these changes in our food supply, many people argue that we should take a good high-potency daily multivitamin. There is, however, little scientific evidence that taking isolated single nutrients, even in combination, is as nutritious as eating a good diet. Think of it as a sort of insurance against nutritional deficiencies.

Most quality multis require you to take three to six tablets or capsules with each meal. If you can't tolerate taking that many pills, at least try to get some supplemental vitamin C and magnesium each day. Men should try to get 15 to 20 mg of zinc and selenium daily for prostate health. If you live in a cloudy climate, some supplemental vitamin D is a good idea. If you're getting chronic infections, take a vitamin A supplement. (Now you're starting to see why it might be good to take a multivitamin.)

Although most multis will contain it, we don't necessarily recommend beta-carotene/carotenoids. Green and yellow vegetables contain 600 different carotenes that work in synergy to create their antioxidant effects. Beta carotene by itself does not have the potent effects of the vegetables.

Choosing a multivitamin can be difficult because there are so many out there, but I'm going to try to make it a little easier by giving you some basic guidelines on which vitamins and minerals should be included. I recommend that you choose a multivitamin that contains the following:

Vitamin A: 5,000 to 10,000 IU

This antioxidant is fat-soluble and reserves can be stored in the liver for long periods. This also means that it can have lasting positive effects. However, it also means that it can build up to toxic levels if more than 10,000 IU is taken daily for a long period of time. Fish and fish liver oils are naturally rich in vitamin A.

B Vitamins

Thiamine (B1): 10 to 25 mg
Riboflavin (B2): 10 to 25 mg
Niacin (B3): 50 to100 mg
Pantothenic acid (B5): 10 to 50 mg
Pyridoxine (B6): 50 mg daily
Vitamin B12: 1,000 to 2,000 mcg (micrograms)
Biotin: 100 to 300 mcg
Choline: 50 to 100 mg

Folic acid/folate/folacin: 400 to 800 mcg
Inositol: 150 to 300 mg

The B vitamins play multiple roles in brain function, the transformation of food into energy within the cells, and neutralizing
of a toxic by-product of protein metabolism called *homocysteine*.
The cardiovascular risk of elevated serum or urinary homocysteine was recognized more than 30 years ago and is finally being
accepted as a very substantial risk factor for heart disease because
it directly damages the walls of blood vessels. Treatment involves
folic acid, B6, and B12.

Pantothenic acid is essential for the healthy functioning of
your adrenal glands, and vitamin B12 is necessary for the proper
absorption of some vitamins. B vitamins are found in whole
grains, fruits, vegetables, and meats. It's best to take the B vitamins together because their effects are synergistic.

Vitamin C: 1,000 to 2,000 mg

This super-antioxidant nutrient has been making news for
decades, since Linus Pauling and Ewan Cameron began researching its amazing immunity-boosting effects. Vitamin C
also helps in the building of collagen, the basic building block
of connective tissue. Without sufficient vitamin C, the result
is scurvy, a debilitating disease of degenerating connective tissue. The chemical name of vitamin C is ascorbic acid, meaning an acid that prevents scurvy. It's water-soluble, so you
eliminate what you don't need. The adrenal glands are dependent on adequate vitamin C; they concentrate vitamin C
over 100-fold. When you're sick or stressed, vitamin C is used
up at a much faster rate. It's a good idea to keep a bottle of vitamin C around so that you can take more when you're coming down with a cold or flu bug, or are under the proverbial
stress gun. One or 2 grams (1,000 to 2,000 mg) a day should
suffice when you're feeling your best. Good food sources include citrus fruits, tomatoes, mangoes, kiwi, paprika, and red

peppers. Remember, heat destroys vitamin C, so you don't get it in cooked foods.

Vitamin D: 300 to 400 IU

We make some vitamin D when we go out into the sunshine, but a little extra is a good idea, especially for women. Vitamin D interacts with calcium and phosphorus to build strong, healthy bones. It's fat-soluble and can build up to toxic levels if doses higher than this one are taken for long. Fish and fish liver oil contain vitamin D.

Vitamin E: 400 to 500 IU

The many roles of this fat-soluble antioxidant are the subject of a great deal of research these days. It stops free radicals from damaging cells and repairs other "spent" antioxidant and B vitamins. It helps prevent the blood from being too sticky, relieves *edema* (accumulation of excess fluid), and strengthens blood vessel walls. Vitamin E is found in the "germ" of all grains and nuts.

Other Antioxidants

Powerful, newly discovered antioxidants are showing promise as cancer preventatives. Especially promising are proanthocyanidins (PCOs) from grapeseed extract; resveratrol from purple grape juice and red wine; bioflavonoids such as quercetin, hesperidin, and rutin; and phytochemicals found in green tea. CoQ-10 (coenzyme Q10) is also a powerful antioxidant that has been shown in some studies to help prevent breast cancer growth.

Minerals

The passage of minerals in and out of cells is a delicately balanced operation, dependent on the health of the membrane around each cell. Too-high levels of estrogen coupled with synthetic progestins actually impair the action of cell membranes, whereas natural progesterone heals cell membranes and allows normal mineral balance to be restored. Make sure that your multivitamin contains optimal amounts of the following minerals:

Boron: 1 to 5 mg

This mineral plays a role in the maintenance of healthy bones.

Calcium: 300 mg

I recommend less calcium than most guides because total daily calcium intake should be around 600 to 800 mg per day, which is easily accomplished by any good diet, even without milk. A cup full of spinach contains 300 mg, and a tablespoon of cheese contains 300 mg, for example.

Calcium is well known for its role as a bone and tooth builder, and that's the role of 99 percent of the calcium in the body. The 1 percent left over is an indispensable player in nerve conduction, muscle contraction, heartbeat and blood pressure regulation, clotting of blood, and functioning of the thyroid gland. Tofu, black-eyed peas, leafy green vegetables, dairy products, and broccoli are good sources of calcium in the diet.

Chromium: 200 to 400 mcg (as chromium picolinate)

This trace mineral helps keep blood sugars steady so you can fight off cravings for sugar and refined flour. It also helps manufacture needed nutrients like cholesterol and fatty acids. It's found naturally in mushrooms, beef, beets, liver, whole wheat, brewer's yeast (used often as a nutritional supplement), and molasses made from beet sugar. Low-fat, processed food diets often result in chromium deficiency.

Copper: 1 to 5 mg

Copper has many roles in the body, including wound healing, transport of oxygen through the blood (it's a component of the body's oxygen-carrying molecule, *hemoglobin*), and maintaining the integrity of nerves, skin, and bones. Seafood, beans, al-

monds, whole grains, and green leafy vegetables are good
sources of this mineral.

Magnesium: 300 to 400 mg

Magnesium is involved in just about every aspect of our physiology. It makes up 0.05 percent of our body weight and is incorporated into bones as well as being distributed throughout
our other tissues. Its action occurs within cells, being the most
common cofactor for intracellular enzymes, usually sharing that
role with vitamin B6. Being an intracellular mineral means that
conventional serum levels of magnesium are totally irrelevant. If
a relevant level is desired, a good alternative is red blood cell
magnesium testing. Calcium and magnesium need each other to
fulfill their roles. Intravenous magnesium has been used to treat
heart arrhythmias, high blood pressure, heart failure, and
asthma with great success. It's also an effective laxative.

Because of soil depletion, our plant food is deficient in magnesium. Most Americans are sorely deficient in magnesium. It's
found in nuts, seeds, figs, corn, apples, milk, soybeans, milk,
and wheat germ. Just as iron is what makes hemoglobin red,
magnesium makes chlorophyll green.

If you have asthma, chronic muscle cramps, or high blood
pressure, or are at high risk of osteoporosis or heart disease, take
300 mg in the morning and evening for a total of 600 mg daily.
Reduce the dose if it causes diarrhea.

Manganese: 10 mg

The B vitamins and vitamin C need manganese to do their jobs.
This mineral also helps the thyroid gland and ovaries make their
hormones, and participates in the synthesis of carbohydrates,
fatty acids, cholesterol, and protein. It's an important one for
hormone balance as well as for prevention of heart disease and
diabetes. Egg yolks, green veggies, seeds, whole grains, and nuts
contain generous amounts of manganese.

Selenium: 60 to 100 mcg

This mineral is a major water-soluble antioxidant. Selenium and vitamin E work together to prevent the oxidation of polyunsaturated fats in the bloodstream. Prostaglandins can't be produced without selenium. It plays a role in cellular energy production, has great potential as a cancer fighter, and has antiviral properties. Those parts of the world where the soil is depleted of selenium tend to have higher rates of cancer.

Vanadyl Sulfate: 10 to 25 mcg

Vanadyl is another blood sugar balancing mineral that works cooperatively with chromium.

Zinc: 10 to 20 mg

Zinc aids the immune system, works in synergy with vitamin A, and in men is required for healthy prostate function.

Note the absence of iron in this recommendation. Unless you have documented iron deficiency or anemia, there's no reason for you to take extra iron. Excess iron can be very harmful, sparking the formation of free radicals. Iron is the only mineral that is not excreted by urine. Its absorption is determined by an intestinal transfer factor. Excessive iron increases the risk of heart disease, liver and colon cancer, and rheumatoid degeneration of joints. More than 4 percent of the population has hemochromatosis (absorbs too much iron) and about 40 percent of the population carries the recessive gene for this disease. Please turn to page 209 for details.

Your Ideal Diet

Although you now have some guidelines to follow for optimal nutrition, a regimented, written-in-stone plan is not what I have set out to create. I can't tell every woman to eat the same way, because every woman's body is different and will thrive on a different combination of foods. You don't have to rigidly adhere to a specific number of fat grams and carbohydrate grams; you don't have to eat foods that don't agree with you. Learn to listen to your body; it will tell you what is good for you.

For example: Some women do quite well on a diet rich in soy, others get terrible indigestion when they eat soy foods. Some women thrive on a nice cut of red meat a couple of times a week; others feel red meat is too heavy and feel sluggish after eating it. Some women choose a vegetarian diet and find it's the right thing for their bodies; other women always feel hungry if they don't eat protein-rich foods with most meals. Many people are allergic to certain foods, especially wheat, soy, and dairy, and feel better when they eliminate these foods from their diets.

Each woman's ideal diet may change over the years. Foods that agreed with you as a 20-year-old may not cut it when you're pushing 50. The point is not to eat exactly the same diet everyone else is eating, but to find the combination that works best for your particular physiological makeup.

Get Some Exercise

Most of our chronic illnesses, such as heart disease, arthritis, and cancer, can be traced to poor diet, lack of exercise, and the obesity caused by lack of exercise. The human body is built for movement. Every system in your body, from your organs, circulatory and lymph systems, to your muscles and bones, performs best for you when it is moved and stretched regularly. This is especially true of hormone balance. Estrogen is made and stored in fatty tissues, so obesity is a major cause of estrogen dominance. Obese women also tend to become insulin resistant, which means sugar isn't being removed from the blood and utilized properly. This sets up imbalances in the adrenal glands, which affect the reproductive organs. Your body works as a unit—when one part of it is out of balance, the rest tends to follow.

You don't need to take up jogging or go to the gym to get adequate exercise. For most people, a brisk 20- to 30-minute walk every day or so will do the job. I have horses, cows, chickens, geese, cats, and dogs, so I get my exercise doing the chores twice a day. Gardening, raking leaves, mowing the lawn, and shoveling snow are all good exercise. Swimming, bike riding, tennis, and golf also work well. Yoga and the Chinese movement exercises such as tai chi and qi gong are excellent for keeping the body toned and supple. Some people dance, some take aerobics classes, some use exercise videos, and some have exercise machines. What's important is to find a form (or forms) of exercise that you enjoy, and then make it a near daily habit. (For most people, planning daily exercise results in actually getting it three to four days a week!)

How Are Your Adrenal Glands Working?

As you discovered earlier in the book, having healthy adrenal glands is essential for proper hormone balance.

Lack of adrenal reserve or adrenal exhaustion is caused by chronic, unremitting stress, a common scenario in industrialized cultures. It can be the cause of debilitating fatigue. The key to healthy adrenal glands is de-stressing your life, getting plenty of sleep, and eating a balanced diet of healthy, whole foods. If your stress is largely mental, I recommend you take up some form of meditation that induces a relaxation response. Exercise can also be relaxing, but if you have adrenal insufficiency, exercise probably makes you even more tired. Because sugar stimulates the adrenals, one of the first steps you can take to support yourself is to eliminate sugar and alcohol from your diet. Progesterone is a precursor to the cortical hormones, so using it may also help significantly.

If you have followed the above guidelines for six months and still feel tired most of the time, ask your doctor about using some hydrocortisone for a few months to support your adrenal function. This is a natural form of cortisone (the same molecule as is found in the body), and in small, physiologic doses does not have the side effects of large doses of the synthetic cortisones. In fact, the history of the use of cortisone in the United

States is very similar to progesterone: It's a very effective medicine in small doses in its natural form, but since there were no profits to be made from the natural cortisones, the drug companies turned to synthetic versions with all their awful side effects. Research on hydrocortisone was halted and it faded into oblivion as a medicine for the most part. It boggles my mind that millions of people taking large doses of synthetic cortisone may be suffering needlessly because mainstream medicine has forgotten how well the real thing works. If you or your doctor would like to know more about this subject, I highly recommend the book *The Safe Uses of Cortisol*, by William McK. Jefferies.

Digestion

Digestion is an important key to good health and hormone balance. Indigestion interferes with the absorption of nutrients, makes you more susceptible to disease, and can cause food allergies or intolerances. It's nearly impossible to have good overall health without having good digestion as a foundation. If you aren't absorbing your nutrients properly, you won't have the vitamins and minerals necessary to convert one hormone into another.

The most common triggers for indigestion and heartburn are too much fat or fried food, processed meats with nitrates or nitrites in them; too much sugar, alcohol, chocolate, and drugs (especially antibiotics); and stress. If your digestive tract is already irritated, substances such as coffee, citrus fruits, tomato-based foods, and spicy foods will only irritate it more. If you have heartburn, you may be able to cure it simply by eliminating coffee.

If you have heartburn, please do not reach for antacids; they will temporarily suppress the symptoms for an hour or so, but in the long run they will make matters worse. You may even become dependent on them. Antacids also contain aluminum, silicone, sugar, and a long list of dyes and preservatives, none of which will help you and may even harm you. And no matter what the new advertising strategies are, I definitely do not recommend you get extra calcium by chewing on antacid tablets! The side effects of the antacids far outweigh any advantage you might get from the calcium, which is in a poorly absorbed form.

H2 blockers such as Pepcid, Zantac, and Tagamet, which the FDA has allowed to be sold over the counter, are even worse; they suppress the secretion of stomach acid and in many people create a distressingly long list of side effects. They interfere with the absorption of nutrients, especially calcium. Tagamet, one of the best-selling drugs in the United States, has the worst side effects: It can cause breast enlargement in men because it interferes with estrogen metabolism and excretion in the liver. Tagamet enhances the effects of many drugs, which can have deadly side effects. Your stomach acid is also one of your front line defenses against harmful bacteria. Suppress it, and the rest of your systems have to work overtime to protect you.

In spite of what the makers of Tums, Rolaids, Mylanta, Pepcid, Zantac, and Tagamet would have you believe, in my opinion, heartburn is rarely caused by too much stomach acid. In fact, I believe it's most often caused by *too little* stomach acid. As we age, we tend to produce less stomach acid. Without enough stomach acid, our food isn't properly digested in the stomach and tends to sit there. This is especially true of fatty foods. The longer food sits undigested in the stomach, the better the chance it will be burped back up to irritate the esophagus—the real source of heartburn pain. That feeling of having something stuck in your throat is an almost sure sign of too little stomach acid. Chronic heartburn is usually caused by an esophagus that's irritated by constant exposure to stomach acid.

PREVENTING HEARTBURN

- Don't lie down right after you eat. If your esophageal muscle is already too relaxed or weak, your semidigested meal will escape back up your throat.
- Eat small meals and chew your food thoroughly. Overeating and eating on the run are two of the most common causes of heartburn.

- Lose excess weight; obesity can cause heartburn.
- If you drink a lot of alcohol, cut down (no more than two drinks daily); this will almost certainly help long-term, and abstaining while you have symptoms will make healing much faster.
- Avoid sweets, a potential culprit. For some reason, chocolate is particularly aggravating to many people.
- Examine your prescription medications; many cause heartburn. Ask your doctor or pharmacist if you're taking a drug that causes heartburn.
- In case you need another reason to give up cigarettes, stop smoking and your heartburn may disappear. Nicotine relaxes the sphincter muscle that separates the esophagus from the stomach, allowing stomach acid to reflux (burp) up.
- Reduce stress, which greatly aggravates heartburn by suppressing stomach acid.

Most people with chronic heartburn, especially those over the age of 50, have low levels of hydrochloric acid (HCl), the main digestive acid in the stomach. The most common symptoms of a stomach acid deficiency show up after eating, in the form of heartburn, belching, bloating, or a heavy feeling. If you feel that most of your meal is still in your stomach more than 45 minutes after eating a normal meal, your stomach is working inefficiently. One way to stimulate your digestive juices is to drink a glass of water half an hour before eating. Other people swear by a tablespoon of apple cider vinegar in ⅓ of a cup of water before a meal. Vinegar is highly acidic and may provide your stomach with enough acidity for quick, easy digestion.

If none of the other heartburn prevention and treatment suggestions work, you can try taking betaine hydrochloride (HCl) supplements. But please don't take vinegar or start HCl supplements while you have an active case of heartburn. This will only irritate your esophagus even more. Wait until you feel better, then try taking one tablet with food. You can increase your dose up to two to three tablets per meal, but if you get a burning feeling in your stomach, you're taking too much. You can buy HCl supplements at health food stores and at some pharmacies.

Taking Care of the Large Intestine: Probiotics

During the last stages of digestion in the large intestine and colon, what was once food is now mostly waste products, fiber, and water. The colon, in contrast to the germ-free stomach, is heavily populated with both "good" and "bad" bacteria. In a healthy system, the good bacteria run the show in the colon, keeping the bad bacteria under control. Probiotics are the good bacteria found in your intestines as well as other parts of the body, such as the mouth, the urinary tract, and the vagina. Your overall health is closely tied to the health of these bacteria. If they are sick, often so are you. Along with our digestive enzymes, they play a major role in digesting food and moving it out of the body.

The three most common families of friendly bacteria are called *Lactobacillus acidophilus*, *Lactobacillus bulgaricus*, and *Bifidobacterium bifidum*. These versatile bugs change and adapt rapidly, depending on geographic location, individual biochemistry, and what types of unfriendly bacteria are invading the body at the moment. Probiotics are the ultimate antibiotics, elegantly crafted by nature to fight off unfriendly bacteria without killing the friendly ones. It's simple—take care of your friendly bacteria and they will take care of you.

Probiotics play other roles as well: The immune system depends on them; they manufacture the B vitamins, which play a major role in adrenal hormone production; they reduce cholesterol and help keep all hormones in balance.

The surest way to get in trouble with your friendly bacteria is to take antibiotics, which kill the friendly bacteria along with the unfriendly ones. Always follow antibiotic treatment with at least two weeks of probiotics. Other factors are a poor diet, stress, and poor digestion in the stomach and small intestine. Probiotics also decline as we age, so if you're having digestive problems or working to bring your hormones back into balance, it's important to add probiotic supplements to your diet or eat yogurt with *live cultures* (check the label) daily. Many super-markets and health food stores also sell acidophilus, a milk product containing live cultures. Probiotics are "alive" and have a relatively short shelf life of a few months. If you want to try probiotic supplements, buy the refrigerated capsules or liquid. You can find them at your health food store.

Herbs for Hormone Balance

Although I did not use herbs in my medical practice because I wasn't trained in their proper use, I'm sure they have a place in treating hormone imbalances. A number of physicians and other health care practitioners have successfully used herbs to help their patients balance their hormones, in conjunction with a balanced diet, some vitamin and mineral supplements, and exercise. Some herbs contain relatively high levels of plant sterols, and others contain a combination of substances that seem to help balance hormones by bringing the whole body into better balance.

Overall, herbal tinctures (the herb extracted and preserved in a liquid form with alcohol) seem to work better than capsules or tablets, and tinctures made from the fresh plant seem to be preferable to the dried plant.

Although herbs are generally safer and gentler than pharma-ceutical drugs in their actions, they should be used only as pre-scribed. Taking high doses of any medicine can be harmful. Please be sensible and moderate in your use of herbs. None of these herbs should be used by pregnant women, except under the supervision of a health care practitioner experienced in their use. As you will discover as you read about these herbs, the fact that they contain plant sterols doesn't necessarily mean they all have the same effect. For example, fenugreek can stimulate a miscarriage, while unicorn root can prevent one. They can also have very different effects on different people. If you want to use herbs to help balance your hormones, I recommend you work with an experienced herbalist, such as a Chinese medicine doc-tor or a naturopathic doctor. I am including the following list of herbs more to clear up some of the misconceptions about them than to provide a guide for using them.

Dong quai or angelica (*Angelica sinensis, Angelical polymorpha*) might best be called a woman's tonic. We have recently rediscovered it in the West thanks to the Chinese, who use it extensively in their medicine. Contrary to popular opinion, Dong quai does not contain any estrogen or phytoestrogens, or have any type of estrogenic activity. What it does do is affect the uterine muscles by contracting or relaxing them, enhances metabolism, improves liver function (which improves the excretion of hormones), aids in the utilization of vitamin E, stabilizes heart rhythm, lowers blood pressure by dilating blood vessels, and has a mild sedative activity. Overall, Dong quai might best be labeled an adaptogen, as ginseng is, meaning it tends to bring the entire organism into greater balance. The Chinese use it to bring on menstrual periods, as a tonic for women who have just given birth, as a mild sedative, and for stomachaches.

Angelica archangelica is another type of angelica, in a different plant family (*Apiaceae*) from the Dong quai angelica (*Umbelliferae*), which does appear to have some hormonal activity. It is also known as masterwort. This plant is more a stimulant than a sedative and in folklore is used to bring on menstrual periods.

Fenugreek (*Trigonella foenum-graecum*) is best known as an herbal tea with a maple syrup–like flavor. Fenugreek seeds contain plant sterols, including diosgenin, in relatively large amounts. Fenugreek has oxytocin-like properties, which means it can induce uterine contractions. This can be helpful when a menstrual period is late, but it could theoretically end a pregnancy. Fenugreek also lowers blood sugar and cholesterol, and the seeds, when eaten, can act as a laxative.

Unicorn root (*Aletris farinosa*) is not well researched, but we do know it contains a form of diosgenin and has some type of hormonal activity. Herbalists use it to alleviate menopausal symptoms, to prevent miscarriage, and to stimulate menstrual flow, which seems contradictory, but the adaptogenic herbs seem to work by bringing what is out of balance into balance. Since unicorn root is one of the most popular menopausal herbs, it may be worth trying, especially in combination with other herbs.

Sarsaparilla (*Smilax spp.*) used to be sold as a soda or tonic that was supposed to "cleanse the blood" and cure whatever ailed you. It does contain plant sterols called "saponins," and in fact a component of it, called "sarsasapogenin," has a structural similarity to some of the human steroid hormones. Male athletes have tried using it as a steroid replacement, but I don't know of any studies showing it actually worked. According to herbalist Michael Moore, it is a gentle adrenocortical stimulant, which could make it useful for balancing hormones, particularly if there is adrenal insufficiency.

Licorice (*Glycyrrhiza glabra and uralensis*) is said to be the most common ingredient in Chinese herbal formulas. We know it works well in the treatment of ulcers, probably by encouraging the production of the protective mucosa that lines the stomach. It also has hormonal effects that seem to vary from person to person. The Chinese use licorice extensively to treat any type of adrenal insufficiency. A component of licorice called "glycyrrhizin," if taken in large doses over a long period of time, can raise blood pressure by causing sodium retention and potassium loss. Many licorice tinctures come deglycyrrhizinized, thus eliminating that concern, but also possibly eliminating many of the therapeutic effects they might have in balancing hormones.

Wild yam (*Dioscorea villosa*) was and still is used extensively by pharmaceutical companies to manufacture steroid hormones from its diosgenin, including pregnenolone, progesterone, DHEA, estrogen, testosterone, and the cortisones. It is this use that has caused the progesterone in many progesterone creams to be labeled "wild yam extract." This, unfortunately, has become misleading, as companies seeking to jump onto the progesterone bandwagon have (out of ignorance or the desire for profit) added diosgenin to a cream, and claim it does the same thing as progesterone. Diosgenin does *not* equal progesterone.

CHAPTER 22

COMMONLY ASKED QUESTIONS ABOUT USING NATURAL PROGESTERONE

After giving hundreds of talks around the world about progesterone and receiving thousands of letters and e-mails, I've found that the same questions tend to come up over and over again. While all these questions have been thoroughly answered in the preceding chapters, I hope this list of questions and succinct answers will provide a useful refresher and guide.

Q: I had a hysterectomy but still have my ovaries. How should I use progesterone cream?

A: Removing the uterus appears to interfere with blood flow to the ovaries, and they tend to stop functioning within a year or two (at the most) of having a hysterectomy. If you know that you're still ovulating, you can use progesterone as recommended for women who are still having periods, but if you're unsure, follow the guidelines for menopausal women. If you've had both your uterus and your ovaries removed, you are by definition menopausal can use progesterone accordingly.

Q: I had a bone density test that shows I have osteoporosis, and my doctor wants me to start using Fosamax. Will this help my bones?

A: First, you should make sure that your low bone density isn't simply a result of having small bones. If you're petite, chances are that any given bone density test is going to show you as having osteoporosis, because most of the tests don't take smaller bones into account. That's why I recommend that women have a bone mineral density (BMD) test in their 40s, so they'll have something to compare against in their 50s. Then, I recommend that you review the chapter in this book on osteoporosis and make sure you're doing everything recommended there to build and maintain good bones.

Fosamax doesn't build bone, it slows bone resorption. This will make bone density tests look better for a few years, but bone needs to be constantly replaced to stay healthy. In other words, old, brittle bone needs to be taken away, or resorbed, so that new and stronger bone can replace it. If you're only stopping bone resorption without building new bone, what's left will eventually be of poor quality and more prone to fracture.

Q: How long should I stay on progesterone supplementation?

A: Since progesterone has so many positive benefits, and no known side effects when used as I recommend, there is no reason to discontinue it. I tell postmenopausal women to continue until age 96 and then we'll reevaluate. If you're premenopausal and still having periods, use it only if needed. If you get your hormones back in balance, and you are ovulating and producing enough progesterone every month, then there's no need to use supplemental progesterone.

Q: How do I know how much progesterone to use?

A: The goal is to restore normal physiologic progesterone levels for at least two to three weeks a month. An ovulating woman makes about 20 to 24 milligrams a day for about 12 days each month after ovulation, or about 240 milligrams a month. Let's say a progesterone cream supplies 480 milligrams of progesterone per ounce (960 milligrams per 2-ounce jar). That jar would last for three to four months. One of the most frequent problems I encounter is women who are taking a much higher dose of progesterone. This is very counterproductive because it suppresses progesterone receptors, and as a result the progesterone cannot get into the cells, and within a few months estrogen dominance has returned. More is not better!

Q: Who should use estrogen supplements?

A: Estrogen works especially well for hot flashes and vaginal dryness. These symptoms can generally be taken as a sign of estrogen deficiency. Progesterone receptors help to sensitize estrogen receptors (and vice versa), progesterone alone is often sufficient to restore estrogen levels to normal and eliminate these symptoms. If a three-month trial of progesterone plus proper diet and supplements of magnesium and B6 do not relieve hot flashes or vaginal dryness, then low-dose *natural* estrogen may be helpful. (Estrogen is not recommended in those women with a history of breast or uterine cancer, obesity, diabetes, or a history of clotting or vascular disorders.) If used for hot flashes, find the lowest dose of estrogen that works. If vaginal dryness is the problem, I usually recommend vaginal gels or creams containing estriol. Often, a small dose applied vaginally only twice a week, three weeks a month, will do wonders.

Q: I'm still having periods, but I have problems with hot flashes, water retention, poor sleep, and mood swings. What is wrong with me?

A: During the years before actual menopause, estrogen may be decreasing slightly and, more often, ovulation has ceased or is rare. Without ovulation, progesterone production is essentially zero, and estrogen receptors become less sensitive to the estrogen still being made. You are actually estrogen dominant. Your doctor, however, will probably prescribe estrogen, but the results are only partially effective and many of the problems, such as fluid retention, become worse. When a synthetic progestin (e.g., birth control pill) is added, the results are usually not good because progestins are not the same as natural progesterone and also cause undesirable side effects. The best treatment is a diet low in sugar and refilled carbohydrates, vitamin E, magnesium, and vitamin B6 supplements, plus natural progesterone. In these cases, progesterone can be added during the "luteal" phase, that is, from day 12 (ovulation time) to day 26 (48 hours before the expected period). Please read my book *What Your Doctor*

May Not *Tell You About Premenopause* for more detailed information about hormone balance prior to menopause.

Q: My periods are sometimes scant, sometimes heavy, and sometimes come early or late. What should I do?

A: Irregular periods in the years before menopause are another sign that menopause is approaching, and you are most probably deficient in progesterone due to not ovulating every month. Remember, shedding of the bloody endometrial lining is triggered primarily by the fall of progesterone levels 12 days or so after ovulation. If you are not ovulating, you are not making much progesterone, and therefore there will be no fall of progesterone to trigger a proper shedding. Follow the advice of the previous question for at least three cycles and your periods should become more regular again.

Q: I'm 43 years old and still having periods, but I've lost interest in sex. What's wrong?

A: Libido (the desire for sex) is mistakenly thought by most doctors to come from estrogen. The fact that you are still having periods means you are making plenty of estrogen. But you are most probably low in progesterone. Progesterone is an important factor in libido. Testosterone also improves libido. Since most doctors are unaware of this role of progesterone, some are tempted to give women testosterone for their flagging libido. However, this choice is not desirable unless you have a measurable testosterone deficiency. Follow the advice of the two previous questions and your libido will most probably return to normal. Don't worry; you will not become a sex maniac—the guy across the room will just become a little better looking, that's all. If the progesterone doesn't help, get a saliva hormone level test and find out if you're deficient in testosterone.

Q: Help! My hair is falling out by the handful.

A: When progesterone levels fall as a result of ovarian follicle failure (lack of ovulation or simply by follicle dysfunction), the body responds by increasing its production of the adrenal cortical steroid, androstenedione, an alternative precursor for the production of other adrenal cortical hormones. Androstenedione conveys some androgenic (male-like) properties, in this case, male pattern hair loss. When progesterone levels are raised by progesterone supplements, the androstenedione level will gradually fall, and your normal hair growth will eventually resume. Since hair growth is a slow process, it may take four to six months for the effects to become apparent.

Q: My sister developed breast cancer when she was 45 and still menstruating. I'm now 43 and my periods are changing. What should I do?

A: Excess estrogen unopposed by progesterone is the primary cause of breast cancer. In industrialized countries, it has become epidemic that progesterone deficiency and estrogen dominance among women occur during their mid-30s. (This is probably due to xenobiotic [petrochemical] toxins affecting ovary development during the embryo stage.) Estrogen dominance increases the risk of breast cancer. Please read *What Your Doctor May* Not *Tell You About Breast Cancer* for detailed information about how your hormone balance affects your risk of breast cancer.

Q: My own doctor doesn't seem to know much about natural progesterone, and in fact makes fun of the whole idea. What should I do?

A: Your doctor is making fun of the idea out of ignorance, discomfort at his or her own ignorance, or both. I have found over and over again that once a doctor is introduced to the science and logic behind the idea of using physiologic doses of natural hormones, they can't jump on the bandwagon fast enough. Furthermore, *all* of the doctors I know who are using natural hormones in the dosages and timing that I recommend have busy practices and very happy patients.

You can either find another doctor or attempt to educate the one you have. I'm all for educating doctors! You can also give your doctor a copy of this book or my book written for doctors, *Natural Progesterone: The Multiple Roles of a Remarkable Hormone*. (See the Resources section for more information.)

Q: What progesterone cream should I use?

A: Use a progesterone cream that contains at least 400 milligrams of progesterone per ounce. Some creams on the market contain less than 10 milligrams an ounce, and these won't do the job. Neither will the creams that contain so-called precursors to progesterone, such as diosgenin or ground up wild yam. Calling a progesterone cream a "wild yam" cream is confusing and misleading to the consumer. It either contains real progesterone or it doesn't, and if the company can't or won't tell you exactly how much progesterone is in their cream, find another one. I prefer the creams that contain only progesterone as their active ingredient, and I recommend against mixing a number of hormones (e.g., estrogen and testosterone) into one cream.

Q: Why do you prefer creams instead of pills or capsules for progesterone?

A: Mother Nature guides us in this: The ovary never puts its hormones into the stomach, and for good reason. Progesterone is fat-soluble and, when absorbed from the stomach or intestines, is taken by the portal vein directly to the liver, where it is efficiently metabolized for excretion in bile. When taken orally, about 85 to 90 percent of progesterone is lost via the bile or converted into metabolites that are not the same as real progesterone. Thus, oral doses must be 100 to 200 milligrams per day, 10 to 20 times greater than transdermal doses, just to get the 20 to 24 milligrams needed daily. I see no reason to put the liver to all this work just to get 10 to 15 percent of the progesterone into the bloodstream.

Natural progesterone is well absorbed through the skin and then into the bloodstream, riding on fatty components such as chylomicrons and red blood cell membranes. (Being fat-soluble, very little of the skin-absorbed progesterone is found in the watery blood serum.) An Australian study by researchers Waddell and O'Leary found that transdermal progesterone absorption is equivalent to progesterone by intravascular injection.

Our goal is to achieve equivalence with normal physiologic progesterone levels. Transdermal progesterone does this easily. There is no need to take oral doses of 100 to 200 milligrams per day.

Q: How can I check my hormone levels?

A: In the past, blood serum levels were used, but these don't measure progesterone taken transdermally (through the skin). When the ovaries make estrogen and progesterone for circulation in the watery blood serum, they bind them to protein (sex hormone–binding globulin in the case of estrogen or cortisol-binding globulin in the case of progesterone) to make them more water-soluble. Protein-bound hormones are not biologically active, but they represent over 90 percent of the hormones found in the serum. Thus the serum results do not accurately reflect the biologically available hormones. Transdermal progesterone is immediately biologically available. Saliva hormones reflect only the biologically available hormones. Saliva hormone assays are less expensive, very accurate, easier to obtain, and more relevant than serum assays. Check the Resources section for more information on getting a saliva hormone level test.

Since progesterone levels are apt to be highest two or three days after ovulation, it is wise to check hormone levels around day 18 to 21 of the menstrual month, counting day 1 as the first day of the preceding period. If the levels are found to be low at that time, you are probably not ovulating that month and your body progesterone level will be low.

Q: Can I use progesterone for birth control?

A: Folklore describes herbal and other plant sources (including Mexican wild yam) as being effective for birth control. Theoretically, progesterone or progestational effects are the key mechanism since, if taken early in the cycle, they could inhibit ovulation as the progestins in birth control pills do. However, I have no clinical experience using natural progesterone for this purpose and am unaware of any scientific studies testing this hypothesis, and therefore cannot recommend it.

Q: I quit HRT last year and now I have hot flashes. What should I do?

A: It's a mistake to suddenly quit taking Premarin or any other type of estrogen. Conventional medicine tends to grossly overdose estrogen and your brain gets used to the high doses. If you suddenly stop taking the estrogen, you will have a withdrawal reaction that can include severe hot flashes and night sweats, irritability, mood swings, depression, and foggy thinking. A better approach is to very gradually reduce your dose of estrogen over a period of anywhere from two to six months, depending on how high your dose has been.

I do not teach that women have no need of some hormone supplementation. I teach that conventional HRT (e.g., Prem-Pro) is a mistake. About 66 percent of postmenopausal women have sufficient fat for making sufficient estrogen during their postmenopausal years up to at least age 80. Thin women make less estrogen (because of less body fat) and therefore may need some supplemental estrogen. Some will do well using phyto-estrogens, as in herbs. Some will require real estrogen such as estrone, estradiol, and/or estriol. All of these can be safely used by making sure that low physiological doses are used, and progesterone is given along with them. The usual optimal dose is one-eighth of that used by conventional HRT. (See Chapter 4 for instructions on estrogen dosing.)

Q: I've had a mastectomy for breast cancer and I am using tamoxifen. Can I take progesterone along with the tamoxifen?

A: I believe that achieving correct hormone balance using progesterone is far more important than tamoxifen. Yes, they can be used together but I believe there is no need for tamoxifen—the proof of benefit is questionable and the risks of harm are too great. Please read my book *What Your Doctor May* Not *Tell You About Breast Cancer* for more detailed information about breast cancer and tamoxifen.

Q: I had breast cancer and my doctor wants me to take Arimidex, what should I do?

A: Arimidex inhibits aromatase, an enzyme in the body fat of both men and women that converts adrenal androgens (male hormones) into estrone, an estrogen. The doctor prescribes Arimidex to eliminate that source of estrogen in the hope of preventing recurrent breast cancer. However, we all need some estrogen; the question is—how best to create hormone balance? In most cases, the answer is (1) transdermal progesterone and (2) saliva hormone assays to find the desired balance between estradiol and progesterone. Again, please read my book *What Your Doctor May* Not *Tell You About Breast Cancer* for more detailed information about breast cancer and hormone balance.

Q: My mother is taking medication for her high blood pressure, low thyroid, and arthritis. If she uses progesterone cream will that interact or interfere with the medication?

A: I often get mail from people wondering if progesterone will interfere with their medication. Small, physiologic doses of progesterone per se won't interfere with nonhormonal medications, any more than ovulating every month will interfere with them. However, progesterone often improves conditions such as high blood pressure, low thyroid and arthritis, so it would be a good idea for your mother to keep track of her blood pressure for a month or two and to have her thyroid function checked to make sure she still needs the medication. Progesterone also tends to have an antianxiety effect, so many women find they no longer need sleeping pills or antidepressants once they begin using it. On the other hand, excessively high doses of progesterone taken over a long period of time can have a wide range of drug-like effects, so I don't recommend mixing medications and high doses of progesterone without a doctor's supervision.

GLOSSARY

amenorrhea	absence of menstruation
androgenic	producing masculine characteristics
anovulatory	suspension or cessation of ovulation
carcinogen	any cancer-producing substance
catalyst	any substance that enhances the rate or velocity of a chemical reaction
chromosome	a molecule that comprises the gene (genome), or hereditary factor, composed of DNA or RNA
conjugated	in biochemistry, one compound combined with another
corpus luteum	small yellow glandular mass in the ovary formed by an ovarian follicle after ovulation (release of its egg [ovum])
corticosteroid	hormone produced by the adrenal cortex
cytoplasm	the watery protoplasm of a cell, excluding the nucleus
diuretic	substance that increases urine production
DNA	deoxyribonucleic acid, the basic molecular subunit of chromosomes
dysmenorrhea	painful menstruation
endocrine	refers to organs (glands) that secrete hormones
endogenous	developing or originating within the body
endometrium	the inner lining of the uterus
enzyme	an organic compound, usually a protein, capable of facilitating a specific chemical reaction
exogenous	originating outside of the body

follicle	a very small sac or cavity composed of cells, e.g., the ovarian follicle that produces the ovum
gonadal	refers to the gamete-producing glands, i.e., ovaries and testes
gonadotropic	refers to hormones that affect or stimulate gonads
gram	unit of mass (weight); about one twenty-eighth of an ounce
homeostasis	the body's ability to maintain a stable internal environment
hydroxylation	the addition of a hydroxyl radical (—OH) to a compound
hypermenorrhea	excessive bleeding with menses
hypothalamus	neural centers of the limbic brain just above the pituitary that control visceral activities, water balance, sleep, and hormone production by the pituitary
hysterectomy	surgical removal of the uterus
libido	sex drive
limbic brain	brain cortex below the corpus callosum and above the pituitary that contains neural centers controlling autonomic functions, homeostasis, and emotional sensation and responses, and regulates immune responses
luteinizing	refers to the maturation of ovarian follicles following ovulation, during which the follicle become the corpus luteum producing progesterone
mastodynia	painful breasts
metabolism	the biochemical process of living organisms by which substances are produced and energy is made available to the organism
microgram	one millionth (10^{-6}) of a gram
milligram	one thousandth (10^{-3}) of a gram
mineralcorticoid	an adrenal hormone that regulates sodium, potassium, and water balance

mitochondria	small organelles within the cytoplasm that are the site of converting sugar into energy
nanogram	one billionth (10^{-9}) of a gram
oocyte	the cell that produces the ovum
oophorectomy	surgical removal of an ovary or ovaries
osteoblast	bone cell that forms new bone
osteoclast	bone cell that resorbs old bone
osteocyte	means bone cell; may become an osteoclast or an osteoblast
osteoid	the noncellular, collagenous matrix of bone
peptide	a class of low-molecular-weight compounds composed of several amino acids; a miniprotein
perimenopausal	referred to as premenopausal in this book—refers to the time preceding menopause when hormone changes are occurring
phyto-	denotes relationship to plants
premenopausal	prior to menopause, also called "perimenopausal"
resorption	the loss or dissolving away of a substance
serum	the watery, noncellular liquid of the blood
steroid	group name for compounds based on the cholesterol molecule, e.g., sex hormones and corticosteroids
sterol	compounds with a single hydroxyl group (—OH) soluble in fats, widely found in plants and animals. Cholesterol is a sterol.
synovial	referring to the inner lining of a joint
thermogenic	capable of inducing a rise in temperature
trans-	prefix referring to something altered from the natural state, such as trans-fatty acids
xeno-	combining form meaning strange or foreign

RESOURCES

Dr. Lee's Website

www.johnleemd.com

This is where you can find Dr. Lee's other books and booklets, as well as back issues of his newsletter and timely articles about hormones in the news.

How to Find Natural Progesterone Cream

You can find progesterone cream in most health food stores these days, but a few contain little to no real progesterone—buyer beware. If you have any doubt, call the company and ask how many milligrams of progesterone per ounce the cream contains.

Regardless of the source, please be sure you're getting the real thing. If the label says "wild yam extract" don't buy the product without confirming that it contains progesterone and not the so-called precursors such as diosgenin (see page 301 for details). The following are progesterone creams that we know contain real progesterone.

Neither of the authors endorse any one progesterone cream or company, or make any money from the sale of any progesterone cream.

Many natural progesterone creams contain ingredients other than progesterone that may be active, including "wild yam extract" which is usually diosgenin, a variety of herbs, and aromatic oils. We do not know which are active and which aren't, or what biochemical effects these ingredients may or may not have, nor do we know what effect they may have when used by women who are pregnant or nursing.

The following list changes regularly. Please visit Dr. Lee's website (www.johnleemd.com) for the most up-to-date list.

AIM International, Inc.
3904 East Flamingo Ave.
Nampa, ID 83687
(208) 465-5116

Renewed Balance progesterone cream.

Alternative Medicine Network
601 16th St. #C-#105
Golden, CO 80401
Toll-free (877) 753-5424
www.altmednetwork.net
e-mail: sales@altmednetwork.net

They make Awakening Woman Natural Progesterone Cream, which contains only progesterone as its active ingredient.

Arbonne International, Inc.
P.O. Box 2488
Laguna Hills, CA 92654
(800) ARBONNE
www.arbonne.com
e-mail: customerservice@arbonne.com

They make PhytoProlief and Prolief Natural Balancing Creams.

Better Health Naturally by Helen Pensanti, M.D.
P.O. Box 5033
Irvine, CA 92616
(877) 880-0170
www.askdrhelen.com, www.doctortodoctor.com
e-mail: info@askdrhelen.com

Dr. Pensanti has developed ProHELP natural progesterone creme and Menopause Relief Creme.

Bio-Nutritional Formulas
106 E. Jericho Tpke.
P.O. Box 311
Mineola, NY 11501
(800) 950-8484

Fem-Gest cream.

Broadmoore Labs, Inc.
3875 Telegraph Road/294
Ventura, CA 93003
(800) 822-3712

Makers of Natra-Gest progesterone creams.

Easy Way International
5340 Commerce Circle, #E
Indianapolis, IN 46237
(800) 267-4522

They make Gentle Changes progesterone cream.

Elan Vitale
P.O. Box 13990
Scottsdale, AZ 85267
(800) 527-5898, or (602) 483-5650

They make BioBalance progesterone cream.

Emerita, Pro-Gest
621 SW Alder, Suite 900
Portland, OR 97205-3627
(800) 648-8211, or (503) 226-1010
www.transitionsforhealth.com, www.progest.com

The original natural progesterone cream. A Division of Transitions for Health, Inc.

The Health and Science Research Inst.
661 Beville Rd., Suite 101
Daytona Beach, FL 32119
(888) 222-1415, fax (904) 267-9005
www.health-science.com

Serenity for Women progesterone cream.

HM Enterprises
2622 Bailey Dr.
Norcross, GA 30071
(800) 742-4773
www.hmenterprises.com, or
www.paulbunyan.net/users/mlzeller

They make Happy PMS progesterone cream.

International Health
8704 E. Mulberry St.
Scottsdale, AZ 85251
(800) 481-9987, or (480) 874-1419
e-mail: nopms@doitnow.com

Makers of EssPro'Leve Plus Progesterone Cream with Essential
Oils.

Kevala, a division of Karuna
42 Digital Drive #7
Novato, CA 94949
(888) 749-8643
www.kevalahealth.com
e-mail:info@kevalahealth.com

They make PureGest Lotion, which is free from additional hormones, herbs, and alcohols.

Kokoro, LLC
P.O. Box 597
Tustin, CA 92781
(800) 599-9412, (714) 836-7749
www.kokorohealth.com

They offer Kokoro Women's Balance Crème.

Life-flo Health Care Products
8146 N. 23rd Ave., Suite E
Phoenix, AZ 85021
(888) 999-7440
www.life-flo.com, or www.sheld.com/lifeflo/
e-mail care@life-flo.com

They make Progestacare cream.

Matol Botanical International
Quebec, Canada
(514) 639-3347
www.matol.com

Makers of Botanelle Progesterone Cream.

Natural Pause—Natural Menopause Solutions
11683 Noguera Ave.
Ventura, CA 93001
(888) 267-5032
www.naturalpause.com

Makers of Natural Pause Cream.

Nature's Sunshine Products, Inc.
75 E. 1700 S.
Provo, UT 84606
(800) 223-8225
www.naturessunshine.com
e-mail, questions@natr.com

Pro-G-Yam 500 Progesterone Cream with wild yam extract.

Neways
150 E. 400 North
P.O. Box 651
Salem, UT 84653
(801) 423-2800

They make Endau cream.

Products of Nature
54 Danbury Road
Ridgefield, CT 06877
(800) 665-5952
www.pronature.com—Connecticut, or
www.prodnature.com—Texas

Maker of Natural Woman progesterone cream.

Pure Essence Labs, Inc.
1999 Whitney Mesa Drive, Suite A
Henderson, NV 89014
(888) 254-8000

www.pureessencelabs.com
Online distributors: www.getleaner.com, www.vitaminlady.com

Makers of FemCreme.

Restored Balanced Inc.
42 Meadowbridge Dr. SW
Cartersville, GA 30120
(800) 865-7499
www.restoredbalanceusa.com
e-mail restoredbalance@adelphia.net

They make Restored Balance PMS/Menopausal progesterone cream.

Sarati International
Rt. 3, Box 385
Ted Hunt Rd.
Los Fresno, TX 78566
(800) 900-0701
www.sarati.com. Online distributors: www.sunrisewd.com, or
www.progestnet.com

They make Natural Progesterone Cream.

Springboard
3115 Stoney Oak Drive
Spring Valley, CA 91978
Toll-free (866) 882-6868, or (619) 670-3860,
fax (619) 670-4149
www.springboard4health.com, or
www.naturalprogesterone.com

They make ProBalance progesterone cream.

Vitality Lifechoice
Carson City, NV
(800) 423-8365

They make Balance Cream.

Vitamin Research Products, Inc.
3579 Highway 50 East
Carson City, NV 89701
(800) 877-2447, (775) 884-1300
www.advancedmenopauserelief.com

Makers of HerBalance Cream.

Women's Medicine, Inc.
Toll-free (866) 628-6337 or (904) 249-3743
www.womens-medicine.com or www.safesthormones.com

This is Dr. C. W. Randolph's Natural Progesterone Cream. Formulated by a gynecologist who is also a pharmacist.

Compounding Pharmacists

If your doctor is interested in natural hormones but hesitant about prescribing over-the-counter cream, you can put him or her in touch with a compounding pharmacist skilled in the use of natural hormone supplements, who can educate your physician and provide dosing guidelines. For a referral in your area contact IACP (International Academy of Compounding Pharmacists), (800) 927-4227, ext. 300, or go online to www.iacprx .org.

Saliva Hormone Testing

State-of-the-art saliva hormone level testing with analysis, plus blood spot testing.

ZRT Laboratory
1815 NW 168th Place, Suite 5050
Beaverton, OR 97006
(503) 466-2445, fax (503) 466-1636
www.salivatest.com
e-mail infor@zrtlab.com

How to Find a Health Care Professional in Your Area Who Practices Alternative Medicine

Of course we can't guarantee that any given individual you might contact is knowledgeable, competent, and willing to work in partnership with you, but the following resources will give you a good jump-start on your search. One of the best sources of information is your local health food store. You can also look in your Yellow Pages under "Physicians." Those who practice alternative medicine often advertise themselves as wholistic or holistic physicians.

Dr. Lee's website (www.johnleemd.com) has a selection called Resources, with a heading, "Suggestions for Finding a Doctor in

Your Area." It contains the following list plus other websites that have doctor referrals.

Organizations you can contact that will give you a referral in your area are:

American College for Advancement in Medicine
P.O. Box 3427
Laguna Hills, CA 92654
(800) 532-3688, or (949) 583-7666

American Association of Naturopathic Physicians
8201 Greensboro Drive, Suite 300
McLean, VA 22102
(703) 610-9037, fax (703) 610-9005
www.aanp.com

Send $5 for a Natural Referral Directory and brochure, or fax your request with credit card information.

American Holistic Medical Association
Resources for Natural HRT
6728 Old McLean Village Drive
McLean, VA 22101
(703) 556-9245, fax (703) 556-8729
www.holisticmedicine.org

Professional Referral Network: www.healthreferral.com

Natural Pest Control

The Bio-Integral Resource Center
P.O. Box 7414
Berkeley, CA 94707
(510) 524-2567, fax (510) 524-1758
www.birc.org

A nonprofit educational organization that provides information and services in the area of "least toxic" pest control, also known as integrated pest management (IPM).

Rachel Carson Council, Inc.
8940 Jones Mill Road
Chevy Chase, MD 20815
(301) 652-1877, fax (301) 587-3863
www.members.aol.com/rccouncil/ourpage

Provides information on pesticides and chemicals, as well as a newsletter. They have an excellent list of low-cost books and pamphlets on natural lawns and gardens.

Northwest Coalition for Alternatives to Pesticides (NCAP)
P.O. Box 1393
Eugene, OR 97440
(541) 344-5044, fax (541) 344-6923
www.pesticide.org

An informative service on the hazards of pesticides and alternatives to their use. They have an extensive library and offer information packets, books, and a newsletter.

National Coalition Against the Misuse of Pesticides (NCAMP)
701 E Street, SE, Suite 200
Washington, DC 20003
(202) 543-5450, fax (202) 543-4791
www.beyondpesticides.org

A voice for pesticide safety and alternatives. Publishes a quarterly newsletter, and has a good list of books and pamphlets.

Exercise

Find a reputable trainer in your area through:

The American College of Sports Medicine (ACSM)
(317) 637-9200
www.acsm.org

or

The National Academy of Sports Medicine (NASM)
(800) 656-2739

If you're hiring a gym trainer, be sure the gym trainer is certified by one of these organizations, or by the American Council of Exercise (ACE).

RECOMMENDED READING

Creating a Toxin-Free Environment

Schultz, Warren. *The Chemical-Free Lawn: The Newest Varieties and Techniques to Grow Lush, Hardy Grass with No Pesticides, No Herbicides, No Chemical Fertilizers.* Emmaus, Penn.: Rodale Press.

Steinman, David. *Diet for a Poisoned Planet: How to Choose Safe Foods for You and Your Family.* New York: Ballantine Books, 1990.

Steinman, David, and Michael R. Wisner. *Living Healthy in a Toxic World.* New York: A Perigee Book, 1996.

Women's Health

The Boston Women's Health Collective. *The New Our Bodies, Ourselves.* New York: Simon & Schuster, 1992.

Love, Susan, MD. *Dr. Susan Love's Breast Book.* Redding, Mass. Addison Wesley, 1990.

Northrup, Christiane, MD. *Women's Bodies, Women's Wisdom.* New York: Bantam Books, Revised Edition, 1998.

————. *The Wisdom of Menopause: Creating Physical and Emotional Health and Healing During the Change.* New York: Bantam Books, 2001.

Alternative Medicine and Nutrition

Batmanghelidj, F., MD. *Your Body's Many Cries for Water.* Falls Church, Va.: Global Health Solutions, 1995.

Braverman, Eric R., MD. *The Healing Nutrients Within: How to Use Amino Acids.* North Bergen, N.J.: Basic Health Publications, 2003.

Enig, Mary, PhD. *Know Your Fats: The Complete Primer for Understanding the Nutrition of Fats, Oils and Cholesterol.* Silver Spring, Md.: Bethesda Press, 2000.

Fallon, Sally. *Nourishing Traditions.* San Diego: ProMotion Publishing, 1995.

Galland, Leo, MD. *The Four Pillars of Healing.* New York: Random House, 1997.

Golan, Ralph, MD. *Optimal Wellness.* New York: Ballantine Books, 1995.

Kristal, Harold J., DDS. *The Nutrition Solution: A Guide to Your Metabolic Type.* Berkeley, Calif: North Atlantic Books.

Mindell, Earl, RpH, PhD, and Virginia Hopkins. *Prescription Alternatives.* Chicago, Ill.: Keats Publishing, 1998.

Pizzorno, Joseph N. *Total Wellness.* Roseville, Calif.: Prima Publishing, 1996.

Raffelock, Dean, DC, Robert Rountree, MD, et al. *A Natural Guide to Pregnancy and Postpartum Health: The First Book by Doctors That Really Addresses Pregnancy Recovery.* New York: Avery/Penguin Putnam, 2002.

Rose, Marc, MD and Michael Rose, MD.*Save Your Sight.* New York: Warner Books, 1998.

Sears, Barry. *The Zone.* New York: HarperCollins, 1996.

Todd, Gary Price, MD. *Nutrition, Health and Disease.* West Chester, Penn.: Whitford Press, 1985.

Wilson, James L. ND, DC. *Adrenal Fatigue: The 21st Century Stress Syndrome.* Petaluma, Calif.: Smart Publications, 2001.

Hormones

Barnes, Broda. *Hypothyroidism: The Unsuspected Illness.* New York: Harper & Row, 1976.

Jefferies, William McK., MD. *Safe Uses of Cortisol.* Springfield, Ill.: Charles C Thomas Publishers, 1996.

Khalsa, Dharma Singh, MD. *Brain Longevity.* New York: Warner Books, 1997.

Lee, John R., MD, and Virginia Hopkins. *What Your Doctor May Not Tell You About Premenopause: Balance Your Hormones and Your Life from Thirty to Fifty.* New York: Warner Books, 1999.

Lee, John R., MD, David T. Zava, PhD, and Virginia Hopkins. *What Your Doctor May Not Tell You About Breast Cancer: How Hormone Balance Can Help Save Your Life.* New York: Warner Books, 1996.

Sahelian, Ray. *DHEA: A Practical Guide.* Garden City Park, N.Y.: Avery Publishing, 1996.

———. *Pregnenolone: A Practical Guide.* Marina del Rey, Calif.: Melatonin/DHEA Research Institute, 1996.

Drugs

Breggin, Peter. *Talking Back to Prozac.* New York: St. Martin's Press, 1994.

Fried, Stephen. *Bitter Pills: Inside the Hazardous World of Legal Drugs.* New York: Bantam Books, 1998.

Lappe, Marc. *When Antibiotics Fail: Restoring the Ecology of the Body.* Berkeley, Calif.: North Atlantic Books, 1995.

Schmidt, Michael, Lendon Smith, and Keith Sehnert. *Beyond Antibiotics.* Berkeley, Calif.: North Atlantic Books, 1994.

REFERENCES

Chapter 1: The Crux of the Matter: Menopausal Politics and Women's Hormone Cycles

Goodman, Louis S., and Alfred Gilman. *The Pharmacological Basis of Therapeutics*, 8th edition. Toronto: The Macmillan Company, 1990: Chapter 58.

Kolata, Gina. Hormone replacement study a shock to the medical system. *New York Times*, July 10, 2002.

Premarin Statistics: *Business Week Online*: September 27, 2002.

Textbook of Clinical Chemistry. Norbert W. Tietz, PhD., ed. Philadelphia: W.B. Saunders Co., 1986:1085–1171.

Thomas, J. Hywel, and Brian Gillham. *Will's Biochemical Basis of Medicine,* 2d edition. Oxford: Butterworth-Heinemann Ltd., 1989: Chapter 17.

Chapter 2: The Dance of the Steroids

Goodman, Louis S., and Alfred Gilman. *The Pharmacological Basis of Therapeutics*, 8th edition. Toronto: The Macmillan Company, 1990: Chapter 58.

Morley, John E., M.B., 1994. Nutrition modulation of behavior and immunocompetence. *Nutrition Reviews* August, 52(8):S6–S8.

Textbook of Clinical Chemistry. Norbert W. Tietz, PhD., ed. Philadelphia: W.B. Saunders Co., 1986:1085–1171.

Will's Biochemical Basis of Medicine, 2d edition. Oxford: Butterworth-Heinemann Ltd., 1989: Chapter 17.

Chapter 3: The History of Hormone Replacement Therapy and the Estrogen Myth

Albright, F. 1936. Studies in ovarian function III: The menopause. *Endocrinology* 20:24.

Barret-Conner, E. 1991. Postmenopausal estrogen and prevention bias. *Annals of Internal Medicine* 115:455–56.

Byyny, R. L., and L. Speroff. *A Clinical Guide for the Care of Older Women.* Baltimore: Williams & Wilkins, 1990.

Coney, Sandra. *The Menopause Industry.* Alameda, Calif.: Hunter House, 1994.

Coronary Drug Project Rsearch Group. 1973 Coronary drug project: Findings leading to the discontinuation of the 2.5 mg/day estrogen group. *Journal of American Medical Association* (hereafter cited as *JAMA*) 226:652–57.

———.1978. Coronary Drug Project: estrogens and cancer (letter). *JAMA* 239:2758–59.

Gallagher, J. C., W. T. Kable, and D. Goldgar. 1991. The effect of progestin therapy on cortical and trabecular bone: Comparison with estrogen. *American Journal of Medicine* 90:171–78.

Jaszman, I., N. D. Van Lith, and J. C. Saat. 1969. The perimenopausal symptoms: The statistical analysis of a survey. Parts A and B. *Medical Gynecology Sociology* 4:268–76.

Jayo, M. J., D. S. Weaver, M. R. Adams, and S. E. Rankin. 1990. Effects on bone of surgical menopause and estrogen therapy with or without progesterone replacement in cynomolgus monkeys. *American Journal of Obstetrics and Gynecology* 614:618.

Kaufert, P. A., P. Gilbert, and R. Tate. 1987. Defining menopausal status: The impact of longitudinal data. *Maturitas* 9:217–26.

Lacey, J. V., P. J. Mink, J. H. Lubin, et al. Menopausal hormone replacement and risk of Ovarian cancer. *JAMA*, July 17, 2002, vol. 288, no. 3.

Leather, A. T., M. Savras, and J. W. Stuidd. 1991. Endometrial histology and bleeding patterns after eight years of continuous combined estrogen and progestin therapy in postmenopausal women. *Obstet Gynecol* 78:1008–10.

McKinlay, S. M., D. J. Brambilla, and J. G. Posner. 1992. The normal menopausal transition. *Maturitas* 14:103–15.

Neugarten, B. L., and R. J. Kraines. 1964. Menopausal symptoms in women of various ages. *Psychom Med* 27:266–73.

Prior, J. C. One Voice on Menopause. *JAMWA* 49, no. 1 (January/February 1994):27–29.

———.1990. Progesterone as a bone-trophic hormone. *Endocr Rev* 11:386–98.

———.1991. Postmenopausal estrogen therapy and cardiovascular disease (letter). *New England Journal of Medicine* 326:705–706.

Prior, J. C., B. Ho Yuen, P. Clement, et al. 1992. Reversible luteal phase changes and infertility associated with marathon training. *Lancet* 1:269–70.

Prior, J. C., and Y. M. Vigna. 1991. Ovulation disturbances and exercise training. *Clin Obstet Gynecol* 26:180–90.

Prior, J. C., and Y. M. Vigna, N. Alojado, et al. 1987. Conditioning exercise decreases premenstrual symptoms: A prospective controlled six-month trial. *FertilSteril* 47:402–406.

Prior, J. C., and Y. M. Vigna, M. T. Schechter, and A. E. Burgess. 1990. Spinal bone loss and ovulatory disturbances. *New England Journal of Medicine* 323:1221–27.

Reyes, F. L., J. S. Winter, and C. Paiman. 1977. Pituitary ovarian relationships preceding the menopause: a cross-sectional study of serum follicle-stimulating hormone, lutenizing hormone, prolactin, estradiol and progesterone levels. *American Journal of Obstetrics and Gynecology* 129:557–64.

Rinzler, Carol Ann. *Estrogen and Breast Cancer.* New York: MacMillan Publishing Co., 1993:31–32.

Seaman, Barbara, and Gideon Seaman. *Women and the Crisis in Sex Hormones.* New York: Rawson Associates, 1977:82.

Sherman, B. M., J. H. West, and S. G. Korenmam. 1976. The menopausal transition: Analysis of LH, FSH, estradiol and progesterone concentrations during menstrual cycles of older women. *J Clin Endocrinol Metab* 42:629–36.

Strauss, S. 1988. A capsulated history of drug law in the U.S. *U.S. Pharmacist.* November.

Tilt, E. J. *The Change of Life in Health and Disease. A Practical Treatise on the Nervous and Other Affections Incidental to Women at the Decline of Life.* Philadelphia: Lindsay and Blakiston, 1871.

Trial of HRT to prevent CHD halted early because of increased harm. *Lancet,* July 13, 2002, vol. 360, no. 9327.

Vaughn, Paul. *The Pill on Trial.* London: Weidenfeld and Nicolson, 1970:25.

Writing Group for the Women's Health Initiative Investigators, Risks and benefits of estrogen plus progestin in healthy post-menopausal women. *JAMA*, July 17, 2002, vol. 288, no. 3.

Chapter 4: What Is Estrogen?

Campbell, B. C., and P. T. Ellison. 1992. Menstrual variation in salivary testosterone among regularly cycling women. *Horm Res* 37:132–36.

DeMarco, Carolyn, MD. *Take Charge of Your Body.* Winlaw, BC, V0G 2J0, Canada: The Well Woman Press, P.O. Box 66, 1994.

Documenta Geigy. *Scientific Tables.* 6th edition. Ardsley, NY: Geigy Pharmaceuticals: 493.

Ellison, P. T., C. Panter-Brick, S. F. Lipson, and M. T. O'Rourke. 1993. The ecological context of human ovarian function. *Human Reproduction* 8:2248–58.

Greer, Germaine. *The Change: Women, Aging and Menopause.* New York: Fawcett Columbine, 1991.

Hammar, M. L., M. B. Hammar-Henriksson, et al. Few oligo-amenorrheic athletes have vasomotor symptoms. *Maturitas* 2000 Mar 31; 34(3):219–25.

Human Reproduction, December 1993.

Ivarsson, T., A. C. Spetz, and M. Hammar. Physical exercise and vasomotor symptoms in postmenopausal women. *Maturitas* 1998 Jun 3; 29(2):139–46.

Lennon, H. M., H. H. Wotiz, L. Parsons, and P. J. Mozden. 1966. Reduced estriol excretion in patients with breast cancer prior to endocrine therapy. *JAMA* 196:112–20.

Leonetti, H. B., S. Longo, and J. N. Anasti. Transdermal progesterone cream for vasomotor symptoms and postmenopausal bone loss. *Obstetrics and Gynecology* 94 (1999):225–228.

Lipsett, M. P. Steroid hormones, in *Reproductive Endocrinology, Physiology, and Clinical Management*. S. S. C. Yen, and R. B. Jaffe, eds. Philadelphia: W. B. Saunders Co., 1978:80.

Novak's Textbook of Gynecology, 11th edition. Baltimore: Williams & Wilkins, 1987.

Overlie, I., M. H. Moen, A. Holte, and A. Finset. Androgens and estrogens in relation to hot flushes during the menopausal transition. *Maturitas* 2002 Jan 30: 41(1):69–77.

Raloff, J. 1993. Ecocancers. *Science News*, July 3, 144:10–13 and reported in article Sperm-count drop tied to pollution rise. *Medical Tribune*, March 26, 1992.

Raz, R., amd W. E. Stamm. 1993. A controlled trial of intravaginal estriol in postmenopausal women with recurrent urinary tract infections. *New England Journal of Medicine* 329:753–56.

Rose, D. P. *Obstetrics & Gynecology*, 1977.

Vines, Gail. Oestrogen overdose. *British Vogue*.

Yahya, S., and N. Rehan. Age, pattern and symptoms of menopause among rural women of Lahore. *J Ayub Med Coll Abbottabad* 2002 Jul-Sep; 4(3):9–12.

Zhao, G., and L. Wang. Menopausal symptoms: experience of Chinese women. *Climacteric* 2000 Jun; 3(2):135–44.

Chapter 5: Hormone Balance, Xenobiotics, and Future Generations

Baj, Z., et al. The effect of chronic exposure to formaldehyde, phenol and organic chlorohydrocarbons on peripheral blood cells and the immune system in humans. *J Investig Allergol Clin Immunol* 1994 Jul-Aug; 4(4):186–91.

Begley, S., and D. Glick. 1994. The estrogen complex. *Newsweek*, March 21: 76–77.

Colborn, T., F. S. vom Saal, and A. M. Soto. 1993. Developmental effects of endocrine-distrupting chemicals in wildlife and humans. *Environmental Health Perspectives* 10:378–84.

Cone, Marla. 1994. Sexual confusion in the wild. Pollution's effect on sexual development fires debate. Battle looms on chemicals that disrupt hormones. 3-part series. *The Los Angeles Times.* October 2–4.

Faustini, A., et al. Immunological changes among farmers exposed to phenoxy herbicides: preliminary observations. *Occup Environ Med* 1996 Sep; 53(9):583–85.

Fitzgerald, E. F., et al. Polychlorinated biphenyl (PCB) and dichlorodiphenyl dichloroethylene (DDE) exposure among Native American men from contaminated Great Lakes fish and wildlife. *Toxicol Ind Health* 1996 May-Aug; 12(3–4):361–68.

Hagmar, L., et al. High consumption of fatty fish from the Baltic Sea is associated with changes in human lymphocyte subset levels. *Toxicol Lett* 1995 May; 77(1–3):335–42.

Hileman, Beth. 1994. Reproductive estrogens linked to reproductive abnormalities, cancer. *Chemical and Engineering News* January 31:19–23.

Hoy, Claire. *The Truth About Breast Cancer.* Stoddard, 1995.

Lemonick, Michael D. 1994. Not so fertile ground. *Time* September 19:68–70.

McLachlan, John. Diagram "Hormonal mimic" taken from 1993. Functional toxicology: A new approach to detect biologically active xenobiotics. *Environmental Health Perspectives* 10:386–87.

Nagayama, J., et al. Postnatal exposure to chlorinated dioxins and related chemicals on lymphocyte subsets in Japanese breast-fed infants. *Chemosphere* 1998 Oct–Nov; 37(9–12):1781-87.

Raloff, J. 1993. Ecocancers. *Science News* 144, July 3:10–13.

———.1994. The gender benders. *Science News* 145, Jan 8:24–27.

———.1994. That feminine touch. *Science News* 145, Jan 22:56–59.

Roof, R. L. Gender influences outcomes of brain injury: Progesterone plays a protective role. *Brain Research* 1993, April 2; 607(1–2):333–36.

Ross, P. S., et al. Impaired cellular immune response in rats exposed perinatally to Baltic Sea herring oil or 2, 3, 7, 8-TCDD. *Arch Toxicol* 1997; 71(9):563–74.

Svensson, B. G., et al. Parameters of immunological competence in subjects with high consumption of fish contaminated with persistent organochlorine compounds. *Int Arch Occup Environ Health* 1994; 65(6):351–58.

Van Loveren, H., et al. Contaminant-induced immunosuppression and mass mortalities among harbor seals. *Toxicol Lett* 2000 Mar 15; 112–113:319–24.

Weiss, Rick. 1994. Estrogen in the environment. *The Washington Post*, January 25: 10–13.

Chapter 6: What Is Natural Progesterone?

Campbell, B. C., and P. T. Ellison. 1992. Menstrual variation in salivary testosterone among regularly cycling women. *Horm Res* 37:132–36

DeBold, J. F., and C. A. Frye. 1994. Progesterone and the neural mechanisms of hamster sexual behavior. *Psychoneuroendocrinology* 19:563–66.

Elks, M. L. 1993. Peripheral effects of sex steroids implications for patient management. *JAMWA* 48:41–45.

Goodman, Louis S., and Alfred Gilman. *The Pharmacological Basis of Therapeutics*, 8th edition. Toronto: The Macmillan Company, 1990: Chapter 58.

History of progesterone as described by Goodman & Gilman. *The Pharmacological Basis of Therapeutics*, 6th edition, 1980: chapter 61 (Estrogens and Progestins: 1420), and *Textbook of Clinical Chemistry*. Norbert W. Tietz, Ph.D., ed. Philadelphia. W.B. Saunders Co., 1986:1085–1171.

Roof, Robin, et al. of Rutgers University. 1993. Reported in *The Economist*, December 11, 329:35.

Stampfer, M. J., G. A. Colditz, W. C. Willett, et al. 1991. Postmenopausal estrogen therapy and cardiovascular disease—Ten-year follow-up from the Nurses' Questionnaire Study. *New England Journal of Medicine* 325:756–62.

Swerdloff, R. S., and C. Wang. 1993. Androgen deficiency and aging in men. *WJM* 159:579–84.

Textbook of Clinical Chemistry. Norbert W. Tietz, Ph.D., ed. Philadelphia: W. B. Saunders Co., 1986:1085–1171.

Thomas, J. Hywel, and Brian Gillham. *Will's Biochemicol Basis of Medicine*, 2d edition. Oxford: Butterworth-Heinemann Ltd., 1989: Chapter 17.

Witt, D. M., L. J. Young, and D. Crews. 1994. Progesterone and sexual behavior in males. *Psychoneuroendocrinology* 19:553–56.

Chapter 7: The Dramatic Difference Between Progesterone and Progestins

Bergkvist, L., H.-O. Adami, I. Persson, R. Hoover, and C. Schairer. 1989. The risk of breast cancer after estrogen and estrogen-progestin replacement. *New England Journal of Medicine* 321:293–97.

Crane, M. G., and J. J. Harris. Effects of gonadal hormones on plasma renin activity and aldosterone excretion rate. In *Metabolic Effects of Gonadal Hormones and Contraceptive Steroids*, H. A. Salhanick, D. M. Kipnis, and R. L. Vande Weile, eds. New York: Plenum Press, 1969:446–46, and discussion: 736.

Crane, M. G., J. J. Harris, and W. Winsor III. 1971. Hypertension, oral contraceptive agents, and conjugated estrogens. *Annals of Internal Medicine* 74:13–21.

Edgren, R. A. Progestagens. Reprinted from *Clinical Use of Sex Steroids*. Chicago: Year Book Medical Publishers, Inc., 1980.

Gambrell, R. D. 1982. The menopause: Benefits and risks of estrogen-progesterone replacement therapy. *Fertil Steril* 37:457–74.

Hargrove, J. T., W. S. Maxson, A. C. Wentz, and L. S. Burnett. 1989. Menopausal hormone replacement therapy with continuous daily oral micronized estradiol and progesterone. *Obstetrics & Gynecology* 71:606–12.

Landau, R. L., and K. Lugibihl. 1961. The catabolic and natriuretic effects of progesterone in man. *Recent Progress in Hormone Research* 17:249–81.

Medical Times. 1989. Sept:35–43.

Ottoson, U. B., B. G. Johansson, and B. von Schoultz. 1985. Subfractions of high-density lipoprotein cholesterol during estrogen replacement therapy: A comparison between progestogens and natural progesterone. *American Journal of Obstetrics and Gynecology* 151:746–50.

Scientific American Medicine, updated 1992. New York: *Scientific American*, chapter 15 (X):9.

Stevenson, J. C., K. F. Ganger, et al. 1990. Effects of transdermal versus oral hormone replacement therapy on bone density in spine and proximal femur in postmenopausal women. *Lancet* 336:265–69.

Whitehead, M. I., D. Fraser, L. Schenkel, D. Crook, and J. C. Stevenson. 1990. Transdermal administration of oestrogen/progestagen hormone replacement therapy. *Lancet* 335:310–12.

The Writing Group for the PEPI Trial, 1995. Effects of estrogen or estrogen/progestin regimens on heart disease risk factors in postmenopausal women: The postmenopausal estrogen/progestins interventions (PEPI) trial. *JAMA*, January 18. 273(3):240–41.

———. 1995. *JAMA* 273:199–208.

Chapter 8: Sex Hormones and the Brain

Backstrom, T., 1962. Epileptic seizures in women related to plasma oestrogen and progesterone during the menstrual cycle. *Acta Neurol Scand* 54:312–47.

Backstrom, T., et al. 1974. Estrogen and progesterone in plasma in relation to premenstrual tension. *J Steroid Biochem Mol Biol* 5:257–260.

Backstrom, T., et al. Effects of ovarian steroid hormones on brain excitability and their relation to epilepsy seizure variation during the menstrual cycle. *Advances in Epileptology*, XVth Epilepsy International Symposium, New York, Raven Press, 1993.

Braverman, Eric. 1993. New era in hormone therapy. *Total Health* 7, no. 4 (August):31.

———. 1991. Natural estrogen and progesterone research indicates health benefits of natural vs. synthetic hormones. *Total Health* 13, no. 5 (October): 55.

Gonzalez, Deniselle M. C., et al. 2002. Basis of progesterone protection in spinal cord neurodegeneration. *J Steroid Biochem Mol Biol* Dec; 83(1–5):199–209.

Harris, Brian. 1994. Maternity blues and major endocrine changes: Cardiff puerperal mood and hormone study II, Wales. *British Medical Journal*, April 19, 308:949–53.

Leary, Warren E. 1995. Progesterone may play major role in the prevention of nerve disease. *New York Times*, June 27, C3.

Peat, Ray, Ph.D. *Progesterone in Orthomolecular Medicine*. Self-published.

Roof, R. L., et al. 1993. Gender influences outcome of brain injury: Progesterone plays a protective role. *Brain Res.* April 2, 607(1–2):333–36.

———. 1994. Progesterone facilitates cognitive recovery and reduces secondary neuronal loss caused by cortical contusion injury in male rats. *Exp Neurol*, September, 129(1):64–69.

Chapter 9: What Are Androgens?

The Biologic Role of Dehydroepiandrosterone. M. Kalimi and W. Regelson, ed. Walter de Gruyter, 1990.

Ebeling, P., and V. A. Koivisto. 1994. Physiological importance of dehydroepiandrosterone. *Lancet* 343:1479–81.

Greenblatt, R. B. 1987. The use of androgens in the menopause and other gynetic disorders. *Obstet Gynecol Clin North Am. Mar*; 14(1):251–68.

Lissoni, P., et al. 1998. Dehydroepiandrosterone sulfate (DHEAS) secretion in early and advanced solid neoplasms: Selective deficiency in metastatic disease. *Int J Biol Markers*. Jul–Sep; 13(3):154–57.

Chapter 10: Hormone Balance and the Menstrual Cycle

Campbell, B. C., and P. T. Ellison. 1992. Menstrual variation in salivary testosterone among regularly cycling women. *Horm Res* 37:132–36.

Kaplan, Abraham, M.D. *The Nervous System*, Volume I, The Hypothalamus Supplement. Illustrated by Frank H. Netter, M.D. New York: CIBA, 1957:147–65. (A good presentation of the functions and neural systems of the limbic brain.)

Prior, J. C., Y. M. Vigna, M. T. Schechter, et al. 1990. Spinal bone loss and ovulatory disturbances. *New England Journal of Medicine* 323:1221–27.

Stevenson, J. C., K. F. Ganger, et al. 1990. Effects of transdermal versus oral hormone replacement therapy on bone density in spine and proximal femur in postmenopausal women. *Lancet* 336:265–69.

Chapter 11: Progesterone and Menopause Symptoms

Arafat, E. S., and J. T. Hargrove. 1988. Sedative and hypnotic effects of oral administration of micronized progesterone may be mediated through its metabolites. *American Journal of Obstetrics and Gynecology*, 159:1203–1209.

Belchetz, P. E. 1994. Hormonal treatment of postmenopausal women. *New England Journal of Medicine* 330:1062–71.

Lees, B., T. Molleson, T. R. Arnett, and J. C. Stevenson, 1993. Differences in proximal femur bone density over two centuries. *Lancet* 341:673–75.

Leridon, H. *Human Fertility: The Basic Components.* Chicago: University of Chicago Press, 1977:202.

Textbook of Clinical Chemistry. Philadelphia: W.B. Saunders Co., 1986:1088.

Van Noord-Zaadstra, B. M., C. W. N. Looman, H. Alsback, et al. 1991. Delaying childbearing: Effect of age on fecundity and outcome of pregnancy. *British Medical Journal* 302:1361–65.

Velde, E. R. 1993. Disappearing ovarian follicles and reproductive aging (letter). *Lancet* 341:1125.

Chapter 12: Hormone Balance and the Adrenal and Thyroid Glands

Bower, B. 1998. Stress hormones may speed up brain aging. *Science News*, vol. 153, no. 17:263.

Chapter 13: Hormone Balance, Nutrition, and Osteoporosis

Albright, F., P. H. Smith, and A. M. Richardson. 1941. Postmenopausal osteoporosis: Its clinical features. *JAMA* 116:2465–74.

Aitken, M., D. M. Hart and R. Lindsay. 1973. Oestrogen replacement therapy for prevention of osteoporosis after oopherectomy. *British Medical Journal* 3:515–18.

Barengolts, E. I., D. J. Curry, et al. 1991. Comparison of the effects of progesterone and estrogen on established bone loss in ovariectomized aged rats. *Cells and Materials* supplement 1 (pages 105–111).

Barengolts, E. I., H. F. Gajardo, et al. 1990. Effects of progesterone on post-ovariectomy bone loss in aged rats. *Journal of Bone Mineral Res* 5:1143–1147.

Barzel, U. S. 1988. Estrogens in the prevention and treatment of postmenopausal osteoporosis: a review. *American Journal of Medicine* 85:847–50.

Bayley, T. A., et al. 1990. Fluoride-induced fractures: relation to osteogenic effect. *Journal of Bone Mineral Res* Mar; 5 Suppl 1:S217–22.

Bone, H. G. et al. 2000. Alendronate and estrogen effects in postmenopausal women with low bone mineral density. *J Clin Endocrinol Metab* Feb; 85(2):720–26.

Christiansen, C., M. S. Christiansen, and I. Transbol. 1981. Bone mass in postmenopausal women after withdrawal of oestrogen/progestagen replacement therapy. *Lancet* February 28: 459–61.

Coats, C. 1990. Negative effects of a high-protein diet. *Family Practice Recertification* 12:80–88.

Cooper, C., C. A. C. Wickham, D. J. R. Barker, and S. J. Jacobsen. 1991. Water fluoridation and hip fracture (letter). *JAMA* 266:513–14.

Cummings, S. R., W. S. Browner, D. Bauer, K. Stone, et al. 1998. Endogenous hormones and the risk of hip and vertebral fracture among older women. *NEJM* 339:733–38.

Cummings, S. R., M. C. Nevitt, W. S. Browner, et al. 1995. Risk factors for hip fracture in white women. *New England Journal of Medicine* 332:767–73.

Cundy, T., M. Evans, H. Roberts, et al. 1991. Bone density in women receiving a depot medroxyprogesterone acetate for contraception. *British Medical Journal* 303:13–16.

Dalsky, G. P., K. S. Stocke, A. A. Ehsani, et al. 1988. Weight-bearing exercise training and femoral neck and lumbar spine bone mineral density. *Annals of Internal Medicine* 108:824–28.

Danielson, C., J. L. Lyon, M. Egger, and G. K. Goodenough. 1992. Hip fractures and fluoridation in Utah's elderly population. *JAMA* 268:746–47.

Delmas, P. D., K. E. Ensrud, et al. 2002. Efficacy of raloxifene on vertebral fracture risk reduction in postmenopausal women with osteoporosis: Four-year results from a randomized clinical trial. *Journal of Clinical Endocrinology and Metabolism* Aug; 87(8):3609–17.

Ellison, P. T., C. Panter-Brick, S. F. Lipson, and M. T. O'Rourke. 1993. The ecological context of human ovarian function. *Human Reproduction* 8:2248–58.

Ettinger, B., D. M. Black, B. H. Mitlak, R. K. Knickerbocker, et al. 1999. Reduction of vertebral fracture risk in postmenopausal women with osteoporosis treated with raloxifene. *JAMA* 282:637–45.

Ettinger, B., H. K. Genant, and C. E. Cann. 1985. Long-term estrogen replacement therapy prevents bone loss and fractures. *Annals of Internal Medicine* 102:319–24.

Felson, D. T., Y. Zhang, M. T. Hannan, D. P. Kiel, P. W. F. Wilson, and J. J. Anderson. 1993. The effect of postmenopausal estrogen therapy on bone density in elderly women. *New England Journal of Medicine* 329:1141–46.

Gordon, G. S., J. Picchi, and B. S. Root. 1973. Antifracture efficacy of long-term estrogens for osteoporosis. *Trans Assoc Am Physicians* 86:326–32.

Hammond, C. B., F. R. Jelvsek, K. L. Lee, W. T. Creasman, and R. T. Parker. 1979. Effects of long-term estrogen replacement therapy. I. Metabolic effects. *American Journal of Obstetrics and Gynecology* 133:525–36.

Hedlund, L. R., and J. C. Gallagher. 1989. Increased incidence of hip fracture in osteoporotic women treated with sodium fluoride. *J Bone & Miner Res* 4:223–25.

Hosking, D., C. E. Chilvers, C. Christiansen, P. Ravn, et al. 1998. Prevention of bone loss with alendronate in postmenopausal women under 60 years of age. *NEJM* 19 February 1998; 338:485–92.

Hutchinson, T. A., S. M. Polansky, and A. R. Feinstein. 1979. Postmenopausal oestrogens protect against fractures of hip and distal radius: A case control study. *Lancet* II:705–709.

Israel, E., et al. 2001. Effects of inhaled glucocorticoids on bone density in premenopausal women. *New England Journal of Medicine* 345:941–47.

Jacobsen, S. J., J. Goldberg, T. P. Miles, J. A. Brody, et al. 1990. Regional variation in the incidence of hip fractures: U.S. white women aged 65 years and older. *JAMA* 264:500–501.

Johansen, J. S., S. B. Jensen, B. J. Riis, et al. 1990. Bone formation is stimulated by combined estrogen, progestagen. *Metabolism* 39:1122–26.

Kass-Wolff, J. H. 2001. Bone loss in adolescents using Depo-Provera. *Journal of Society of Pediatric Nursing* Jan–Mar; 6(1):21–31.

Kleerekoper, M. E., E. Peterson, E. Phillips, D. Nelson, et al. 1989. Continuous sodium fluoride therapy does not reduce vertebral fracture rate in postmenopausal osteoporosis (abstract). *J Bone & Miner Res* 4 (Suppl.1):S376.

Lee, J. R. 1990. Osteoporosis reversal: The role of progesterone. *Intern Clin Nutr Rev* 10:384–91.

———. 1990. Osteoporosis reversal with transdermal progesterone (letter). *Lancet* 336:1327.

———. 1991. Is natural progesterone the missing link in osteoporosis prevention and treatment? *Medical Hypothesis* 35:316–18.

Lees, B., T. Molleson, T. R. Arnett, and J. C. Stevenson. 1993 Differences in proximal femur density over two centuries. *Lancet* 341:673–75.

Lees, C. J., T. C. Register, et al. 2002. Effects of raloxifene on bone density, biomarkers, and histomorphometric and biomechanical measures in ovariectomized cynomolgus monkeys. *Menopause* Sep–Oct; 9(5):320–28.

Lindsay, R., D. M. Hart, C. Forrest, and C. Baird. 1980. Prevention of spinal osteoporosis in oophorectomized women. *Lancet* II:1151–54.

Manolagas, S. C., R. L. Jilka, G. Hangoc, et al. 1992. Increased osteoclast development after estrogen loss: Mediation by interleukin-6. *Science* 257:88–91.

Munk-Jensen, N., S. P. Nielsen, E. B. Obel, and P. B. Eriksen. 1988. Reversal of postmenopausal vertebral bone loss by oestrogen and progestagen: A double-blind placebo-controlled study. *British Medical Journal* 296:1150–52.

Nolan, Charles R., M.D., et al. 1994. Aluminum and lead absorption from dietary sources in women ingesting calcium citrate. *Southern Medical Journal.* September; 87(9):894–98.

Osteoporosis prevention, diagnosis, and therapy. 2001. NIH Consensus Conference Report. *JAMA* 285:785–95.

Prior, J. C. 1990. Progesterone as a bone-trophic hormone. *Endocrine Reviews* 11:386–98.

Prior, J. C., and Y. M. Vigna. 1990. Spinal bone loss and ovulatory disturbances. *New England Journal of Medicine* 223:1221–27.

Prior, J. C., Y. M. Vigna, and N. Alojado. 1991. Progesterone and the prevention of osteoporosis. *Canadian Journal of Obstetrics/Gynecology & Women's Health Care* 3:178–84.

Prior, J. C., Y. M. Vigna, and R. Burgess. Medroxyprogesterone acetate increases trabecular bone density in women with menstrual disorder. Presented at the annual meeting of the Endocrine Society, Indianapolis, June 11, 1987.

Riggs, B. L., S. F. Hodgson, W. M. O'Fallon, E. Y. S. Chao, et al. 1990. Effect of fluoride treatment on the fracture rate in postmenopausal women with osteoporosis. *New England Journal of Medicine* 322:802–809.

Riggs, B. L., H. W. Wahner, L. J. Melton, et al. 1986. Rates of bone loss in the appendicular and axial skeleton of women: evidence of substantial vertebral bone loss before menopause. *J Clin Invest* 77:1487–91.

Rudy, D. R. 1990. Hormone replacement therapy. *Postgraduate Medicine* Dec; 157–64.

Schmidt, I. U., G. K. Wakely, et al. 2000. Effects of estrogen and progesterone on tibia histomorphometry in growing rats. *Calcif Tissues Int* 67(1):47–52.

Siris, E., et al. 2002. Effects of raloxifene on fracture severity in postmenopausal women with osteoporosis: results from the MORE study. *Osteoporosis International* Nov; 13(11):907–13.

Sowers, M. F. R., M. K. Clark, M. L. Jannausch, and R. B. Wallace. 1991. A prospective study of bone mineral content and fracture in communities with differential fluoride exposure. *American Journal of Epidemiology* 134:649–60.

Vieth, Reinhold. 1999. Vitamin D Supplementation, 25-hydroxy-vitamin D concentrations, and safety. *American Journal of Clinical Nutrition*, vol. 69, no. 5, 842–856.

Weiss, N. S., C. L. Ure, J. H. Ballard, A. R. Williams, and J. R. Daling. 1980. Decreased risk of fracture of hip and lower forearm with postmenopausal use of estrogen. *New England Journal of Medicine* 303:1195–98.

Chapter 14: Women and Cardiovascular Disease

Barbagallo, M., L. J. Dominguez, et al. 2001. Vascular effects of progesterone: role of cellular calcium regulation. *Hypertension* 37:142–47.

Cheng, W., O. D. Lau, et al. 1999. Two antiatherogenic effects of progesterone on human macrophages: Inhibition of Cholesterol ester synthesis and block of its enhancement by glucocorticoids. *Journal of Clinical Endocrinology & Metabolism* 64:265–71.

ESPRIT team. 2002. Oestrogen therapy for prevention of re-infarction in postmenopausal women: a randomized placebo controlled trial. *Lancet* 360:2001–2008.

Herrington, D. M., D. M. Reboussin, et al. 2000. Effects of estrogen replacement on the progression of coronary-artery atherosclerosis. *NEJM* 343:522–37.

Huley, S., D. Grady, T. Bush, C. Furberg, et al. 1998. Randomized trial of estrogen plus progestin for secondary prevention of coronary heart disease in postmenstrual women. *JAMA* August 19; 280:605–613.

Miyagawa, K., J. Rosch, J. F. Stanczyk, and K. Hermsmeyer. 1997. Medroxyprogesterone acetate interferes with ovarian steroid protection against coronary vasospasm. *Nature Medicine* 3:324–27.

Moura, M. J., and F. K. Marcondes. 2001. Influence of estradiol and progesterone on the sensitivity of rat thoractic aorta to non-adrenaline. *Life Sciences* 68:881–88.

Otsuki, M., and H. Saito. 2001. Progesterone, but not medroy-progesterone, inhibits vascular cell adhesion molecule-1 expression in human endothelial cells. *Arteriosclerosis Thrombosis Vascular Biology* 21:243–48.

Prior, J. C. 1992. Letter. *New England Journal of Medicine* 326:705–706.

Ray, W. A., C. M. Stein, et al. 2002. Non-steroidal anti-inflammatory drugs and risk of serious coronary heart disease: An observational cohort study. *Lancet* 359:118–23.

Rodriguez, I., M. J. Kilborn, et al. 2001. Drug-induced QT prolongation in women during the menstrual cycle. *JAMA* 1322–26.

Rossouw, J. E. 2002. Commentary: Hormones for coronary disease—full circle. *Lancet* 360:1996–97.

Stampfer, M. J., G. A. Colditz, W. C. Willett, et al. 1991. Post-menopausal estrogen therapy and cardiovascular disease—10-year follow-up from the Nurses' Questionnaire Study. *New England Journal of Medicine* 325:756–62.

Tribble, D. L., and E. Frank. 1994. Dietary antioxidants, cancer, and atherosclerotic heart disease. *W J Med* 161:605–12.

Wilson, P. W. F., R. J. Garrison, and W. P. Castelli. 1985. Post-menopausal estrogen use, cigarette smoking, and cardiovascular morbidity in women over 50. *New England Journal of Medicine* 313:1038–43.

Writing Group for the WHI Investigation. 2002. Risks and benefits of estrogen plus progestin in healthy postmenopausal women. *JAMA* 17 July 2002; 288:321–333.

Chapter 15: Hormone Balance and Cancer

A report by Ruby Senie, Ph.D., of the Centers for Disease Control, at the annual science writers seminar sponsored by the American Cancer Society. Reported by the February 5, 1992, issue of *Health* and by the May 7, 1992, issue of *Medical Tribune*.

Astrow, Alan B., M.D. 1994. Rethinking cancer (letter). *Lancet* February 26.

Bergkvist, L., H.-O. Adami, I. Persson, R. Hoover, and C. Schairer. 1989. The risk of breast cancer after estrogen and estrogen-progestin replacement. *New England Journal of Medicine* 321:293–97.

Campbell, B. C., and P. T. Ellison. 1992. Menstrual variation in salivary testosterone among regularly cycling women. *Horm Res* (Switzerland) 37(4–5):132–36.

2002. The Canadian National Breast Screening Study—1: breast cancer mortality after 11 to 16 years of follow-up. A randomized screening trial of mammography in women age 40 to 49 years. *Ann Intern Med* Sep 3; 137(5 Part 1):305–12.

Cauley, J. A. 1999. Elevated serum estradiol and testosterone concentration associated with a high risk for breast cancer: Study of Osteoporotic Fractures Research Group. *Ann Intern Med* Feb 16; 130(4 Pt 1):270–77.

Chang, K. J., et al. 1995. Influences of percutaneous administration of estradiol and progesterone on human breast epithelial cell cycle in vivo. *Fertility and Sterility* 63:785–91.

Cowan, L. D., L. Gordis, J. A. Tonascia, and G. S. Jones. 1981. Breast cancer incidence in women with a history of progesterone deficiency. *American Journal of Epidemiology* 114:209–17.

Ellison, P. T. 1993. Measurements of salivary progesterone. *Annals of the New York Academy of Science* September 20, 694:161–76.

Ellison, P. T., S. F. Lipson, M. T. O'Rourke, et al. 1993. Population variation in ovarian function (letter) *Lancet* August 14, 342:433–34.

Ellison, P. T., C. Panter-Brick, S. F. Lipson, and M. T. O'Rourke. 1993. The ecological context of human ovarian function. *Human Reproduction* 8(12):2248–58.

Foidart, J. M., C. Colin, et al. 1998. Estradiol and progesterone regulate the proliferation of human breast epithelial cells. *Fertility and Sterility* May; 69(5):963–69.

Gruenigen, V. E., and J. R. Karlen. 1995. Carcinoma of the endometrium. *American Family Physician*, May 1:1531–36.

Henderson, B. E., R. K. Ross, M. C. Pike, and J. T. Casagrande. 1982. Endogenous hormones as a major factor in human cancer. *Cancer Research* 42:3232–39.

Hoover, R., L. A. Gray, Sr., P. Cole, and B. MacMahon. 1976. Menopausal estrogens and breast cancer. *New England Journal of Medicine* 295:401–405.

Hiatt, R. A., R. Bawol, G. D. Friedman, and R. Hoover. 1984 Exogenous estrogen and breast cancer after bilateral oophorectomy. *Cancer* 54:139–44.

Kerlikowske, K., D. Grady, S. M. Rubin, et al. 1995. Efficacy of screening mammography. *JAMA* 273:149–54.

La Vecchia, C., A. Decarli, F. Parazzini, A. Gentile, C. Liberati, and S. Franceschi. 1986. Noncontraceptive oestrogens and the risk of breast cancer in women. *International Journal of Cancer* 38:853–58.

Malet, C., P. Spritzer, et al. 2000. Progesterone effect on cell growth, ultrastructural aspect and estradiol receptors of normal human breast epithelial (HBE) cells in culture. *Journal of Steroid Biochemistry and Molecular Biology*, vol. 73, issue 3/4, 171–181.

Miller, A. B., C. J. Baines, and T. Wall. 1992. Canadian national breast screening study 2: Breast cancer detection and death rates among women aged 50 to 59 years. *Canadian Medical Association Journal* 147:1477–88.

Pike, M. C., D. V. Spicer, L. Dahmoush, and M. F. Press. 1993. Estrogens, progestogens, normal breast proliferation, and breast cancer risk. *Epidem Rev* 15:64–82.

Raloff, Janet. 1993. Ecocancers: Do environmental factors underlie a breast cancer epidemic? *Science News*, July 3, 144:10–13.

Willett, W. C., M. J. Stampfer, M. B. Colditz, et al. 1987. Dietary fat and the risk of breast cancer. *New England Journal of Medicine* 316:22–28.

Chapter 17: Natural Hormone Balance and Pelvic Disorders

Bodner, K., and B. Bodner-Adler. 2003. Estrogen and progesterone receptor expression in patients with uterine leiomyosarcoma and correlation with different clinicopathological parameters. *Anticancer Res* Jan–Feb; 23(1B):729–32.

Crane, M. G., and J. J. Harris. Effects of gonadal hormones on plasma rennin activity and aldosterone excretion rate. In H. A. Salhanick, D. M. Kipnis, and R. L. Vande Weile, eds. *Metabolic Effects of Gonadal Hormones and Contraceptive Steroids.* New York: Plenum Press, 1969:446–63, and discussion: 736.

Crane, M. G., J. J. Harris, and W. Widsor III. 1971. Hypertension, oral contraceptive agents and conjugated estrogens. *Annals of Internal Medicine* 74:13–21.

Dalton, K. *The Premenstual Syndrome and Progesterone Therapy.* Chicago: Year Book Medical Publishers, Inc., 1977.

DeBold, J. F., and C. A. Frye. 1994. Progesterone and the neural mechanisms of hamster sexual behavior. *Psychoneuroendocrinology* 19:563–79.

De Leo, V., G. Morgante, et al. 2002. A benefit-risk assessment of medical treatment for uterine leiomyomas. *Drug Safety* 25(11):759–79.

Eisinger, S. H., S. Meldrum, et al. 2003. Low-dose mifepristone for uterine leiomyomata. *Obstetrics and Gynecolgy* Feb; 101(2):243–50.

Harris, B., L. Lovett, et al. 1994. Maternity blues and major endocrine changes: Cardiff puerperal mood and hormone study II. *British Medical Journal* Apr; 308:949–953.

Hodges, L. C., D. S. Hunter, et al. 2001. An in vivo/in vitro model to assess endocrine disrupting activity of xenoestrogens in uterine leiomyoma. *Annals of New York Academy of Sciences* Dec; 948:100–11.

Jeffries, William M.D. *The Safe Uses of Cortisone.* Springfield, IL: Charles C Thomas Publisher, 1981.

Kurachi, O., and H. Matsuo. 2001. Tumor necrosis factor-alpha expression in human uterine leiomyoma and its down-regulation by progesterone. *Journal of Clinical Endocrinology and Metabolism* May; 86(5):2275–80.

Shozu, M., K. Murakami, et al. 2003. Successful treatment of a symptomatic uterine leiomyoma in a perimenopausal woman with a nonsteroidal aromatase inhibitor. *Fertility and Sterility* Mar; 79(3)628–31.

Smith, E. P., J. Boyd, G. R. Frank, et al. 1994. Estrogen resistance caused by a mutation in the estrogen-receptor gene in a man. *New England Journal of Medicine* 331:1056–61.

Stampfer, M. J., G. A. Colditz, W. C. Willett, et al. 1991. Postmenopausal estrogen therapy and cardiovascular disease. *New England Journal of Medicine* 325:756–62.

Walker, C. L. 2002. Role of hormonal and reproductive factors in the etiology and treatment of uterine leiomyoma. *Recent Prog Horm Res* 57:277–94.

Witt, D. M., L. J. Young, and D. Crews. 1994. Progesterone and sexual behavior in males. *Psychoneuroendocrinology* 19:553–62.

Chapter 18: Hormone Balance and Other Common Health Problems

Diaz-Zagoya, J. C., J. Laguna, and J. Guzman-Garcia. 1971. Studies on the regulation of cholesterol metabolism by the use of the structural analogue, diosgenin. *Biochem Pharmacol* 20(12):3473–80.

Juarez-Oropeza, M. A., J. C. Diaz-Zagoya, and J. L. Rabinowitz. 1987. In vivo and in vitro studies of hypocholesterolemic effects of diosgenun in rats. *International Journal of Biochemistry* 19(8):679–83.

Melillo, Mark. 1994. Estrogen use may predispose women to lupus. *Medical Tribune*, November 17.

Odumosu, A. 1982. How vitamin C, clofibrate and diosgenin control cholesterol metabolism in male guinea-pigs. *Int J Vitam Nutr Res* Suppl (Switzerland) 23:187–95.

Tuppala, M., U. Bjorses, T. Wahlstrom, and O. Ylikorkala. 1991. Luteal phase defect in habitual abortion: Progesterone in saliva. *Fertile Steril* 56:41–44.

Chapter 19: How to Use Progesterone Supplementation

Anasti, J. N., H. B. Leonetti, and K. J. Wilson. 2001. Topical progesterone cream has antiproliferative effect on estrogen-stimulated endometrium. *Obstetrics and Gynecology* 97:510.

Beumont, P. J. L., et al. 1972. Lutenizing hormone and progesterone levels after hysterectomy. *BMJ*, 836:363.

Bourgain, C., et al. 1990. Effects of natural progesterone on the morphology of the endometrium in patients with primary ovarian failure. *Hum Repod* 5:537–43.

Chakmakjian, Z. R., and N. Y. Zackariah. 1987. Bioavailabilty of progesterone with different modes of administration. *Journal of Reproductive Medicine* 32:443–48.

Chang, K. J., T. T. Y. Lee, G. Linares-Cruz, S. Fournier, and B. de Lignieres. 1995. Influences of precutaneous administration of estradiol and progesterone on human breast epithelial cell cycle in vivo. *Fertility and Sterility* 63:785–79.

Dabbs, J. 1990. Salivary testosterone measurements: reliability across hours, days and weeks. *Phys Behav* 48:83–86.

de Lignieres, B., L. Dennerstein, and T. Backstrom. 1995. Influence of route of administration on progesterone metabolism. *Maturitas* Apr; 21(3):251–57.

Devenuto, F., et al. 1969. Human erythrocyte membrane. Uptake of progesterone and chemical alterations. *Biochim Biophys Acta* 193:36–47.

Dollbaum, C. M., and G. F. Duwe. Absorption of progesterone after topical applications: serum and saliva levels. Presented at the 7th Annual Meeting of the American Menopause Society.

Foidart J.M., C. Colin, X. Denoo, and J. Desroux, et al. 1998. Estradiol and progesterone regulate proliferation of human breast epithelial cell. *Fertility and Sterility* 69:963–69.

Johnson, M. E., et al. 1995. Permeation of steroids through human skin. *Journal of Pharmaceutical Science* 84:1144–46.

Koefoed, P., and J. Brahm. 1994. The permeability of the human red cell membrane to steroid sex hormones. *Biochim Biophys Acta* 1195:55–62.

Leonetti, H. B., S. Longo, and J. N. Anasti. 1999. Transdermal progesterone cream for vasomotor symptoms and post-menopausal bone loss. *Obstetrics and Gynecology* 94:225–28.

Levine, H., and N. Watson. 2000. Comparison of the pharma-cokinetics of crinone 8% administered vaginally versus Prometrium administered orally in postmenopausal women. *Fertil Steril* Mar; 73(3):516–21.

Nahoul, K., and D. de Ziegler 1993. "Validity" of serum pro-gesterone levels after oral progesterone. *Fertil Steril* Jul; 60(1):26–33.

O'Leary P., P. Feddema, K. Chan, et al. 2000. Salivary, but not serum or urinary levels of progesterone are elevated after topical application of progesterone cream to pre- and postmenopausal women. *Clinical Endocrinology* 53:615–20.

Waddell B. J., and P. C. O'Leary. 2002. Distribution and me-tabolism of topically applied progesterone in a rat model. *Journal of Steroid Biochemistry and Molecular Biology* 80:449–55.

Wren, B. G., K. McFarland, L. Edwards, et al. 2000. Effect of sequential transdermal progesterone cream on endometrium, bleeding pattern, and plasma progesterone levels in post-menopausal women. *Climateric* 3:155–60.

Chapter 20: How to Use Estrogen, DHEA, Pregnenolone, the Corticosteroids, Testosterone, and Androstenedione

Aardal-Eriksson, E., B. Karlberg, and A. Holm. 1998. Salivary cortisol- and alternative to serum cortisol determinations in dynamic function tests. *Clin Chem Lab Med* 36:215–222.

Andrews, R. V. Influence of adrenal gland on gonadal function. in R.A. Thomas and R. L. Singhal, eds. *Advances in Sex Hormones Research, Vol. 3: Regulatory Mechanisms Affecting Gonadal Hormone Action.* Baltimore, University Park, MD, 1976:197–215.

The Biologic Role of Dehydroepiandrosterone. M. Kalimi and W. Regelson, eds. Walter de Gruyter, 1990.

Christiansen, K., and R. Knussmann. 1987. Androgen levels and components of aggressive behavior in men. *Hormones and Behavior* 21:170–80.

Navarro M., J. Nolla, M. Machuca, A. Gonzalaz, L. Mateo, R. Bonnin, and D. Roig-Escofet. 1998. Salivary testosterone in postmenopausal women with rheumatoid arthritis. *Journal of Rheumatology* 25:1059–62.

Shifren, J. L. 2000. Transdermal testosterone treatment in women with impaired sexual function after oophorectomy. *NEJM* Sep 7; 343(10):682–88.

Steptoe, A., M. Cropley, J. Griffith, and C. Kirschbaum. 2000. Job strain and anger expression predict early morning elevation in salivary cortisol. *Psychosomatic Medicine* 62:286–92.

Vedhara, K., J. Hyde, I. Gilchrist, M. Tytherleigh, and S. Plummer. 2000. Acute stress, memory, attention and cortisol. *Psychoneuroendocrinology* 25:535–49.

Young, M., R. Walker, Riad-Fahmy, and I. Hughes. 1988. Androstenedione rhythms in saliva in congenital adrenal hyperplasia. *Arch Dis Child* 63:624–28.

Chapter 21: Nutrition for Healthy Hormones

Austoker, Joan. 1994. Diet and cancer. *British Medical Journal* 308:1610–14.

Blaylock, Russell L., M.D. *Excitotoxins: The Taste That Kills.* Santa Fe: Health Press, 1994.

Davies, N. T., and H. Reid. 1979. An evaluation of the phytate, zinc, copper, iron and manganese contents of, and zinc availability from, soya-based textured-vegetable-protein meat-substitutes or meat-extenders. *Br J Nutr* 41(3):579–89.

Diaz-Zagoya, J. C., J. Laguna, and J. Guzman-Garcia. 1971. Studies on the regulation of cholesterol metabolism by the use of the structural analogue, diosgenin. *Biochem Pharmacol* 20(12):3473–80.

Erasmus, Udo. *Fats That Heal, Fats That Kill.* Burnaby, BC, Canada: Alive Books, 1993.

Fallon, S. W., and M. G. Enig. 1995. Soy products for dairy products? Not so fast. *Health Freedom News*, September.

Foods that may prevent breast cancer: Studies are investigating soybeans, whole wheat and green tea among others. *Primary Care and Cancer* 14(2):10–11.

Fotsis, T. 1993. Genistein, a dietary-derived inhibitor or in vitro angiogenesis. *Proc Natl Acad Sci* 90:2690–94.

Hargreaves, D. F. et al. 1999. Two-week dietary soy supplementation has an estrogenic effect on normal premenopausal breast. *J Clin Endocrinol Metab* Nov; 84(11):4017–24.

Juarez-Oropeza, M. A., J. C. Diaz-Zagoya, and J. L. Rabino-witz. 1987. In vivo and in vitro studies of hypocholesterolemic effects of diosgenin in rats. *International Journal of Biochemistry* 19(8):679–83.

Kushi, L. H. 1997. Physical activity and mortality in post-menopausal women. *JAMA* Apr 23/30; 277(16):1287–92.

LaPierre, A., et al. 1994. Exercise and psychoneuroimmunology. *Medicine and Science in Sports and Exercise* 26(2):182–190.

Laino, C. 1994. Trans-fatty acids in migraine can increase MI risk. *Circulation*, 89:94–101.

Leiner, I. E. 1994. Implications of antinutritional components in soybean foods. *Crit Rev Food Sci Nutr* 34:31–67.

Miller, A. B., et al. 1994. Diet in the etiology of cancer: A review. *European Journal of Cancer* 30A(2):207–28.

Odumosu, A. 1982. How vitamin C, clofibrate and diosgenin control cholesterol metabolism in male guinea-pigs. *Int J Vitam Nutr Res* Suppl (Switzerland) 23:187–95.

Rogers, Adrianne E., et al. 1993. Diet and carcinogenesis. *Carcinogenesis* 14(11):2205–17.

Sandberg, A. S. 1991. The effect of food processing on phylate hydrolysis and availability of iron and zinc. *Adv Exp Med Biol* 289:499–508.

Sandstrom, B., B. Kivisto, and A. Cederblad. 1987. Absorption of zinc from soy protein meals in humans. *J Nutr* 117:321–327.

Schell, O. *Modern Meat.* New York: Vintage Books, Random House, 1985:283–84 and 287.

Schmidt, Erik Berg, and Jorn Dyerberg. 1994. Omega-3 fatty acids—Current status in cardiovascular medicine. *Drugs* 47(3):405–24.

Semplicini, Andrea and Valle. 1994. Fish oils and their possible role in the treatment of cardiovascular disease. *Pharmac Ther* 61:385–97.

Slavin, J. L. 2000. Mechanisms for the impact of whole grain foods on cancer risk. *J Am Coll Nutr* June; 19(3 Suppl): 300S–307S.

Toniolo, Paolo, et al. 1994. Consumption of meat, animal products, protein and fat and risk of breast cancer: A prospective cohort study in New York. *Epidemiology* July; 5(4):391–96.

Trichopoulous, Antonia, M.D., et al. 1995. Consumption of olive oil and specific food groups in relation to breast cancer risk in Greece. *Journal of the National Cancer Institute* Jan 18; 87(2):110–16.

Trichopoulous, A., et al. 2000. Cancer and the Mediterranean dietary traditions. *Cancer Epidemiol Biomarkers Prev* Sep; 9(9):869–73.

Verschuren, Monique W. M., et al. 1995. Serum total cholesterol and long-term coronary heart disease mortality in different cultures. *JAMA* July 12, 274(2).

Wilgus, H. S. Jr., et al. 1941. Goitrogenicity of soybeans. *J Nutr* 22:43–52.

Willett, W. C., M. J. Stampfer, G. A. Colditz, and F. E. Speizer, et al. 1993. Intake of trans-fatty acids and risk of coronary heart disease among women. *Lancet* 341:581–85.

Zava, D. T., and G. Duwe. 1997. Estrogenic and antiproliferative properties of genistein and other flavonoids in human breast cancer cells in vitro. *Nutrition and Cancer* 27:31–40.

APPENDIX: THE STRUCTURE OF STEROID HORMONES

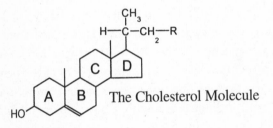

The Cholesterol Molecule

Figure 16: Notice the four rings, labeled A, B, C, and D, that make up the main chassis of the molecule. These are the four rings that characterize all the steroid hormones. In the following figure are three such hormones.

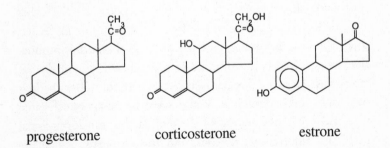

progesterone   corticosterone   estrone

Figure 17: Notice how the basic structure of cholesterol, the precursor to the steroid hormones, remains the same in three different steroid hormones. Slight molecular variations produce hormones that create enormous variations in humans.

Note that all of these steroid hormones retain the similar four-ring structure of the cholesterol molecule. (See Figures 16 and 17.) They differ, however, in the atoms attached at various places to the basic structure. The differences appear minor, though their actions are thereby changed considerably. Others, like estrone (and all estrogens), have a different A-ring. This ring, depicted with a circle inside, indicates it has had three hydrogens removed, leaving three sets of double bonds circulating around the ring of carbon atoms making up the six-sided ring. This is what chemists call a benzene ring. However, with the presence of the —OH group at the side of the ring farthest away from the rest of the molecule, this ring is called a phenol ring. Among the steroid hormones, only estrogen molecules have a phenol ring. Nearly all of the xenoestrogens have phenol rings.

The body does not build these various important steroid hormones on different assembly lines. Cholesterol is the main building block. Tiny energy packets (mitochondria) within each and every cell of the body can substitute and rearrange some atoms at the top of cholesterol's D-ring, creating a new version called pregnenolone. As it passes through the bloodstream to the ovaries and adrenal glands, pregnenolone can then be transformed into progesterone or (almost identical) 17-OH-pregnenolone. Then, from these two steroids, all the other steroid hormones can be made by relatively minor molecular modifications, depending on body need. In this sort of production, one steroid is transformed into another. Many of the intermediate steps in this pathway are active hormones in their own right, even though they also serve by being transformed into still other hormones. At the end of the transformational paths are aldosterone, cortisol, and the estrogens, which are fated to be metabolized and excreted from the body.

Although the steroid hormones are remarkably similar in shape, each of them has markedly different effects, and these differences arise from very slight variations in their molecular structure. (See Figure 18.)

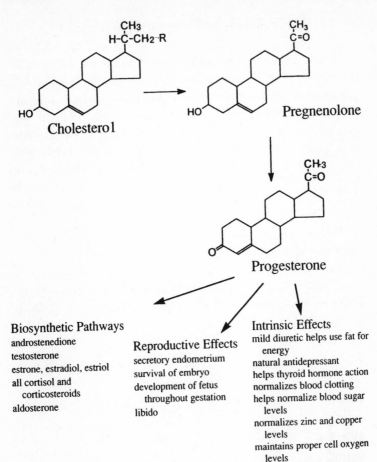

Figure 18: The multiple roles of progesterone.

DHEA (Dehydroepiandrosterone)

DHEA is an adrenal-produced steroid hormone whose functions are not well known at this time despite the fact that it is produced in greater quantity than any other adrenal hormone. DHEA circulates in blood primarily as DHEA-S, a sulfated version which is not, in itself, biologically active. When blood tests for DHEA are done, the test results do not usually discriminate between the 95 percent which is DHEA-S and the 5 percent that is DHEA. Radioimmune assay of saliva, however, can be used to measure the concentration of the biologically active hormone, DHEA.

Plasma DHEA-S can be considered a circulating reservoir from which the active form can be derived. Conversely, DHEA can be converted back into DHEA-S. Regulators of this conversion process are not known. The enzymes that accomplish the conversions are known and are indicated on the diagram shown in Figure 19.

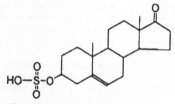

Dehydroepiandrosterone sulfate
DHEA-S

Dehydroepiandrosterone
DHEA

Figure 19: The enzymes that accomplish the transformations, labeled as 1 and 2 at the arrows, are the following:

1. *Sulfatases*
2. *Sulfokinases*

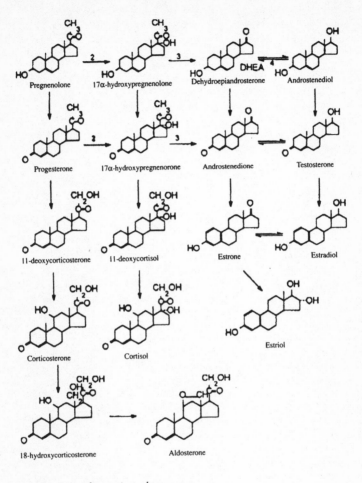

Figure 20: Steroidogenesis pathways.

INDEX

ABOUT THE AUTHORS

John R. Lee, M.D. (1929–2003), is internationally acknowledged as a pioneer and expert in the study and use of the hormone progesterone, and on the subject of hormone replacement therapy for women. He used transdermal progesterone extensively in his clinical practice for nearly a decade, doing research that showed that it can reverse osteoporosis. Dr. Lee had a distinguished medical career, including graduating from Harvard and the University of Minnesota Medical School. He retired from a 30-year family practice in Northern California and began writing and traveling around the world speaking to doctors, scientists, and laypeople about progesterone. Dr. Lee taught a very popular course on Optimal Health at the College of Marin for 15 years. He is the author of *Optimal Health Guidelines, Natural Progesterone: The Multiple Roles of a Remarkable Hormone* (written for doctors) and the bestsellers *What Your Doctor May Not Tell You About Menopause, What Your Doctor May Not Tell You About Premenopause,* and *What Your Doctor May Not Tell You About Breast Cancer* and was editor-in-chief of the *John R. Lee, M.D., Medical Letter.*

Virginia Hopkins, M.A., has been a writer and editor since she graduated from Yale University in 1976. She has a master's degree in applied psychology from the University of Santa Monica. She is the coauthor, with John R. Lee, M.D., of *What Your Doctor May Not Tell You About Menopause: The Breakthrough Book on Natural Progesterone* (Warner Books, 1996), *What Your Doctor May Not Tell You About Premenopause* (Warner Books, 1999), *What Your Doctor May Not Tell You About Breast Cancer* (Warner Books, 2003), and *Prescription Alternatives* (Keats Publishing, 1998), which she coauthored with Earl Mindell, R.Ph., Ph.D. She was the executive editor of the *John R. Lee, M.D., Medical Letter,* and has written or coauthored more than 30 books on alternative health and nutrition.

FIBROMYALGIA FATIGUE
The Powerful Program That Helps You Boost Your Energy
and Reclaim Your Life

HPV AND ABNORMAL PAP SMEARS
Get the Facts on This Dangerous Virus—Protect Your Health
and Your Life!

HYPERTENSION
The Revolutionary Nutrition and Lifestyle Program to Help
Fight High Blood Pressure

HYPOTHYROIDISM
A Simple Plan for Extraordinary Results

KNEE PAIN AND SURGERY
Learn the Truth About MRIs and Common Misdiagnoses—
and Avoid Unnecessary Surgery

MIGRAINES
The Breakthrough Program That Can Help End Your Pain

OSTEOPOROSIS
Help Prevent—and Even Reverse—the Disease
That Burdens Millions of Women

PARKINSON'S DISEASE
A Holistic Program for Optimal Wellness

PEDIATRIC FIBROMYALGIA
A Safe, New Treatment Plan for Children

PREMENOPAUSE
Balance Your Hormones and Your Life from Thirty to Fifty